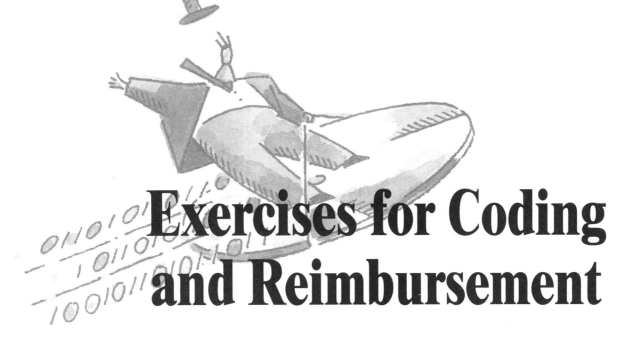

Exercises for Coding and Reimbursement

Second Edition

ICDC Publishing, Inc.

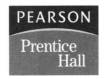

PEARSON

Prentice Hall

Upper Saddle River, New Jersey 07458

Publisher: Julie Levin Alexander
Publisher's Assistant: Regina Bruno
Executive Editor: Joan Gill
Assistant Editor: Bronwen Glowacki
Director of Marketing: Karen Allman
Senior Marketing Manager: Harper Coles
Marketing Coordinator: Michael Sirinides
Marketing Assistant: Wayne Celia, Jr.
Managing Production Editor: Patrick Walsh
Production Liaison: Julie Li
Production Editor: Assunta Petrone, Preparé, Inc.
Manufacturing Manager: Ilene Sanford
Manufacturing Buyer: Pat Brown
Senior Design Coordinator: Maria Guglielmo
Interior Designer: Amy Rosen
Cover Designer: Solid State Graphics
Composition: Preparé, Inc.
Printing and Binding: Edwards Brothers, Inc.
Cover Printer: Phoenix Color Corporation

Pearson Education Ltd.
Pearson Education Singapore Pte. Ltd.
Pearson Education Canada, Ltd.
Pearson Education—Japan
Pearson Education Australia Pty. Limited

Pearson Education North Asia Ltd.
Pearson Educación de Mexico, S.A. de C.V.
Pearson Education Malaysia Pte. Ltd.
Pearson Education Inc., Upper Saddle River, New Jersey

12 11   10 9 8 7 6

ISBN 0-13-172253-0

Disclaimer

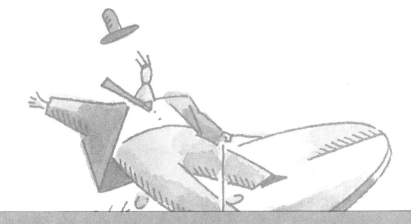

This text is an exercise book for learning medical billing and health claims examining. Decisions should not be based solely on information within this guide. Decisions impacting the practice of medical billing or health claims examining must be based on individual circumstances including legal/ethical considerations, local conditions, and payer policies.

The information contained in this exercise book is based upon experience and research. However, in the complex, rapidly changing medical and insurance environments, this information may not always prove correct. The data used is widely variable and can change at any time. Readers should follow current coding regulations as outlined by official coding organizations. Any five-digit numeric *Physicians' Current Procedural Terminology*, (CPT®) codes, services descriptions, instructions and/or guidelines are copyright (or such other date of publication of CPT® as defined in the federal copyright laws) by the American Medical Association. All Rights Reserved.

The American Medical Association assumes no responsibility for the consequences attributable to, or related to, any use or interpretation of any information or views contained in or not contained in this Publication.

CPT® is a listing of descriptive terms and five-digit numeric identifying codes and modifiers for reporting medical services performed by physicians. This presentation includes only CPT® descriptive terms, numeric identifying codes and modifiers for reporting medical services and procedures that were selected by ICDC Publishing, Inc. for inclusion in this Publication. The most current CPT® is available from the American Medical Association. No fee schedules, basic unit values, relative value guides, conversion factors or scales or components thereof are included in the CPT®.

ICDC Publishing, Inc. has selected certain CPT® codes and service/procedure descriptions and assigned them to various specialty groups. The listing of a CPT® service or procedure description and its code number in this Publication does not restrict its use to a particular specialty group. Any procedure or service in this Publication may be used to designate the services rendered by any qualified physician.

Information contained in this text are examples only. The publisher and author do not accept responsibility for any adverse outcome from undetected errors, opinion, and analysis contained in this manual that may prove inaccurate or incorrect, or from the reader's misunderstanding of an extremely complex topic. All names used in this book are completely fictitious. Any resemblance to persons or companies, current or no longer existing, is purely coincidental.

Contents

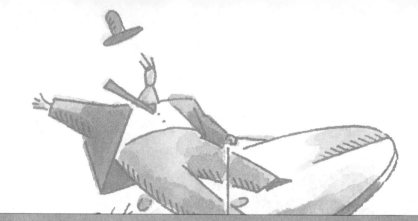

3 Diagnostic X-Ray and Laboratory Services   23

4 Surgery Services   38

5 Multiple Surgery Services 53

6 Assistant Surgery Services 64

7 Anesthesia Services 79

8 Hospital Services 89

9 Coordination of Benefits   193

10 Medicare and Medicaid Services   243

Preface

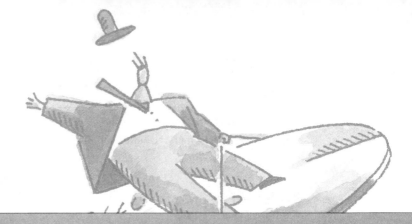

Introduction

Welcome to the exciting world of medical billing and health claims examining. This book is designed to help the student gain the real life experience of a medical biller and health claims examiner through a simulated work practice.

Writing Style

The straightforward easy-to-understand writing style presents information clearly and concisely. Patient and provider names, diagnoses, exercises and examples in this training material have been designed to incorporate a light-hearted humorous context. We have found that humorous writing improves the ability to comprehend and retain information.

Text Features

Special features of the text, such as medical billing exercises, health claims examining exercises, and simulated work practice, enhance understanding and retention of the material.

Medical Billing Exercises

Exercises for medical billers are located in the front of the chapters.

Health Claims Examining Exercises

Exercises for health claims examiners are located at the end of the chapters.

Simulated Work Practice

This exercise book allows the student to stay focused on the task of medical billing and coding or health claims examining. The often-quoted "practice makes perfect" rings true with this exercise book designed for the purpose of practicing medical billing and coding, and health claims examining.

Organization of the Text

This book is created for use in conjunction with ICDC Publishing's *Guide to Medical Billing and Coding,* and *Guide to Health Claims Examining.* The exercises are based upon concepts learned in the *Guide to Medical Billing and Coding,* and *Guide to Health Claims Examining.* This book should not be considered a complete text for learning medical billing or health claims examining.

This text may be used by students who are using a pegboard or manual system, as well as those using a computerized medical billing and/or health claims examining program. Many schools have used this book with the MediSoft Patient Accounting program, as well as with Medical Manager and various other computerized medical billing programs.

This book uses an innovative case scenario format to provide students with an opportunity to bill and process claims as they would in a work setting. Chapters Two through Eleven include the claim information (encounter forms) for billing and processing claims for a variety of services and providers. Chapters Twelve and Thirteen provide the students with Contracts, a UCR Conversion Factor Report, and a Relative Value Study to be used to complete the exercises. This text is designed to enable the student to work through the material at their own pace.

Ancillary and Program Material

When designing a curriculum and related materials, ICDC does extensive research regarding the skills employers consider essential for job performance. The curriculum and related books and materials are then written to ensure that students learn each of these essential skills. Many schools have gained state and accrediting agency approval with these materials. ICDC's material provides instructors and training institutions with all the materials needed to quickly and easily start and run a new program.

The *Exercises for Coding and Reimbursement Instructor Resource Guide*, the *Guide to Medical Billing and Coding,* and the *Guide to Health Claims Examining* are all designed to reinforce the concepts learned in the *Exercises for Coding and Reimbursement* and also provide the student an opportunity to practice and sharpen their skills.

Exercises for Coding and Reimbursement Instructor Resource Guide The Instructor Resource Guide (IRG) for the *Exercises for Coding and Reimbursement* is an all inclusive combined performance evaluator and curriculum. This Guide provides the instructors with the necessary tools to both run and manage a medical billing program, and to also assess the student's progress at critical points.

The Instructor Resource Guide includes the following components:

- **IRG Overview**—Provides the instructor with general information on structuring a medical billing program, and details how to obtain maximum benefits from the program materials.
- **Chapter Syllabi**—Outlines the main points of the chapters. The Syllabi includes the following:
  - Objectives.

- Prerequisites.
- Sections Covered.
- **Forms and Transparency Masters**—Forms and documents are provided for in-class presentations.
- **Professional Achievement of Certification and Educational Requirements (PACER™) Curriculum**—Provides the instructor with all the necessary materials needed to quickly and easily start a new program. The PACER™ curriculum is categorized by chapter, and includes the following:
  - **Daily Lesson Plans which include**:
    - Topics/Lessons Covered.
    - Performance Objectives.
    - Required Materials.
    - Discussion and Investigation Questions.
    - Teaching Methodologies/Evaluation.
- **Performance Evaluators and Answer Keys (PEAK™)**—Provides the instructor with the necessary tools to assess the student's progress at critical stages. The PEAKs™ are categorized by chapter, and include the following:
  - Chapter Exercise Answers.
  - Completed Forms.

Additional Resources

The following additional resources are available to accompany this text:

- *Guide to Medical Billing and Coding* is an **Honors Certification™** text and provides the student with all the theoretical knowledge needed to achieve success as a medical biller. This knowledge base is necessary preparation for students moving on to *Exercises for Coding and Reimbursement* medical billing exercises. The material is designed to be comprehensive, yet user-friendly. The text follows a logical learning format by beginning with a broad base of information and then, step-by-step, provides the student with specific information to build and gain proficiency as a medical biller.
- *Guide to Health Claims Examining* is an **Honors Certification™** text and provides the student with all the theoretical knowledge and practice skills needed to achieve success as a health claims examiner. This knowledge base is

necessary preparation for students moving on to *Exercises for Coding and Reimbursement,* claims examining exercises. The material is designed to be comprehensive, yet user-friendly. The text follows a logical learning format by beginning with a broad base of information and then, step-by-step, following the course for learning the specific health claims examiner job duties.

- *CPT© (Current Procedural Coding) Manuals*
- *ICD-9-CM (International Classification of Diseases–9th Revision) Manuals*
- *HCPCS (Healthcare Common Procedure Coding System) Manual*
- *Taber's Medical Dictionary*
- *PDR (Physician's Desk Reference)*
- *Merck Manual*

For more information, please contact Prentice Hall at (800) 526-0485 or www.prenhall.com.

Before You Start

Encounter Forms and Hospital Admission Forms

Encounter Forms and Hospital Admission Forms are located throughout Chapters Two through Eleven. These forms provide a description of the services and other pertinent billing information; however, ICD-9-CM codes and CPT® codes are not included. This allows the students to practice locating the correct codes and unit values as they would in a work environment. Encounter forms normally include services for one day; however, to save space and facilitate learning we have combined several dates on some encounter forms. Additional information for completing and processing claims is also included in the form of itemized hospital billings, Explanation of Benefits, COB Calculation Sheets, and Utilization Review Certification documents. These forms are located after the Encounter Form or Hospital Admission Form to which they apply.

Students are to use the information contained in the Encounter Form and patient chart to properly complete medical billing and claim processing exercises. Information should be placed in the appropriate blocks, fields, items, form locators or spaces on the appropriate billing form.

Additional Information

Occasionally, necessary information (e.g., insured's birth date or hospital address) for a particular claim is includ-

ed in a different scenario, requiring students to check all available resources for the information needed to complete exercises. In other cases, all necessary information is not included in the scenarios. For example, some claims may lack the notation "Authorization to Release Information on File," to give students practice in determining whether or not all necessary information has been provided. In some cases, students should be instructed to complete a Request for Further Information form and submit it to the instructor for additional instructions. The instructor will advise the students how to proceed and once students have requested the proper information and have filed the appropriate letters, they can continue to process the claim as though the necessary form or information were in hand.

Dates Please note that when YY is used in reference to a date, YY indicates the current year (12/01/YY). When PY is used in reference to a date, PY indicates the prior year or last year (12/01/PY). When NY is used in reference to a date, NY indicates the next year (12/01/NY).

Birth Dates Birth dates will be referenced with CCYY-##. This means that the ## should be subtracted from the current year to determine the birth year.

> **Example:** What is the birth date for 10/04/CCYY-14, if **CCYY = 2006**?
>
> **2006 − 14 = 1992**, therefore the birth date is **10/04/1992**

Medical Billing To bill the claims, students will use the CMS-1500 or UB-92 forms supplied by their instructors, or other source. Usage of these forms is explained in the *Guide to Medical Billing and Coding.*

Health Claims Examining Instructors should ensure that students have located and recorded the correct diagnosis and procedure codes prior to processing the claim, as incorrect codes will adversely affect the calculation of the benefit payment.

Upon completion of all of the medical billing exercises in this book the students will use these same claims for the health claims examining exercises. Medical Billing exercises in the entire text should be completed prior to students starting the Health Claims Examining exercises.

Students will use Payment Worksheets and Coordination of Benefits Calculation Worksheets for claims processing exercises. These forms are located in the **Forms** chapter. Usage of these forms is explained in the *Guide to Health Claims Examining.*

Students should process the claims according to the policies set forth in the Contracts found in Chapter 13. Students should also use the UCR Conversion Factor Report and Relative Value Study found in this chapter.

Proper Coding

Correct coding is a vital function of both the medical biller and health claims examiner. The instructor should also ensure that the student is paying the proper amount on the claim, processing it correctly, and issuing the benefit payment to the correct person, whether the insured or provider of services. Periodically checking payment worksheets and COB calculation worksheets will allow the instructor to ensure that students are processing claims correctly and to identify any areas of confusion for the students.

About the Author

ICDC Publishing, Inc. has been writing and creating vocational school materials since 1989. As a training center, Insurance Career Development Center (ICDC) trained students in various vocational occupations. ICDC authors are all professionals who have worked and have extensive training and knowledge in the field of the particular area of study.

Acknowledgements

Many people have contributed to the development and success of *Exercises for Coding and Reimbursement*. We extend our thanks and deep appreciation to the many students and classroom instructors who have provided us with helpful suggestions for this edition of the text.

We would like to express our thanks to the following individuals:

Linda Jepson; Janet Grossfeld, Adelante Career Institute, Van Nuys, CA; Hollis Anglin and Michael Coffin, Dawn Training Institute, New Castle, DE; Michael Williams and Timothy McGraw, 4-D College, Colton, CA; Anna McCracken and Lynn Russell, American Career College, Los Angeles, CA; Evelyn S. Wyskiel CPC, Branford Hall Institute, Southington, CT; Annie Rackley, Western Technical Institute, El Paso, TX; Tabari Jeffries; Krisia J. Hernandez; Sean Adams; Sydney Adams; Floree Brown; Nathaniel Brown Sr.; Celia R. Luna; Teresa Aguilar; Anita M. Garcia; Alexandra Fratkin, and CarolAnn Jeffries, PA-C, MHS.

Thanks to the CPA firm of Miller, Kaplan, Arase and Company, LLP.

We would also like extend our appreciation to the following reviewers for providing valuable feedback throughout the review process:

Beverly Giteles, CPC, CMM
Gibbs College
Livingston, NJ

Jessica Holtsberry
Ohio Institute of Health Careers
Columbus, OH

Kay Nave, CMA, MRT
Hagerstown Business College
Hagerstown, MD

1 Introduction

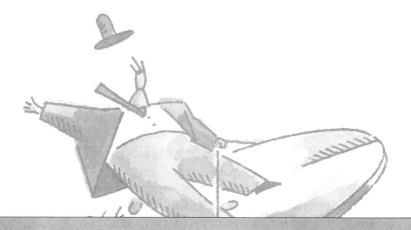

Welcome to the exciting world of medical billing and health claims examining. This text allows you to gain experience by taking you through a number of tasks, similar to what you will face in the everyday working world. It is intended to simulate the atmosphere and environment of a real medical or insurance office.

This text is intended to be included in a medical billing and health claims examining course. This text will reinforce the skills which you have learned and allow you to practice them in a controlled setting. You will have the opportunity to code, bill, and process numerous types of claims, including physician's services, lab, surgery, assistant surgery, anesthesia, hospital, durable medical equipment, and ambulance claims. During this simulated work program be sure to use the dates indicated in the text. In each case the year CCYY or YY should be replaced with the current year. The year PY should be replaced with the prior year (i.e., if you are completing exercises in 2006, YY = 2006 and PY = 2005).

This text is set up so that you can progress at your own pace. All exercises should be completed, and the exercise numbers should be placed in the upper right-hand corner of any forms or printouts.

Feel free to use other available resources to complete the exercises. On the job you will often have many of these resources available to you. These can include CPTs®, ICD-9-CMs, and HCPCS manuals, medical dictionaries, medical terminology books, medical billing instruction books, reference books on completing forms, etc. If you have difficulty remembering how to complete an exercise, consult your *Guide to Medical Billing and Coding* or *Guide to Health Claims Examining* textbook.

In order to save paper, we have included information for dependents on the same form as the insured. This prevents duplication of items such as address, phone number, insurance plan information, etc.

Go through the exercises step by step. Do not skip any exercises or move on until you have fully completed an exercise. If you skip exercises, completion of future exercises may be affected.

Getting Started

You are now ready to start the simulated work program. If you are using computerized software, you should first become familiar with it. You need not become proficient right away, as you will get plenty of practice using the software during the simulated work program. However, you should be familiar with how the program operates and the correct screen for entering various data.

When entering transactions (charges or payments), be sure to link the payment(s) to the proper charge(s). Doing this allows you to keep track of the amount which has been paid.

The directions provided in this exercise text are for a manual billing and claims processing system. However, the materials may be adapted for usage with a computerized billing or claims processing program.

Entering a Claim "Into A Computer System"

It is important to not only learn to enter data into a computer program, but also to understand the concepts behind what is being entered. At various times patients will need to be billed for services rendered, and claims will have to be processed for payment. The provider's office will complete a superbill, charge slip, or encounter form for the patient that shows the services performed and the related diagnoses. These documents will be presented to the patient for payment or sent to the insurance for payment. If you are using a computerized program, you will need to understand the dynamics of your program and process information accordingly.

To give you practice in coding procedures and diagnoses, the appropriate CPT®, ICD-9-CM, and HCPCS codes have not been listed on the Encounter forms. To complete the billing on a claim, use the CPT®, ICD-9-CM, and HCPCS manuals to code the procedures and diagnoses. To "enter a claim into the computer system" means to complete each of the following steps.

Medical Billing

a. Enter the patient and any other family members into the Patient Information database.

b. Enter the CPT® and HCPCS codes into the Procedure Information screens. Some procedures may have been previously entered. If so, these proce-

dures do not need to be reentered. If a procedure has already been entered, the data will appear on the screen when you enter the code into the Procedure Code field.

c. Enter the ICD-9-CM codes into the Diagnosis Code Information screen. Some diagnoses may have been previously entered. If so, these diagnoses do not need to be reentered. If a diagnosis has already been entered, the data will appear on the screen when you enter the code into the Diagnosis Code field.

d. Enter the charges as shown on the Encounter and Hospital Admission Forms. If a payment was made, enter the payment and print a walkout receipt before saving the data.

e. Create a CMS-1500 or UB-92 Form for the patient visit. If you are not using two-part CMS-1500 forms, write up two forms or make a copy of the form when it is completed. One copy will be placed in the patient chart; the other will be mailed to the insurance carrier (given to your instructor). Many computer systems allow you to print out all patient claims which were entered in a single day. For this reason, at the end of each day computerized billing users should print out the CMS-1500s or UB-92s which have been entered for that day. Using two-part forms is suggested.

Health Claims Examining

a. Enter the patient and any other family members into the Member Information or Eligibility database.

b. Enter the CPT® and HCPCS codes into the Procedure Information screens. Some procedures may have been previously entered. If so, these procedures do not need to be reentered. If a procedure has already been entered, the data will appear on the screen when you enter the code into the Procedure Code field.

c. Enter the ICD-9-CM codes into the Diagnosis Code Information screen. Some diagnoses may have been previously entered. If so, these diagnoses do not need to be reentered. If a diagnosis has already been entered, the data will appear on the screen when you enter the code into the Diagnosis Code field.

d. Enter the charges as shown on the CMS-1500 or UB-92 Forms.

e. Create an Explanation of Benefits, Remittance Advice, or Payment Worksheet for claims. If you are not using two-part forms, create two forms or make a copy. One copy will be placed in the Family File; the other will be mailed to the member or the provider of service. Many computer systems allow you to print out all claims which were entered in a single day; check your program's specifications to determine if it has this feature.

Let's Begin Medical Billing

You have just begun working for All Billing Services, 123 Any Way, Anytown, USA 12345. As a medical biller, you keep patient accounts for a number of doctors. It is your responsibility to handle all billing for services rendered by providers and to maintain patient accounts. You will bill the appropriate patients, insurance carriers, Medicare, or other entities responsible for payment; keep track of all patient accounts; write collection letters; and prepare bank deposits.

Each Encounter Form and Hospital Admission Form has been assigned a claim number. To help keep track of documents for this program, place the appropriate claim number in the upper right-hand corner of each CMS-1500, UB-92, or other documents created or completed.

Medical Billing Guidelines

- **Family Data Tables**—are to be used to abstract pertinent information to create patient charts and bill for services rendered.

- **Encounter and Hospital Admission Forms**—are to be used to abstract information to create the appropriate billing form.

- **CMS-1500 and UB-92 Forms**—your instructor will provide you with the appropriate number of CMS-1500 and UB-92 forms for billing claims; or they may be purchased from a stationery store.

- **Insurance Coverage Forms**—information to complete the Insurance Coverage Forms should be obtained from the Contracts in Chapter 13, the Patient Data Table, and from the Beginning Financials at the end of Chapters 2 through 11.

- **Services**—should be listed in date order. If information is not available to complete a certain item, that item should be left blank on the billing form. Students should never create information to fill in a field or block.

- **Reference Books**—you will need to reference the CPT®, ICD-9-CM, and HCPCS manuals when completing the billing forms and processing claims.

- **Proper Coding**—it is imperative that you ensure that your claims have been coded properly prior to completing any claims processing worksheets. If claims are incorrectly coded, the unit values and, therefore, your calculations, will be incorrect. Correct coding is a vital function for both medical billers and health claims examiners. If you are incorrectly coding more than 10% of the diagnoses or procedures, the need for more practice is indicated.

- **Signatures on Claims**—each completed claim form should be signed by the provider's representative.

- **Dates**—Please note that when YY is used in reference to a date the YY indicates the current year (12/01/YY). When PY is used in reference to a date the PY indicates the prior year or last year (12/01/PY). When NY is used in reference to a date NY indicates the next year (12/01/NY).

- **Birth Dates**—Birth dates will be referenced with CCYY-##. this indicates to subtract the ## from the current year to determine the birth year.

   Example: Birth date 10/04/CCYY-14, if **CCYY = 2006**; 2006 – 14 = 1992 Birth year.

- **Blank Forms and Stationery**—are included in Chapter 12. These forms are to be used as instructed to complete or create forms and/or write correspondence.

- **Anesthesia Time**—convert hours into minutes and enter the total minutes in block 24G of the CMS-1500 form.

- **Block 23**—should be used to place notations such as "Prescription on File" for DME and Pharmacy claims; "SSO Performed" for claims for which an SSO was performed; and Pre-Authorization or Pre-Certification numbers or a notation that it was performed for those claims requiring it.

Setting Up Your "Office"

As you work through this text, you will be responsible for setting up your office and completing each of the exercises. For this reason it is important to maintain a set of files and other work items which can be used day to day. Setting up your "office" with the following items will help to keep them neat and ensure that items are easily accessible.

You will need the following items to properly complete the exercises in this book:

- One envelope for copies of Patient Receipts to calculate deposit to be made.
- 30 Family/Patient File folders (see **Patient Files** section below).
- One "Practice" folder for keeping all daily charts and forms which are generated for the practice.
- One folder for all completed claims which would be sent to the insurance carrier.
- 125 + CMS-1500 forms for billing.
- 40 + UB-92 forms for billing.
- One expanding file folder for keeping all of the above items together.
- Pens and pencils.

Additionally, you will need access to the following:

- CPT®, ICD-9-CM, and HCPCS coding books.
- Scissors.
- Two-hole punch.
- Medical dictionary and/or other reference books.

Place the cash and deposit envelopes in the front of the expanding folder, followed by the practice folder and then the patient charts. As you are introduced to each patient and/or their family, create a family chart and place it in your expanding file folder. All other forms for setting up your office are located in the Forms chapter.

Deposit Envelope

As a medical biller, you are responsible for depositing the payments collected from patients. At the end of each chapter you will prepare a deposit slip/ticket with all payments received during that chapter.

It is suggested that you keep all deposit and payment receipts in a single envelope. When a patient makes a payment, place a copy of the payment receipt in the patient's chart and a copy in the deposit envelope. Clearly label the envelopes **DEPOSITS**.

Patient Files

The patient files are also kept in your office. All billing services keep family files for their patients, instead of individual files. Each family file consists of a three or four page file folder with pronged paper fasteners at the top for holding information (**see Figure 1–1**). Each file should contain information in the following order:

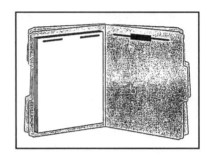

■ Figure 1–1

Fastener 1

1. Patient Information Sheet. These forms will be completed during the exercises in this text.
2. Insurance Coverage Sheet. These forms will be completed during the exercises in this text.
3. Any other forms or information which pertains to the entire family.

Fastener 2

1. Billing information (CMS-1500 claims and patient statements) in chronological order (most recent date first) for the insured. These forms will be completed during the exercises in this text.

Fasteners 3, 4, and 5

1. Billing information, CMS-1500 claims and patient statements in chronological order (most recent first) for dependents. Each dependent should have their own separate fastener. These forms will be completed during the exercises in this text.
2. If there are more than three dependents in the family, insert a divider or folder with fasteners to accommodate the additional family members.

Last Fastener

1. For training purposes, this page will be used to attach all items which are given to the patient or insured. These items can include change for a cash payment, a receipt, or statements which were sent to the patient.

Training tip: For class purposes, you may want to create patient files by placing one manila folder inside another and securing them together at the fold. Then attach a two pronged paper fastener at the top of each page to hold the papers in place. Keep all of your files in an expanding file folder. Patient files should be kept available at all times.

GOOD LUCK as you venture into a challenging, but fulfilling medical billing career.

Let's Begin Health Claims Examining

You have just been hired to work as a claims examiner for Any Insurance Carriers, Inc., P.O. Box 1111, Anywhere, USA 12345. As a health claims examiner you are responsible for the adjudication of claims. It is your responsibility to handle all claims processing activities for claims submitted. You will verify eligibility, calculate reasonable and customary charges, make claim payments, and write correspondence.

If additional information is needed from a provider or other party, complete a Request for Additional Information form which can be found in the Forms chapter and give it to your instructor; who will advise you as to how to proceed.

You should handle all situations as you would in a normal office. Therefore, if you pay a claim incorrectly, do not just erase your figures and correct them; process the claim on a second Payment Worksheet and make an adjustment. If you send payment to the wrong party, make an adjustment to send the payment to the correct party, then write a letter requesting repayment (or the original check back) from the first (incorrect) payee.

Each claim has been assigned a claim number. To help keep track of documents for this program, place the appropriate claim number in the upper right-hand corner of each Payment Worksheet created or other document created or completed.

Health Claims Examining Guidelines

- **Dates**—please note that when YY is used in reference to a date the YY indicates the current year (12/01/YY). When PY is used in reference to a date the PY indicates the prior year or last year (12/01/PY). When NY is used in reference to a date NY indicates the next year (12/01/NY).

- **Birth Dates**—will be referenced with CCYY-## this indicates to subtract the ## from the current year to determine the birth year.

  Example: What is the birth date 10/04/CCYY-14, if **CCYY = 2006**

  2006 – 14 = 1992 therefore the birth date = **10/04/1992**

- **Family Data Tables**—are to be used to verify eligibility for claimants and other pertinent informational usage.

- **Beginning Financials**—are included for individuals and families covered within the exercises. When processing claims, these financials should be incorporated as payment history, and claims calculations should be adjusted accordingly. Deductible information should be included in the current year deductible for that person. Therefore, in figuring current year deductible, subtract the listed deductible from the current year amount. The lifetime maximum listed should be added to the accumulated amount.

- **Insurance Coverage Forms**—information to complete the Insurance Coverage Forms should be obtained from the Contracts in Chapter 13, the Patient Data Table, and from the Beginning Financials at the end of Chapters 2 through 11.

- **Signature on File**—in block 13 is acceptable for the assignment of benefits.

- **Contracts**—are included in Chapter 13. These are the contracts to be used for claims processing.

- **UCR Conversion Factor Report**—is included in Chapter 13. This is the UCR Conversion Factor Report to be used for claims processing.

- **Relative Value Study**—is included in the **Forms** chapter. This is the Relative Value Study to be used for claims processing.

- **By Report Procedures**—when a By Report procedure is encountered a Request for Additional Information Form should be completed. This form should be given to the instructor who in turn will provide the allowable units or dollar amount to be used for the processing of that specific claim.

- **Multiple Surgery Claims**—global claims processing guidelines should be used for multiple surgery claims. Secondary, tertiary, and so on, procedures should be reduced to 50% if applicable.

- **Basic Benefits**—do not accumulate toward the lifetime maximum; however, supplemental accident benefits do accumulate toward the lifetime maximum.

- **Block 23**—may contain notations on them such as "Prescription on File;" Network Provider;" "SSO Performed;" or "Pre-Certification Received", etc. These notations have been placed on the claim to facilitate claims processing and inform the claims examiner that the necessary documents and/or information noted has been received by the insurance carrier. The claims should be processed based on the information noted, and it is not necessary for the claims examiner to request this information. In addition, any associated penalties for noncompliance should not be taken.

- **Anesthesia Time**—will be listed in block 24G of the CMS-1500. Refer to the specific contract for computation of anesthesia time.

- **Assistant Surgeon Procedures List**—is included in Chapter 13. This list should be checked to determine whether an assistant is required for the listed procedure.

- **Network Provider List**—is included in Chapter 13. This list should be checked to determine whether a provider is network or nonnetwork.

- **Payment Worksheets**—are provided in Chapter 12 and are to be used for processing claims. More than one payment worksheet may be needed per claim. This will be the case when an error is made and you need to start over; when the number of services provided exceeds six (the number of available spaces on the payment worksheet).

- **Additional Information Requests Forms**—are included in Chapter 12. This form should be used to request any additional information needed to process claims properly.

- **Coordination of Benefits Calculation Worksheets**—are included in Chapter 12. This form should be used when processing claims as the secondary carrier, thus requiring coordination of benefits.

- **Family Benefits Tracking Sheet**—should be used to keep track of benefits for the family.

- **Blank Forms and Stationery**—are included to be used when you are instructed to complete or create forms and/or write correspondence.

- **Prescription Drugs**—should be allowed as billed (for UCR) if the item is a covered expense under the plan.

Setting Up Your "Desk"

As you go through this text you will be responsible for setting up your desk and completing each of the exercises. For this reason it is important to maintain a set of files and other work items that can be used from day to day. Setting up your "desk" with the following items will help to keep things neat and ensure that items are easily accessible.

You will need the following items to properly complete the exercises in this book:

Quantity	Item
30	Family File folders—(manila folder) (see Family Files section below).
3	Contract folders—(manila folder)—one for each contract.
1	Expanding file folder—for keeping all of the above items together.
1	Miscellaneous folder—(manila folder) for keeping Conversion Factor Report, Beginning Financials, RVS Schedules, etc.

Additionally, you will need the following items:

- Prong fasteners.
- Pens and pencils.
- Two-hole punch.

Optional:
- Plastic sleeves to protect contracts.

As you are introduced to each insurance carrier contract and each insured and/or their dependent(s), create a family folder for all pertinent data relating to that contract or family.

Family Files

Any Insurance Carrier, Inc. keeps family files that contain information on all the family members. The family files are also kept at your desk. Each family file consists of a three- or four-page file folder with pronged paper fasteners at the top for holding the papers in place.

Each file should contain information in the following order:

Fastener 1—Entire Family

1. Insurance Coverage Sheet. This form will be completed during the exercises in this text.
2. Any other forms or information that pertains to the entire family or to more than one individual in the family. This can include:
   * Copy of Marriage Certificate
   * Deductible Payment Information

Fastener 2—Insured

1. Claims, payment worksheets, and any other data pertaining to claims in reverse date order (most recent date first) for the insured. These forms will be completed during the exercises in this text.

In addition to claims and payment worksheets, additional data which may be collected include:

* Copy of Adoption Paperwork
* Preexisting Investigations Paperwork
* Third Party Subrogation or Workers' Compensation Information
* Accident Benefit Payment Information

Fastener 3—Spouse

1. Claims, payment worksheets, and any other data pertaining to the spouse, kept in reverse date order (most recent date first). These forms will be completed during the exercises in this text.

Fasteners 4, 5, and 6—Dependent Data

1. Claims, payment worksheets, and any other data pertaining to the dependents in reverse date order (most recent date first). These forms will be completed during the exercises in this text.
2. Full-time Student Status documents.
3. Birth Certificates.

Each dependent should have their own separate page. If there are more than three dependents in the family, insert a divider or an additional folder inside the file to create additional pages.

Training Tip: For class purposes, you may want to create family files by placing one manila folder inside another and securing them together at the fold. Then attach a two-pronged paper fastener at the top of each page to hold the papers in place. Keep all of your files in an expanding file folder.

Once you have all the items you will need, you are ready to begin the simulated work program.

GOOD LUCK as you venture into a challenging, but fulfilling health claims examining career.

2
Physicians' Services

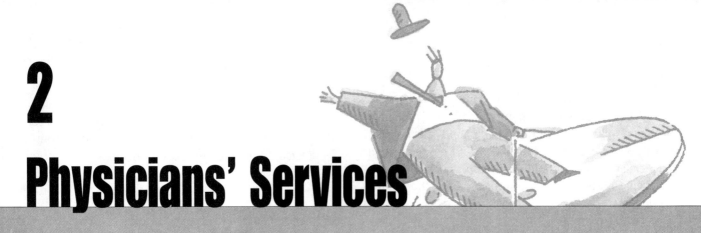

Medical Billing Exercises
Exercise 2-1

Directions: Complete Patient Information Sheets (leave **Assigned Provider** field blank), Ledger Cards and Insurance Coverage Forms and set up patient charts for the following families using copies of the forms in the **Forms** chapter. Refer to the Family Data Tables **(Documents 1–3)** for information.

Individual folders with dividers may be used to store information for each family. One Patient Information Sheet and Insurance Coverage Form should be filled out for the entire family.

DOCUMENT 1

FAMILY DATA TABLE

ESPINOSA FAMILY	INSURED'S INFORMATION	SPOUSE'S INFORMATION	CHILD #1	CHILD #2	CHILD #3
Name	Evelyn Espinosa		Elisa Espinosa	Eva Espinosa	Evan Espinosa
Address	621 Espinaza Ave. Los Angeles, CA 90012		621 Espinaza Ave. Los Angeles, CA 90012	621 Espinaza Ave. Los Angeles, CA 90012	621 Espinaza Ave. Los Angeles, CA 90012
Email Address	evelyne@espinosa.com				
TELEPHONE #					
Home:	(213) 555-9001		(213) 555-9001	(213) 555-9001	(213) 555-9001
Work:	(213) 555-9002				
Cell:	(213) 555-9003				
Date of Birth	08/18/CCYY-53		08/15/CCYY-18	10/08/CCYY-17	02/11/CCYY-16
Social Security #	999-99-9993		999-99-9994	999-99-9995	999-99-9996
Marital Status/Gender	Single/Female		Single/Female	Single/Female	Single/Male
Student Status			Full-time	Full-time	Full-time
Patient Account #	10001		10002	10003	10004
Allergies/Medical Conditions	None		None	None	None
PRIMARY INSURANCE CARRIER					
Name Address	Winter Insurance Company 9763 Western Way Whittier, CO 82963		Winter Insurance Company 9763 Western Way Whittier, CO 82963	Winter Insurance Company 9763 Western Way Whittier, CO 82963	Winter Insurance Company 9763 Western Way Whittier, CO 82963
Effective Date	01/01/CCPY		01/01/CCPY	01/01/CCPY	01/01/CCPY
Member's ID #	99-9993 ABC		99-9993 ABC	99-9993 ABC	99-9993 ABC
Group Policy #	36928		36928	36928	36928
Policy/Employer	ABC Corporation 1234 Whitaker Lane Colter, CO 81222				
OTHER INSURANCE CARRIERS					
Name Address					
Effective Date					
Member's ID #					
Group Policy #					
Policy/Employer					
Responsible Party	Self		Insured	Insured	Insured
EMERGENCY CONTACT					
Name	Eve Espinoli		Eve Espinoli	Eve Espinoli	Eve Espinoli
Telephone #	(213) 555-9004		(213) 555-9004	(213) 555-9004	(213) 555-9004
Address	126 Espinaza Ave. Los Angeles, CA 90012		126 Espinaza Ave. Los Angeles, CA 90012	126 Espinaza Ave. Los Angeles, CA 90012	126 Espinaza Ave. Los Angeles, CA 90012

FAMILY DATA TABLE

SMITH FAMILY	Insured's Information	Spouse's Information	Child #1	Child #2	Child #3
Name	Steve Smith	Sharon Smith	Sam Smith		
Address	1121 Schmidt Road Sortlete, CA 91733	1121 Schmidt Road Sortlete, CA 91733	1121 Schmidt Road Sortlete, CA 91733		
Email Address	steves@smith.com				
TELEPHONE #					
Home:	(415) 555-9173	(415) 555-9173	(415) 555-9173		
Work:	(415) 555-9174				
Cell:	(415) 555-9175				
Date of Birth	08/16/CCYY-56	11/11/CCYY-55	06/16/CCYY-18		
Social Security #	888-88-8888	888-88-8889	888-88-8880		
Marital Status/Gender	Married/Male	Married/Female	Single/Male		
Student Status			Full-time		
Patient Account #	10006	10005	10007		
Allergies/Medical Conditions	None	None	None		
PRIMARY INSURANCE CARRIER					
Name Address	Rover Insurers, Inc. 5931 Rolling Road Ronson, CO 81369	Rover Insurers, Inc. 5931 Rolling Road Ronson, CO 81369	Rover Insurers, Inc. 5931 Rolling Road Ronson, CO 81369		
Effective Date	01/01/CCPY	01/01/CCPY	01/01/CCPY		
Member's ID #	88-8888 NIN	88-8888 NIN	88-8888 NIN		
Group Policy #	21088	21088	21088		
Policy/Employer	Ninja Enterprises 1234 Nockout Road Newton, NM 88012				
OTHER INSURANCE CARRIER					
Name Address					
Effective Date					
Member's ID #					
Group Policy #					
Policy/Employer					
Responsible Party	Self	Self	Insured		
EMERGENCY CONTACT					
Name	Sammy Stone	Sammy Stone	Sammy Stone		
Telephone #	(415) 555-9176	(415) 555-9176	(415) 555-9176		
Address	1211 Schmidt Road Sortlete, CA 91733	1211 Schmidt Road Sortlete, CA 91733	1211 Schmidt Road Sortlete, CA 91733		

DOCUMENT 3

FAMILY DATA TABLE

PARKER FAMILY	INSURED'S INFORMATION	SPOUSE'S INFORMATION	CHILD #1	CHILD #2	CHILD #3
Name	Patricia Parker	Peter Parker	Pauline Parker		
Address	1501 Pea Pod Drive Princeton, CA 90021	1501 Pea Pod Drive Princeton, CA 90021	1501 Pea Pod Drive Princeton, CA 90021		
Email Address	patriciap@parker.com				
TELEPHONE #					
Home:	(626) 555-9012	(626) 555-9012	(626) 555-9012		
Work:	(626) 555-9022				
Cell:	(626) 555-9032				
Date of Birth	01/12/CCYY-60	03/20/CCYY-60	07/05/CCYY-18		
Social Security #	777-77-7771	777-77-7772	777-77-7773		
Marital Status/Gender	Married/Female	Married/Male	Single/Female		
Student Status			Full-time		
Patient Account #	10008	10009	10010		
Allergies/Medical Conditions	None	None	None		
PRIMARY INSURANCE CARRIER					
Name Address	Ball Insurance Carriers 3895 Bubble Blvd. Ste. 283 Boxwood, CO 85926	Ball Insurance Carriers 3895 Bubble Blvd. Ste. 283 Boxwood, CO 85926	Ball Insurance Carriers 3895 Bubble Blvd. Ste. 283 Boxwood, CO 85926		
Effective Date	01/01/CCPY	01/01/CCPY	01/01/CCPY		
Member's ID #	77-7771 XYZ	77-7771 XYZ	77-7771 XYZ		
Group Policy #	62958	62958	62958		
Policy/Employer	XYZ Corporation 9817 Bobcat Blvd. Bastion, CO 81319				
OTHER INSURANCE CARRIER					
Name Address					
Effective Date					
Member's ID #					
Group Policy #					
Policy/Employer					
Responsible Party	Self	Self	Insured		
EMERGENCY CONTACT					
Name	Paul Parks	Paul Parks	Paul Parks		
Telephone #	(626) 555-9033	(626) 555-9033	(626) 555-9033		
Address	1051 Pea Pod Drive Princeton, CA 90021	1051 Pea Pod Drive Princeton, CA 90021	1051 Pea Pod Drive Princeton, CA 90021		

Exercise **2-2**

Directions: Complete a CMS-1500 for each of the Encounter Forms **(Documents 5–9, 11–15, and 17–21)** in this chapter. CMS-1500 forms may be provided by your instructor or purchased from a stationery store.

After completion of each CMS-1500 form complete a Patient Receipt (if a payment was made), and post the transaction(s) to the patient Ledger Card/Statement of Account previously created.

Exercise **2-3**

Directions: Upon completion of all of the activities in Exercise 2–2 complete a Bank Deposit Slip/Ticket (located in the **Forms** chapter) for all payments made on the patient's account in this chapter.

Exercise **2-4**

Directions: Using an Insurance Claims Register (located in the **Forms** chapter) list all claims that have been fully prepared and are ready for submission to the insurance carrier for payment. Enter the date that you created the CMS-1500 in the **Date Claim Filed** column.

Exercise **2-5**

Directions: Using the stationery or Request for Additional Information Form (located in the **Forms** chapter), write a letter or request information for the following scenario. In each case, you are the medical biller working for Any Billing Services.

Addresses and personal information are contained in the patient files that were previously set up. Also, refer to the Family Data Table **(Document 3)** for required information.

1. Create a correspondence for Patricia Parker requesting her to send a copy of her latest insurance card.

Physicians' Claims Beginning Financials
ESPINOSA FAMILY

Insurance Plan	Winter Insurance Company—ABC Corporation				
Patient:	**EVELYN**	**ELISA**	**EVA**	**EVAN**	
C/O DEDUCTIBLE	0.00	0.00	0.00	0.00	
DEDUCTIBLE	0.00	75.00	100.00	0.00	
COINSURANCE	0.00	0.00	475.00	0.00	
ACCIDENT BENEFIT	0.00	0.00	0.00	0.00	
LIFETIME MAXIMUM	1,750.00	0.00	6,000.00	1,275.05	
M/N OFFICE VISITS					
OFFICE VISITS					
HOSPITAL VISITS					
DXL					
SURGERY					
ASSISTANT SURGERY					
ANESTHESIA					

Encounter Form

Provider Information

Name:	Espana Salud Clinic				
Address:	5555 Espana Avenue				
City:	Espana	State:	CA	Zip Code:	90270
Telephone #:		Fax #:			
Medicare ID#:		UPIN #:	W00001		
Tax ID #:	95-3322298	Accepts Medicare Assignment:	☒		
Provider's Signature:	Ervin Erlow, MD		Date: 7/14/CCYY		

Appointment Information

Appointment Date:		Time:	
Next Appt. Date:		Time:	
Date of First Visit:	07/14/CCYY	Date of Injury:	
Referring Physician:			

Patient Information

Name:	Evelyn Espinosa				
Address:	621 Espinaza Avenue				
City:	Los Angeles	State:	CA	Zip Code:	90012
Telephone #:	(213) 555-9001	Account #:	10001		
Date of Birth:	08/18/CCYY-53	Gender:	Female		
Marital Status:	Single	Relationship to Guarantor:	Self		
Student Status:	☐ Full-time	☐ Part-time			
Insurance Type:	☒ Pvt ☐ M/care ☐ M/caid ☐ WC ☐ Other				
Hospitalization Date:					
Hospital Information:					

Guarantor Information

Name:	Evelyn Espinosa
Address:	621 Espinaza Avenue
City: Los Angeles State: CA Zip Code: 90012	
Insurance ID #:	99-9993 ABC
Insurance Name:	Winter Insurance Company
Insurance Group #:	36928
Employer Name:	ABC Corporation

Authorization

☒ Authorization to Release Information
☐ Authorization for Assignment of Benefits
☐ Authorization for Consent for Treatment
☐ My insurance will be billed but there may be a balance due.

Signature: Evelyn Espinosa   Date: 7/14/CCYY

Clinical Information

	DOS	POS	CPT® /HCPCS Description	ICD-9-CM (*Indicates diagnosis for all lines)	Amount
1	07/14/CCYY	Office	New pt, detailed exam with history, low complexity	*Otitis media; *1 Acute pharyngitis	$ 75.00
2	07/14/CCYY	Office	Intramuscular injection of orphenadrine citrate 60 mg	*; *1	$ 30.00
3	07/14/CCYY	Office	Intramuscular, therapeutic injection of ciproflaxin	*; *1	$ 20.00
4					
5					
6					
Remarks:	Services performed by Ervin Erlow, M.D. UPIN #: A12345				

Previous Balance:		Payment:	$20.00	Copay:		Adjustment:			
Total Fee:	$125.00	Cash ☒ Check ☐ Credit ☐		Cash ☐ Check ☐ Credit ☐		Reason:		New Balance:	$105.00

Encounter Form

Provider Information

Name:	Eitsum Estobar, M.D.
Address:	P.O. Box 4666
City:	Espana	State: CA	Zip Code: 90270
Telephone #:	Fax #:
Medicare ID#:	UPIN #: B23456
Tax ID #:	95-2867890	Accepts Medicare Assignment: ☒
Provider's Signature:	*Eitsum Estobar, MD*	Date: *6/11/CCYY*

Patient Information

Name:	Elisa Espinosa
Address:	621 Espinaza Avenue
City:	Los Angeles	State: CA	Zip Code: 90012
Telephone #:	(213) 555-9001	Account #: 10002
Date of Birth:	08/15/CCYY-18	Gender: Female
Marital Status:	Single	Relationship to Guarantor: Child
Student Status:	☒ Full-time	☐ Part-time
Insurance Type:	☒ Pvt ☐ M/care ☐ M/caid ☐ WC ☐ Other _____
Hospitalization Date:	
Hospital Information:	Espana Community Hospital, P.O. Box 1234, Espana, CA 90270

Appointment Information

Appointment Date:		Time:
Next Appt. Date:		Time:
Date of First Visit:	06/11/CCYY	Date of Injury:
Referring Physician:	Saky Shameen, M.D.	

Guarantor Information

Name:	Evelyn Espinosa
Address:	621 Espinaza Avenue
City:	Los Angeles	State: CA	Zip Code: 90012
Insurance ID #:	99-9993 ABC
Insurance Name:	Winter Insurance Company
Insurance Group #:	36928
Employer Name:	ABC Corporation

Authorization

☒ Authorization to Release Information
☐ Authorization for Assignment of Benefits
☐ Authorization for Consent for Treatment
☐ My insurance will be billed but there may be a balance due.

Signature: *Evelyn Espinosa*   Date: *6/11/CCYY*

Clinical Information

	DOS	POS	CPT® /HCPCS Description	ICD-9-CM (*Indicates diagnosis for all lines)	Amount
1	06/11/CCYY	Otpt Hosp	Init consult expand prob focused hist & exam, straight	Ovarian Cyst; Pelvic Adhesions	$ 75.00
2					
3					
4					
5					
6					

Remarks:	Referring Physician: Saky Shameen, M.D. UPIN #: C33322				
Previous Balance:		Payment:	Copay:	Adjustment:	
Total Fee:	$75.00	Cash ☐ Check ☐ Credit ☐	Cash ☐ Check ☐ Credit ☐	Reason:	New Balance: $75.00

Encounter Form

Provider Information

Name:	Emergency Physician Services
Address:	199 E. Foothill Blvd.
City:	Los Angeles	State: CA	Zip Code: 90270
Telephone #:	Fax #:
Medicare ID#:	UPIN #: W00002
Tax ID #:	95-3334086	Accepts Medicare Assignment: ☒
Provider's Signature:	*Eric Elliot, MD*	Date: *7/6/CCYY*

Patient Information

Name:	Eva Espinosa
Address:	621 Espinaza Avenue
City:	Los Angeles	State: CA	Zip Code: 90012
Telephone #:	(213) 555-9001	Account #: 10003
Date of Birth:	10/08/CCYY-17	Gender: Female
Marital Status:	Single	Relationship to Guarantor: Child
Student Status:	☒ Full-time	☐ Part-time
Insurance Type:	☒ Pvt ☐ M/care ☐ M/caid ☐ WC ☐ Other _____
Hospitalization Date:	
Hospital Information:	

Appointment Information

Appointment Date:		Time:
Next Appt. Date:		Time:
Date of First Visit:	07/06/CCYY	Date of Injury: 07/06/CCYY
Referring Physician:		

Guarantor Information

Name:	Evelyn Espinosa
Address:	621 Espinaza Avenue
City:	Los Angeles	State: CA	Zip Code: 90012
Insurance ID #:	99-9993 ABC
Insurance Name:	Winter Insurance Company
Insurance Group #:	36928
Employer Name:	ABC Corporation

Authorization

☒ Authorization to Release Information
☒ Authorization for Assignment of Benefits
☐ Authorization for Consent for Treatment
☐ My insurance will be billed but there may be a balance due.

Signature: *Evelyn Espinosa*   Date: *7/6/CCYY*

Clinical Information

	DOS	POS	CPT® /HCPCS Description	ICD-9-CM (*Indicates diagnosis for all lines)	Amount
1	07/06/CCYY	Otpt Hosp	ER eval; expanded exam and hist; low	Friction Burn	$ 55.00
2					
3					
4					
5					
6					

Remarks:	Services performed by Eric Elliot, M.D. UPIN #: C34567	Parent states child fell while skating at home, scraping knee.			
Previous Balance:		Payment: $55.00	Copay:	Adjustment:	
Total Fee:	$55.00	Cash ☐ Check ☒ Credit ☐	Cash ☐ Check ☐ Credit ☐	Reason:	New Balance: $0.00

Encounter Form

DOCUMENT 8

Provider Information

Name:	Ed Epman, M.D.
Address:	124 N. East Drive

City:	Eldorado	State:	CA	Zip Code:	91236

Telephone #:		Fax #:	

Medicare ID#:		UPIN #:	D45678

Tax ID #:	556-67-9900	Accepts Medicare Assignment:	☒

Provider's Signature:	*Ed Epman, MD*	Date: 1/11/CCYY

Patient Information

Name:	Evan Espinosa
Address:	621 Espinaza Avenue

City:	Los Angeles	State:	CA	Zip Code:	90012

Telephone #:	(213) 555-9001	Account #:	10004

Date of Birth:	02/11/CCYY-16	Gender:	Male

Marital Status:	Single	Relationship to Guarantor:	Child

Student Status:	☒ Full-time ☐ Part-time
Insurance Type:	☒ Pvt ☐ M/care ☐ M/caid ☐ WC ☐ Other _____
Hospitalization Date:	
Hospital Information:	

Appointment Information

Appointment Date:		Time:	
Next Appt. Date:		Time:	
Date of First Visit:	01/07/CCYY	Date of Injury:	
Referring Physician:			

Guarantor Information

Name:	Evelyn Espinosa
Address:	621 Espinaza Avenue

City:	Los Angeles	State:	CA	Zip Code:	90012

Insurance ID #:	99-9993 ABC
Insurance Name:	Winter Insurance Company
Insurance Group #:	36928
Employer Name:	ABC Corporation

Authorization

☒ Authorization to Release Information
☒ Authorization for Assignment of Benefits
☐ Authorization for Consent for Treatment
☐ My insurance will be billed but there may be a balance due.

Signature: *Evelyn Espinosa*   Date: 1/11/CCYY

Clinical Information

	DOS	POS	CPT® /HCPCS Description	ICD-9-CM (*Indicates diagnosis for all lines)	Amount
1	01/11/CCYY	Office	Est pt, prob focused hist and exam, straightforward	Scarlet Fever; Acute URI	$ 35.00
2					
3					
4					
5					
6					

Remarks:						
Previous Balance:		Payment:		Copay:		Adjustment:
Total Fee:	$35.00	Cash ☐ Check ☐ Credit ☐		Cash ☐ Check ☐ Credit ☐		Reason:

New Balance: $35.00

Encounter Form

DOCUMENT 9

Provider Information

Name:	Edgardo Ealua, M.D.
Address:	777 E. Espania Road

City:	Conoga	State:	CA	Zip Code:	91306

Telephone #:		Fax #:	

Medicare ID#:		UPIN #:	E56789

Tax ID #:	95-4277829	Accepts Medicare Assignment:	☒

Provider's Signature:	*Edgardo Ealua, MD*	Date: 8/11/CCYY

Patient Information

Name:	Evan Espinosa
Address:	621 Espinaza Avenue

City:	Los Angeles	State:	CA	Zip Code:	90012

Telephone #:	(213) 555-9001	Account #:	10004

Date of Birth:	02/11/CCYY-16	Gender:	Male

Marital Status:	Single	Relationship to Guarantor:	Child

Student Status:	☒ Full-time ☐ Part-time
Insurance Type:	☒ Pvt ☐ M/care ☐ M/caid ☐ WC ☐ Other _____
Hospitalization Date:	From: 08/10/CCYY To: 08/12/CCYY
Hospital Information:	Espana Community Hospital, P.O. Box 1234, Espana, CA 90270

Appointment Information

Appointment Date:		Time:	
Next Appt. Date:		Time:	
Date of First Visit:	08/11/CCYY	Date of Injury:	
Referring Physician:	Eric Enos, M.D.		

Guarantor Information

Name:	Evelyn Espinosa
Address:	621 Espinaza Avenue

City:	Los Angeles	State:	CA	Zip Code:	90012

Insurance ID #:	99-9993 ABC
Insurance Name:	Winter Insurance Company
Insurance Group #:	36928
Employer Name:	ABC Corporation

Authorization

☒ Authorization to Release Information
☒ Authorization for Assignment of Benefits
☐ Authorization for Consent for Treatment
☐ My insurance will be billed but there may be a balance due.

Signature: *Evelyn Espinosa*   Date: 8/11/CCYY

Clinical Information

	DOS	POS	CPT® /HCPCS Description	ICD-9-CM (*Indicates diagnosis for all lines)	Amount
1	08/11/CCYY	Inpt Hosp	Init inpt consul, comp hist and exam, moderate compl	Calculus of gallbladder with other cholecystitis	$250.00
2					
3					
4					
5					
6					

Remarks:	Referring Physician: Eric Enos, M.D. UPIN #: K33102					
Previous Balance:	$35.00	Payment:		Copay:		Adjustment:
Total Fee:	$250.00	Cash ☐ Check ☐ Credit ☐		Cash ☐ Check ☐ Credit ☐		Reason:

New Balance: $285.00

Physicians' Claims Beginning Financials

SMITH FAMILY

Insurance Plan	Rover Insurers, Inc.—Ninja Enterprises			
Patient:	**STEVE**	**SHARON**	**SAM**	
C/O DEDUCTIBLE	0.00	0.00	0.00	
DEDUCTIBLE	0.00	145.00	0.00	
COINSURANCE	0.00	0.00	0.00	
ACCIDENT BENEFIT				
LIFETIME MAXIMUM	0.00	54,000.00	0.00	
M/N OFFICE VISITS	0-vts	3-vts	0-vts	
OFFICE VISITS				
HOSPITAL VISITS				
DXL				
SURGERY				
ASSISTANT SURGERY				
ANESTHESIA				

Encounter Form

Provider Information

Name:	Shereville Good Health
Address:	P.O. Box 3456
City:	Shereville	State: CA	Zip Code: 91208
Telephone #:	Fax #:
Medicare ID#:	UPIN #: W00003
Tax ID #:	95-1178215	Accepts Medicare Assignment: ☒
Provider's Signature:	*Sharon Shaver, MD*	Date: 8/29/CCYY

Appointment Information

Appointment Date:		Time:
Next Appt. Date:		Time:
Date of First Visit:	12/25/CCPY	Date of Injury:
Referring Physician:		

Guarantor Information

Name:	Steve Smith
Address:	1121 Schmidt Road
City: Sortlete	State: CA	Zip Code: 91733
Insurance ID #:	88-8888 NIN
Insurance Name:	Rover Insurers, Inc.
Insurance Group #:	21088
Employer Name:	Ninja Enterprises

Patient Information

Name:	Sharon Smith
Address:	1121 Schmidt Road
City:	Sortlete	State: CA	Zip Code: 91733
Telephone #:	(415) 555-9173	Account #: 10005
Date of Birth:	11/11/CCYY-55	Gender: Female
Marital Status:	Married	Relationship to Guarantor: Spouse
Student Status:	☐ Full-time ☐ Part-time
Insurance Type:	☒ Pvt ☐ M/care ☐ M/caid ☐ WC ☐ Other
Hospitalization Date:	
Hospital Information:	

Authorization

☒ Authorization to Release Information
☒ Authorization for Assignment of Benefits
☐ Authorization for Consent for Treatment
☐ My insurance will be billed but there may be a balance due.

Signature: *Sharon Smith*   Date: 8/29/CCYY

Clinical Information

	DOS	POS	CPT® /HCPCS Description	ICD-9-CM (*Indicates diagnosis for all lines)	Amount
1	08/07/CCYY	Office	Individual psychotherapy; 50 minutes	*Adjustment Disorder with Depressed Mood	$ 90.00
2	08/21/CCYY	Office	Individual psychotherapy; 50 minutes	*	$ 90.00
3	08/29/CCYY	Office	Psychological testing with interp and report (1 hr)	*	$780.00
4					
5					
6					
Remarks:	Services performed by Sharon Shaver, M.D. UPIN #: F98765				
Previous Balance:		Payment:	Copay:	Adjustment:	
Total Fee:	$960.00	Cash ☐ Check ☐ Credit ☐	Cash ☐ Check ☐ Credit ☐	Reason:	New Balance: $960.00

Encounter Form

Provider Information							Appointment Information				
Name:	Sharla Sayers, M.D.						Appointment Date:			Time:	
Address:	6767 Saratoga Street						Next Appt. Date:			Time:	
City:	Seattle	State:	CA	Zip Code:	90640		Date of First Visit:	07/25/CCYY	Date of Injury:		
Telephone #:		Fax #:					Referring Physician:				
Medicare ID#:		UPIN #:	G87654				**Guarantor Information**				
Tax ID #:	472-02-0164	Accepts Medicare Assignment:	☒				Name:	Steve Smith			
Provider's Signature:	*Sharla Sayers, MD*		Date: *8/6/CCYY*				Address:	1121 Schmidt Road			

Patient Information							City:	Sortlete	State:	CA	Zip Code:	91733
Name:	Steve Smith						Insurance ID #:	88-8888 NIN				
Address:	1121 Schmidt Road						Insurance Name:	Rover Insurers, Inc.				
City:	Sortlete	State:	CA	Zip Code:	91733		Insurance Group #:	21088				
Telephone #:	(415) 555-9173	Account #:	10006				Employer Name:	Ninja Enterprises				
Date of Birth:	08/16/CCYY-56	Gender:	Male				**Authorization**					
Marital Status:	Married	Relationship to Guarantor:	Self				☒ Authorization to Release Information					
Student Status:	☐ Full-time	☐ Part-time					☒ Authorization for Assignment of Benefits ☐ Authorization for Consent for Treatment					
Insurance Type:	☒ Pvt ☐ M/care ☐ M/caid ☐ WC ☐ Other ___						☐ My insurance will be billed but there may be a balance due.					
Hospitalization Date:							Signature: *Steve Smith*		Date: *8/6/CCYY*			
Hospital Information:												

Clinical Information					
	DOS	POS	CPT® /HCPCS Description	ICD-9-CM (*Indicates diagnosis for all lines)	Amount
1	08/06/CCYY	Office	Med exam & eval; diag trmnt and prog; est pt; interm	*Corneal Scar; *1 Pterygium	$100.00
2	08/06/CCYY	Office	Collection of venous blood by venipuncture	*; *1	$ 15.00
3					
4					
5					
6					
Remarks:					
Previous Balance:		Payment:		Copay:		Adjustment:		
Total Fee:	$115.00	Cash ☐ Check ☐ Credit ☐	Cash ☐ Check ☐ Credit ☐	Reason:	New Balance: $115.00

Encounter Form

Provider Information							Appointment Information				
Name:	Sharmin Health Clinic						Appointment Date:			Time:	
Address:	987 Sharmin Avenue						Next Appt. Date:			Time:	
City:	Sharmin	State:	CA	Zip Code:	91208		Date of First Visit:	09/06/CCYY	Date of Injury:		
Telephone #:		Fax #:					Referring Physician:				
Medicare ID#:		UPIN #:	W00004				**Guarantor Information**				
Tax ID #:	95-4204145	Accepts Medicare Assignment:	☒				Name:	Steve Smith			
Provider's Signature:	*Sara Smeen, MD*		Date: *9/6/CCYY*				Address:	1121 Schmidt Road			

Patient Information							City:	Sortlete	State:	CA	Zip Code:	91733
Name:	Sharon Smith						Insurance ID #:	88-8888 NIN				
Address:	1121 Schmidt Road						Insurance Name:	Rover Insurers, Inc.				
City:	Sortlete	State:	CA	Zip Code:	91733		Insurance Group #:	21088				
Telephone #:	(415) 555-9173	Account #:	10005				Employer Name:	Ninja Enterprises				
Date of Birth:	11/11/CCYY-55	Gender:	Female				**Authorization**					
Marital Status:	Married	Relationship to Guarantor:	Spouse				☒ Authorization to Release Information					
Student Status:	☐ Full-time	☐ Part-time					☒ Authorization for Assignment of Benefits ☐ Authorization for Consent for Treatment					
Insurance Type:	☒ Pvt ☐ M/care ☐ M/caid ☐ WC ☐ Other ___						☐ My insurance will be billed but there may be a balance due.					
Hospitalization Date:							Signature: *Sharon Smith*		Date: *9/6/CCYY*			
Hospital Information:												

Clinical Information					
	DOS	POS	CPT® /HCPCS Description	ICD-9-CM (*Indicates diagnosis for all lines)	Amount
1	09/06/CCYY	Office	New pt; comp hist & exam, moderate complexity	*Abdominal Pain; *1 Gastroenteritis	$190.00
2	09/06/CCYY	Office	Collection of venous blood by venipuncture	*; *1	$ 15.00
3					
4					
5					
6					
Remarks:	Services performed by Sara Smeen, M.D. UPIN #: H76543				
Previous Balance:	$960.00	Payment:	$50.00	Copay:		Adjustment:		
Total Fee:	$205.00	Cash ☒ Check ☐ Credit ☐	Cash ☐ Check ☐ Credit ☐	Reason:	New Balance: $1115.00

Encounter Form
DOCUMENT 14

Provider Information

Name:	Sandra Sanchez, M.D.
Address:	4314 Sheatem Avenue
City:	Santa View · State: CA · Zip Code: 90640
Telephone #:	Fax #:
Medicare ID#:	UPIN #: I65432
Tax ID #:	33-3323085 · Accepts Medicare Assignment: ☒
Provider's Signature:	*Sandra Sanchez, MD* · Date: *5/19/CCYY*

Appointment Information

Appointment Date:	Time:
Next Appt. Date:	Time:
Date of First Visit:	Date of Injury:
Referring Physician:	

Patient Information

Name:	Sam Smith
Address:	1121 Schmidt Road
City:	Sortlete · State: CA · Zip Code: 91733
Telephone #:	(415) 555-9173 · Account #: 10007
Date of Birth:	06/16/CCYY-18 · Gender: Male
Marital Status:	Single · Relationship to Guarantor: Child
Student Status:	☒ Full-time ☐ Part-time
Insurance Type:	☒ Pvt ☐ M/care ☐ M/caid ☐ WC ☐ Other
Hospitalization Date:	
Hospital Information:	

Guarantor Information

Name:	Steve Smith
Address:	1121 Schmidt Road
City:	Sortlete · State: CA · Zip Code: 91733
Insurance ID #:	88-8888 NIN
Insurance Name:	Rover Insurers, Inc.
Insurance Group #:	21088
Employer Name:	Ninja Enterprises

Authorization

☒ Authorization to Release Information
☐ Authorization for Assignment of Benefits
☐ Authorization for Consent for Treatment
☐ My insurance will be billed but there may be a balance due.

Signature: *Steve Smith* · Date: *5/19/CCYY*

Clinical Information

	DOS	POS	CPT® /HCPCS Description	ICD-9-CM (*Indicates diagnosis for all lines)	Amount
1	05/19/CCYY	Office	Est pt, comp hist & exam, high complexity	*Acute bronchitis; *1 Chest Pain	$120.00
2	05/19/CCYY	Office	Intramuscular therapeutic injection of ciproflaxin	*; *1	$ 30.00
3					
4					
5					
6					

Remarks:

Previous Balance:		Payment:		Copay:		Adjustment:			
Total Fee:	$150.00	Cash ☐ Check ☐ Credit ☐		Cash ☐ Check ☐ Credit ☐		Remark:		New Balance:	$150.00

Encounter Form
DOCUMENT 15

Provider Information

Name:	Stan Still, M.D.
Address:	P.O. Box 22017
City:	Sortlete · State: CA · Zip Code: 90022
Telephone #:	Fax #:
Medicare ID#:	UPIN #: J54321
Tax ID #:	94-3416985 · Accepts Medicare Assignment: ☒
Provider's Signature:	*Stan Still, MD* · Date: *11/19/CCYY*

Appointment Information

Appointment Date:	Time:
Next Appt. Date:	Time:
Date of First Visit:	11/19/CCYY · Date of Injury:
Referring Physician:	Sandra Sanchez, M.D.

Patient Information

Name:	Sharon Smith
Address:	1121 Schmidt Road
City:	Sortlete · State: CA · Zip Code: 91733
Telephone #:	(415) 555-9173 · Account #: 10005
Date of Birth:	11/11/CCYY-55 · Gender: Female
Marital Status:	Married · Relationship to Guarantor: Spouse
Student Status:	☐ Full-time ☐ Part-time
Insurance Type:	☒ Pvt ☐ M/care ☐ M/caid ☐ WC ☐ Other
Hospitalization Date:	
Hospital Information:	

Guarantor Information

Name:	Steve Smith
Address:	1121 Schmidt Road
City:	Sortlete · State: CA · Zip Code: 91733
Insurance ID #:	88-8888 NIN
Insurance Name:	Rover Insurers, Inc.
Insurance Group #:	21088
Employer Name:	Ninja Enterprises

Authorization

☒ Authorization to Release Information
☒ Authorization for Assignment of Benefits
☐ Authorization for Consent for Treatment
☐ My insurance will be billed but there may be a balance due.

Signature: *Sharon Smith* · Date: *11/19/CCYY*

Clinical Information

	DOS	POS	CPT® /HCPCS Description	ICD-9-CM (*Indicates diagnosis for all lines)	Amount
1	11/19/CCYY	Office	Confirmatory consul, comp hist & exam, mod complex	Calculus of gallbladder, no cholecystitis	$325.00
2					
3					
4					
5					
6					

Remarks: Referring Physician: Sandra Sanchez, M.D. UPIN #: I65432 for Second Surgical Opinion for cholecystectomy.

Previous Balance:	$1115.00	Payment:		Copay:		Adjustment:			
Total Fee:	$325.00	Cash ☐ Check ☐ Credit ☐		Cash ☐ Check ☐ Credit ☐		Remarks:		New Balance:	$1440.00

Physicians' Claims Beginning Financials
PARKER FAMILY

Insurance Plan	Ball Insurance Carriers—XYZ Corporation				
Patient:	**PATRICIA**	**PETER**	**PAULINE**		
C/O DEDUCTIBLE					
DEDUCTIBLE	57.00	125.00	15.00		
COINSURANCE	0.00	375.00	359.50		
ACCIDENT BENEFIT					
LIFETIME MAXIMUM	6,075.00	7,600.00	15,000.00		
M/N LIFETIME					
M/N OFFICE VISITS					
OFFICE VISITS	0.00	0.00	0.00		
HOSPITAL VISITS	0.00	0.00	0.00		
DXL					
SURGERY					
ASSISTANT SURGERY					
ANESTHESIA					

Encounter Form

Provider Information

Name:	Peter Parrer, M.D.			
Address:	1825 Pexa Avenue			
City:	Princeton	State: CA	Zip Code:	90022
Telephone #:		Fax #:		
Medicare ID#:		UPIN #:	K43210	
Tax ID #:	95-3177675	Accepts Medicare Assignment:	☒	
Provider's Signature:	Peter Parrer, MD		Date: 5/4/CCYY	

Appointment Information

Appointment Date:		Time:	
Next Appt. Date:		Time:	
Date of First Visit:	04/25/CCYY	Date of Injury:	
Referring Physician:			

Patient Information

Name:	Patricia Parker			
Address:	1501 Pea Pod Drive			
City:	Princeton	State: CA	Zip Code:	90021
Telephone #:	(626) 555-9012	Account #:	10008	
Date of Birth:	01/12/CCYY-60	Gender:	Female	
Marital Status:	Married	Relationship to Guarantor:	Self	
Student Status:	☐ Full-time	☐ Part-time		
Insurance Type:	☒ Pvt ☐ M/care ☐ M/caid ☐ WC ☐ Other			
Hospitalization Date:				
Hospital Information:				

Guarantor Information

Name:	Patricia Parker		
Address:	1501 Pea Pod Drive		
City:	Princeton	State: CA	Zip Code: 90021
Insurance ID #:	77-7771 XYZ		
Insurance Name:	Ball Insurance Carriers		
Insurance Group #:	62958		
Employer Name:	XYZ Corporation		

Authorization

☒ Authorization to Release Information
☒ Authorization for Assignment of Benefits
☐ Authorization for Consent for Treatment
☐ My insurance will be billed but there may be a balance due.

Signature: Patricia Parker   Date: 5/4/CCYY

Clinical Information

	DOS	POS	CPT® /HCPCS Description	ICD-9-CM (*Indicates diagnosis for all lines)	Amount
1	05/02/CCYY	Office	Evaluation, presenting problem(s) are minimal	*Laryngopharyngitis	$ 35.00
2	05/02/CCYY	Office	Intramuscular therapeutic injection of penicillin	*	$ 15.00
3	05/04/CCYY	Office	Evaluation, presenting problem(s) are minimal	*	$ 30.00
4	05/04/CCYY	Office	Intramuscular therapeutic injection of penicillin	*	$ 15.00
5					
6					
Remarks:					

Previous Balance:		Payment:		Copay:		Adjustment:		
Total Fee:	$95.00	Cash ☐ Check ☐ Credit ☐		Cash ☐ Check ☐ Credit ☐		Remarks:	New Balance:	$95.00

Encounter Form   DOCUMENT 18

Provider Information

Name:	Priscilla Pater, M.D.
Address:	P.O. Box 3456

City:	Princeton	State:	CA	Zip Code:	90022

Telephone #:		Fax #:	

Medicare ID#:		UPIN #:	L12233

Tax ID #:	95-3777777	Accepts Medicare Assignment:	☒

Provider's Signature:	Priscilla Pater, MD	Date: 3/25/CCYY

Patient Information

Name:	Peter Parker
Address:	1501 Pea Pod Drive

City:	Princeton	State:	CA	Zip Code:	90021

Telephone #:	(626) 555-9012	Account #:	10009

Date of Birth:	03/20/CCYY-60	Gender:	Male

Marital Status:	Married	Relationship to Guarantor:	Spouse

Student Status:	☐ Full-time	☐ Part-time

Insurance Type:	☒ Pvt ☐ M/care ☐ M/caid ☐ WC ☐ Other _____

Hospitalization Date:	From: 03/22/CCYY	To: 03/25/CCYY

Hospital Information:	Princeton Community Hospital, P.O. Box 1122, Princeton, CA 90022

Appointment Information

Appointment Date:		Time:	

Next Appt. Date:		Time:	

Date of First Visit:	03/22/CCYY	Date of Injury:	

Referring Physician:	Philip Porter, M.D.

Guarantor Information

Name:	Patricia Parker

Address:	1501 Pea Pod Drive

City:	Princeton	State:	CA	Zip Code:	90021

Insurance ID #:	77-7771 XYZ

Insurance Name:	Ball Insurance Carriers

Insurance Group #:	62958

Employer Name:	XYZ Corporation

Authorization

☒ Authorization to Release Information
☒ Authorization for Assignment of Benefits
☐ Authorization for Consent for Treatment
☐ My insurance will be billed but there may be a balance due.

Signature: Peter Parker   Date: 3/25/CCYY

Clinical Information

	DOS	POS	CPT® /HCPCS Description	ICD-9-CM (*Indicates diagnosis for all lines)	Amount
1	03/22/CCYY	Inpt Hosp	Consult, comp hist & exam, high complexity	*Intestinal obstruction; *1 R/O malignancy	$200.00
2	03/23/CCYY	Inpt Hosp	Subseq hosp care, expand hist & exam, mod complex	*; *1	$ 75.00
3	03/24/CCYY	Inpt Hosp	Subseq hosp care, expand hist & exam, mod complex	*; *1	$ 75.00
4	03/25/CCYY	Inpt Hosp	Hospital discharge, 30 minutes or less	*; *1	$100.00
5					
6					

Remarks:	Referring Physician: Philip Porter, M.D. UPIN #: D33332

Previous Balance:		Payment:		Copay:		Adjustment:		
Total Fee:	$450.00	Cash ☐ Check ☐ Credit ☐	Cash ☐ Check ☐ Credit ☐	Remarks:		New Balance:	$450.00

Encounter Form   DOCUMENT 19

Provider Information

Name:	Parnella Prince, M.D.
Address:	45632 Price Blvd.

City:	Princeton	State:	CA	Zip Code:	90022

Telephone #:		Fax #:	

Medicare ID#:		UPIN #:	M12234

Tax ID #:	95-2743318	Accepts Medicare Assignment:	☒

Provider's Signature:	Parnella Prince, MD	Date: 11/19/CCYY

Patient Information

Name:	Pauline Parker
Address:	1501 Pea Pod Drive

City:	Princeton	State:	CA	Zip Code:	90021

Telephone #:	(626) 555-9012	Account #:	10010

Date of Birth:	07/05/CCYY-18	Gender:	Female

Marital Status:	Single	Relationship to Guarantor:	Child

Student Status:	☒ Full-time	☐ Part-time

Insurance Type:	☒ Pvt ☐ M/care ☐ M/caid ☐ WC ☐ Other _____

Hospitalization Date:	

Hospital Information:	

Appointment Information

Appointment Date:		Time:	

Next Appt. Date:		Time:	

Date of First Visit:		Date of Injury:	

Referring Physician:	

Guarantor Information

Name:	Patricia Parker

Address:	1501 Pea Pod Drive

City:	Princeton	State:	CA	Zip Code:	90021

Insurance ID #:	77-7771 XYZ

Insurance Name:	Ball Insurance Carriers

Insurance Group #:	62958

Employer Name:	XYZ Corporation

Authorization

☒ Authorization to Release Information
☒ Authorization for Assignment of Benefits
☐ Authorization for Consent for Treatment
☐ My insurance will be billed but there may be a balance due.

Signature: Patricia Parker   Date: 11/19/CCYY

Clinical Information

	DOS	POS	CPT® /HCPCS Description	ICD-9-CM (*Indicates diagnosis for all lines)	Amount
1	11/19/CCYY	Office	Supplies and materials	*Delayed menarche	$ 12.00
2	11/19/CCYY	Office	Intramuscular therapeutic injection of prednisone	*	$ 25.00
3	11/19/CCYY	Office	Intramuscular therapeutic injection of calcium glucose	Hyperlipidemia; *	$ 15.00
4					
5					
6					

Remarks:	

Previous Balance:		Payment:	$25.00	Copay:		Adjustment:		
Total Fee:	$52.00	Cash ☒ Check ☐ Credit ☐	Cash ☐ Check ☐ Credit ☐	Remarks:		New Balance:	$27.00

Encounter Form

DOCUMENT 20

Provider Information						Appointment Information			
Name:	Peter Pedro, M.D.					Appointment Date:		Time:	
Address:	5461 Pass Blvd.					Next Appt. Date:		Time:	
City:	Pansy	State:	CA	Zip Code:	90280	Date of First Visit:	12/04/CCYY	Date of Injury:	
Telephone #:		Fax #:				Referring Physician:	Pablo Prode, M.D.		
Medicare ID#:		UPIN #:	A22345			**Guarantor Information**			
Tax ID #:	95-0144440	Accepts Medicare Assignment:	☒			Name:	Patricia Parker		
Provider's Signature:	*Peter Pedro, MD*		Date: *12/6/CCYY*			Address:	1501 Pea Pod Drive		

Patient Information						City:	Princeton	State:	CA	Zip Code:	90021
Name:	Peter Parker					Insurance ID #:	77-7771 XYZ				
Address:	1501 Pea Pod Drive					Insurance Name:	Ball Insurance Carriers				
City:	Princeton	State:	CA	Zip Code:	90021	Insurance Group #:	62958				
Telephone #:	(626) 555-9012	Account #:	10009			Employer Name:	XYZ Corporation				

Date of Birth:	03/20/CCYY-60	Gender:	Male
Marital Status:	Married	Relationship to Guarantor:	Spouse
Student Status:	☐ Full-time	☐ Part-time	
Insurance Type:	☒ Pvt ☐ M/care ☐ M/caid ☐ WC ☐ Other _____		
Hospitalization Date:	From: 12/01/CCYY	To: 12/07/CCYY	
Hospital Information:	Pansy Community Hospital, P.O. Box 2233, Pansy, CA 90280		

Authorization

☒ Authorization to Release Information
☒ Authorization for Assignment of Benefits
☐ Authorization for Consent for Treatment
☐ My insurance will be billed but there may be a balance due.
Signature: *Peter Parker*   Date: *12/6/CCYY*

Clinical Information					
	DOS	POS	CPT® /HCPCS Description	ICD-9-CM (*Indicates diagnosis for all lines)	Amount
1	12/04/CCYY	Inpt Hosp	Comp hist and exam, high complexity	*Urinary Tract Infection	$500.00
2	12/05/CCYY	Inpt Hosp	Consultation, low complexity, problem focused	*	$200.00
3	12/06/CCYY	Inpt hosp	Consultation, low complexity, problem focused	*	$200.00
4					
5					
6					
Remarks:	Referring Physician: Pablo Prode, M.D. UPIN #: E33342				

Previous Balance:	$450.00	Payment:	$350.00	Copay:		Adjustment:				New Balance:	$1000.00
Total Fee:	$900.00	Cash ☐ Check ☐ Credit ☒		Cash ☐ Check ☐ Credit ☐		Remarks:					

Encounter Form

DOCUMENT 21

Provider Information						Appointment Information			
Name:	Pamela Paris, M.D.					Appointment Date:		Time:	
Address:	P.O. Box 46854					Next Appt. Date:		Time:	
City:	Pansy	State:	CA	Zip Code:	90320	Date of First Visit:	12/02/CCYY	Date of Injury:	
Telephone #:		Fax #:				Referring Physician:			
Medicare ID#:		UPIN #:	B23245			**Guarantor Information**			
Tax ID #:	95-5222716	Accepts Medicare Assignment:	☒			Name:	Patricia Parker		
Provider's Signature:	*Pamela Paris, MD*	Date: *12/6/CCYY*				Address:	1501 Pea Pod Drive		

Patient Information						City:	Princeton	State:	CA	Zip Code:	90021
Name:	Pauline Parker					Insurance ID #:	77-7771 XYZ				
Address:	1501 Pea Pod Drive					Insurance Name:	Ball Insurance Carriers				
City:	Princeton	State:	CA	Zip Code:	90021	Insurance Group #:	62958				
Telephone #:	(626) 555-9012	Account #:	10010			Employer Name:	XYZ Corporation				

Date of Birth:	07/05/CCYY-18	Gender:	Female
Marital Status:	Single	Relationship to Guarantor:	Child
Student Status:	☒ Full-time	☐ Part-time	
Insurance Type:	☒ Pvt ☐ M/care ☐ M/caid ☐ WC ☐ Other _____		
Hospitalization Date:	From: 12/02/CCYY	To: 12/06/CCYY	
Hospital Information:	Pansy Community Hospital, P.O. Box 2233, Pansy, CA 90280		

Authorization

☒ Authorization to Release Information
☒ Authorization for Assignment of Benefits
☐ Authorization for Consent for Treatment
☐ My insurance will be billed but there may be a balance due.
Signature: *Patricia Parker*   Date: *12/6/CCYY*

Clinical Information					
	DOS	POS	CPT® /HCPCS Description	ICD-9-CM (*Indicates diagnosis for all lines)	Amount
1	12/02/CCYY	Inpt Hosp	Initial hospital care, detailed history & exam, straight	*Capillary Pneumonia	$325.00
2	12/03/CCYY	Inpt Hosp	Sub hosp care, prob foc hist & exam mod complexity	*	$ 95.00
3	12/04/CCYY	Inpt Hosp	Sub hosp care, prob foc hist & exam mod complexity	*	$ 95.00
4	12/05/CCYY	Inpt hosp	Sub hosp care, prob foc hist & exam mod complexity	*	$ 95.00
5	12/06/CCYY	Inpt Hosp	Hospital discharge; 30 minutes or less	*	$150.00
6					
Remarks:					

Previous Balance:	$27.00	Payment:		Copay:		Adjustment:				New Balance:	$787.00
Total Fee:	$760.00	Cash ☐ Check ☐ Credit ☐		Cash ☐ Check ☐ Credit ☐							

Health Claims Examining Exercises

(**Instructor's Note:** Medical Billing exercises in the entire text should be completed prior to students starting Health Claims Examining Exercise 2–A. New files should be set up for the Health Claims Examining exercises.)

Exercise 2-A

Directions: Complete an Insurance Coverage Form (located in the **Forms** chapter) and set up Family Files for all families in this chapter. Refer to the Family Data Table (**Documents 1–3**), located in the beginning of this chapter, and the Contracts located in the **Contracts, UCR Conversion Factor Report, and Relative Value Study** chapter.

Exercise 2-B

Directions: Complete a Payment Worksheet (located in the **Forms** chapter) for CMS-1500 claims (**Documents 5–9, 11–15, and 17–21**) using the guidelines contained in the **Introduction** chapter and using the UCR Conversion Factor Report, Relative Value Study, and Contracts located in the **Contracts, UCR Conversion Factor Report, and Relative Value Study** chapter.

When processing claims, the Beginning Financials (**Documents 4, 10, and 16**) should be incorporated as payment history and claim calculations should be adjusted accordingly. Any carryover deductible listed should be included in the current year deductible for that individual. Therefore, in figuring current year deductible, students should be instructed to subtract the carryover deductible from the current year's amount.

Upon completion of each claim complete or update the Family Benefits Tracking Sheet (located in the **Forms** chapter) by compiling all of the claims payment data for the family.

3

Diagnostic X-Ray
and Laboratory Services

Medical Billing Exercises

Exercise 3-1

Directions: Complete Patient Information Sheets (leave **Assigned Provider** field blank), Ledger Cards, and Insurance Coverage Forms and set up patient charts for the following families using copies of the forms in the **Forms** chapter. Refer to the Family Data Tables **(Documents 22–24)** for information. Individual folders with dividers may be used to store information for each family. One Patient Information Sheet and Insurance Coverage Form should be filled out for the entire family.

FAMILY DATA TABLE

DOCUMENT 22

GREEN FAMILY	INSURED'S INFORMATION	SPOUSE'S INFORMATION	CHILD #1	CHILD #2	CHILD #3
Name	Greg Green	Gina Green	Greta Green	George Green	
Address	160 Grain Avenue Pasadena, CA 91114	160 Grain Avenue Pasadena, CA 91114	160 Grain Avenue Pasadena, CA 91114	160 Grain Avenue Pasadena, CA 91114	
Email Address	gregg@green.com				
TELEPHONE #					
Home:	(626) 555-9111	(626) 555-9111	(626) 555-9111	(626) 555-9111	
Work:	(626) 555-9112				
Cell:	(626) 555-9113				
Date of Birth	04/04/CCYY-51	04/16/CCYY-49	10/16/CCYY-18	01/24/CCYY-17	
Social Security #	111-11-1111	111-11-1112	111-11-1113	111-11-1114	
Marital Status/Gender	Married/Male	Married/Female	Single/Female	Single/Male	
Student Status			Full-time	Full-time	
Patient Account #	10012	10013	10014	10011	
Allergies/Medical Conditions	None	None	None	None	
PRIMARY INSURANCE CARRIER					
Name Address	Winter Insurance Company 9763 Western Way Whittier, CO 82963	Winter Insurance Company 9763 Western Way Whittier, CO 82963	Winter Insurance Company 9763 Western Way Whittier, CO 82963	Winter Insurance Company 9763 Western Way Whittier, CO 82963	
Effective Date	01/01/CCPY	01/01/CCPY	01/01/CCPY	01/01/CCPY	
Member's ID #	11-1111 ABC	11-1111 ABC	11-1111 ABC	11-1111 ABC	
Group Policy #	36928	36928	36928	36928	
Policy/Employer	ABC Corporation 1234 Whitaker Lane Colter, CO 81222				
OTHER INSURANCE CARRIER					
Name Address					
Effective Date					
Member's ID #					
Group Policy #					
Policy/Employer					
Responsible Party	Self	Self	Insured	Insured	
EMERGENCY CONTACT					
Name	Gray Greeter	Gray Greeter	Gray Greeter	Gray Greeter	
Telephone #	(626) 555-9114	(626) 555-9114	(626) 555-9114	(626) 555-9111	
Address	61 Grain Avenue Pasadena, CA 91114	61 Grain Avenue Pasadena, CA 91114	61 Grain Avenue Pasadena, CA 91114	61 Grain Avenue Pasadena, CA 91114	

FAMILY DATA TABLE

DOCUMENT 23

FRANCISCO FAMILY	INSURED'S INFORMATION	SPOUSE'S INFORMATION	CHILD #1	CHILD #2	CHILD #3
Name	Frank Francisco	Felicia Francisco	Fred Francisco	Freda Francisco	
Address	1540 Farquat Avenue N. Hollywood, CA 91000	1540 Farquat Avenue N. Hollywood, CA 91000	1540 Farquat Avenue N. Hollywood, CA 91000	1540 Farquat Avenue N. Hollywood, CA 91000	
Email Address	frankf@francisco.com				
TELEPHONE #					
Home: Work: Cell:	(818) 555-9100 (818) 555-9101 (818) 555-9102	(818) 555-9100	(818) 555-9100	(818) 555-9100	
Date of Birth	10/04/CCYY-45	11/14/CCYY-44	11/14/CCYY-18	08/25/CCYY-17	
Social Security #	222-22-2222	222-22-2223	222-22-2224	222-22-2225	
Marital Status/Gender	Married/Male	Married/Female	Single/Male	Single/Female	
Student Status			Full-time	Full-time	
Patient Account #	10015	10016	10017	10018	
Allergies/Medical Conditions	None	None	None	None	
PRIMARY INSURANCE CARRIER					
Name Address	Rover Insurers, Inc. 5931 Rolling Road Ronson, CO 81369	Rover Insurers, Inc. 5931 Rolling Road Ronson, CO 81369	Rover Insurers, Inc. 5931 Rolling Road Ronson, CO 81369	Rover Insurers, Inc. 5931 Rolling Road Ronson, CO 81369	
Effective Date	01/01/CCPY	01/01/CCPY	01/01/CCPY	01/01/CCPY	
Member's ID #	22-2222 NIN	22-2222 NIN	22-2222 NIN	22-2222 NIN	
Group Policy #	21088	21088	21088	21088	
Policy/Employer	Ninja Enterprises 1234 Nockout Road Newton, NM 88012				
OTHER INSURANCE CARRIER					
Name Address					
Effective Date					
Member's ID #					
Group Policy #					
Policy/Employer					
Responsible Party	Self	Self	Insured	Insured	
EMERGENCY CONTACT					
Name	Fredrick Fonsi	Fredrick Fonsi	Fredrick Fonsi	Fredrick Fonsi	
Telephone #	(818) 555-9103	(818) 555-9103	(818) 555-9103	(818) 555-9103	
Address	451 Farquat Avenue N. Hollywood, CA 91000	451 Farquat Avenue N. Hollywood, CA 91000	451 Farquat Avenue N. Hollywood, CA 91000	451 Farquat Avenue N. Hollywood, CA 91000	

FAMILY DATA TABLE

HERNANDEZ FAMILY	INSURED'S INFORMATION	SPOUSE'S INFORMATION	CHILD #1	CHILD #2	CHILD #3
Name	Henriquez Hernandez	Hortencia Hernandez	Hector Hernandez		
Address	7931 Harbor Avenue Harbor, CA 90202	7931 Harbor Avenue Harbor, CA 90202	7931 Harbor Avenue Harbor, CA 90202		
Email Address	henriquezh@hernandez.com				
TELEPHONE #					
Home:	(310) 555-9020	(310) 555-9020	(310) 555-9020		
Work:	(310) 555-9021				
Cell:	(310) 555-9022				
Date of Birth	05/16/CCYY-47	10/17/CCYY-45	05/02/CCYY-17		
Social Security #	444-44-4444	444-44-4445	444-44-4446		
Marital Status/Gender	Married/Male	Married/Female	Single/Male		
Student Status			Full-time		
Patient Account #	10021	10020	10019		
Allergies/Medical Conditions	None	None	None		
PRIMARY INSURANCE CARRIER					
Name Address	Ball Insurance Carriers 3895 Bubble Blvd. Ste. 283 Boxwood, CO 85926	Ball Insurance Carriers 3895 Bubble Blvd. Ste. 283 Boxwood, CO 85926	Ball Insurance Carriers 3895 Bubble Blvd. Ste. 283 Boxwood, CO 85926		
Effective Date	01/01/CCPY	01/01/CCPY	01/01/CCPY		
Member's ID #	44-4444 XYZ	44-4444 XYZ	44-4444 XYZ		
Group Policy #	62958	62958	62958		
Policy/Employer	XYZ Corporation 9817 Bobcat Blvd. Bastion, CO 81319				
OTHER INSURANCE CARRIER					
Name Address					
Effective Date					
Member's ID #					
Group Policy #					
Policy/Employer					
Responsible Party	Self	Self	Insured		
EMERGENCY CONTACT					
Name Telephone #	Henry Herrera (310) 555-9023	Henry Herrera (310) 555-9023	Henry Herrera (310) 555-9023		
Address	1397 Harbor Avenue Harbor, CA 90202	1397 Harbor Avenue Harbor, CA 90202	1397 Harbor Avenue Harbor, CA 90202		

Exercise **3-2**

Directions: Complete a CMS-1500 for each of the Encounter Forms (**Documents 26–30, 32–36, and 38–42**) in this chapter. CMS-1500 forms may be provided by your instructor or purchased from a stationery store.

After completion of each CMS-1500 form, complete a Patient Receipt (if a payment was made), and post the transaction(s) to the patient Ledger Card/Statement of Account previously created.

Exercise **3-3**

Directions: Upon completion of all of the activities in Exercise 3–2, complete a Bank Deposit Slip/Ticket (located in the **Forms** chapter) for all payments made on the patient's account in this chapter.

Exercise **3-4**

Directions: Using an Insurance Claims Register (located in the **Forms** chapter) list all claims that have been fully prepared and are ready for submission to the insurance carrier for payment. Enter the date that you created the CMS-1500 in the **Date Claim Filed** column.

Exercise **3-5**

Directions: Using the stationery or Request for Additional Information Form (located in the **Forms** chapter), write a letter or request information for the following scenario. In each case, you are the medical biller working for Any Billing Services. Addresses and personal information are contained in the patient files that were previously set up. Also, refer to the Family Data Table (**Document 23**) for required information.

1. Create a correspondence for Felicia Francisco reminding her of her scheduled appointment on 11/02/CCYY.

DXL Claims Beginning Financials

GREEN FAMILY

Insurance Plan	Winter Insurance Company—ABC Corporation				
Patient:	**GREG**	**GINA**	**GRETA**	**GEORGE**	
C/O DEDUCTIBLE	0.00	0.00	0.00	0.00	
DEDUCTIBLE	100.00	0.00	0.00	50.00	
COINSURANCE	471.96	0.00	0.00	0.00	
ACCIDENT BENEFIT	0.00	0.00	0.00	0.00	
LIFETIME MAXIMUM	7,154.20	6,548.50	24,037.96	2,998.70	
M/N OFFICE VISITS					
OFFICE VISITS					
HOSPITAL VISITS					
DXL					
SURGERY					
ASSISTANT SURGERY					
ANESTHESIA					

Encounter Form

Provider Information

Name:	Gary Greer, M.D.
Address:	1888 Gamp Avenue
City:	Altadena State: CA Zip Code: 91101
Telephone #:	Fax #:
Medicare ID#:	UPIN #: C45468
Tax ID #:	33-3759772 Accepts Medicare Assignment: ☒
Provider's Signature:	Gary Greer, MD Date: 5/1/CCYY

Appointment Information

Appointment Date:	Time:
Next Appt. Date:	Time:
Date of First Visit:	Date of Injury:
Referring Physician:	

Guarantor Information

Name:	Greg Green
Address:	160 Grain Avenue
City: Pasadena	State: CA Zip Code: 91114
Insurance ID #:	11-1111 ABC
Insurance Name:	Winter Insurance Company
Insurance Group #:	36928
Employer Name:	ABC Corporation

Patient Information

Name:	George Green
Address:	160 Grain Avenue
City:	Pasadena State: CA Zip Code: 91114
Telephone #:	(626) 555-9111 Account #: 10011
Date of Birth:	01/24/CCYY-17 Gender: Male
Marital Status:	Single Relationship to Guarantor: Child
Student Status:	☒ Full-time ☐ Part-time
Insurance Type:	☒ Pvt ☐ M/care ☐ M/caid ☐ WC ☐ Other _____
Hospitalization Date:	
Hospital Information:	

Authorization

☒ Authorization to Release Information
☒ Authorization for Assignment of Benefits
☐ Authorization for Consent for Treatment
☐ My insurance will be billed but there may be a balance due.

Signature: Greg Green   Date: 5/1/CCYY

Clinical Information

	DOS	POS	CPT® /HCPCS Description	ICD-9-CM (*Indicates diagnosis for all lines)	Amount
1	05/01/CCYY	Office	Detailed exam with history, low complexity	*Acute URI	$ 90.00
2	05/01/CCYY	Office	Intramuscular injection of antibiotic of penicillin	*	$ 25.00
3	05/01/CCYY	Office	Streptokinase, antibody	*	$ 20.00
4	05/01/CCYY	Office	Urinalysis, by dip stick	*	$ 20.00
5					
6					

Remarks:

Previous Balance:	Payment:	Copay:	Adjustment:	
Total Fee: $155.00	Cash ☐ Check ☐ Credit ☐	Cash ☐ Check ☐ Credit ☐	Remarks:	New Balance: $155.00

Encounter Form

Provider Information

Name:	Ginnie Galil, M.D.
Address:	1435 Grampett Blvd.

City:	S. Whittler	State:	CA	Zip Code:	90605

Telephone #:		Fax #:	

Medicare ID#:		UPIN #:	D54358

Tax ID #:	95-3999477	Accepts Medicare Assignment:	☒

Provider's Signature: _Ginnie Galil, MD_   Date: _7/5/CCYY_

Appointment Information

Appointment Date:		Time:	
Next Appt. Date:		Time:	
Date of First Visit:	06/01/CCYY	Date of Injury:	
Referring Physician:			

Guarantor Information

Name:	Greg Green			
Address:	160 Grain Avenue			
City:	Pasadena	State:	CA	Zip Code:	91114
Insurance ID #:	11-1111 ABC			
Insurance Name:	Winter Insurance Company			
Insurance Group #:	36928			
Employer Name:	ABC Corporation			

Patient Information

Name:	Greg Green
Address:	160 Grain Avenue

City:	Pasadena	State:	CA	Zip Code:	91114

Telephone #:	(626) 555-9111	Account #:	10012

Date of Birth:	04/04/CCYY-51	Gender:	Male

Marital Status:	Married	Relationship to Guarantor:	Self

Student Status:	☐ Full-time	☐ Part-time

Insurance Type: ☒ Pvt ☐ M/care ☐ M/caid ☐ WC ☐ Other _____

Hospitalization Date:	
Hospital Information:	

Authorization

☒ Authorization to Release Information
☒ Authorization for Assignment of Benefits
☐ Authorization for Consent for Treatment
☐ My insurance will be billed but there may be a balance due.

Signature: _Greg Green_   Date: _7/5/CCYY_

Clinical Information

	DOS	POS	CPT® /HCPCS Description	ICD-9-CM (*Indicates diagnosis for all lines)	Amount
1	06/28/CCYY	Office	Est pt, comp exam with history, straightforward	*Hypertension, *1Cardiac dysrhythmia	$ 70.00
2	06/28/CCYY	Office	Collection of venous blood by venipuncture	*, *1	$ 15.00
3	06/28/CCYY	Office	Handling of specimen for transfer	*, *1	$ 10.00
4	07/05/CCYY	Office	Est pt, expand problem exam with history, low compl	*1	$ 60.00
5	07/05/CCYY	Office	EKG monitor for 24 hours with visual superimposition	*1	$380.00
6					

Remarks:							
Previous Balance:		Payment:		Copay:		Adjustment:	
Total Fee:	$535.00	Cash ☐ Check ☐ Credit ☐		Cash ☐ Check ☐ Credit ☐		Remarks:	New Balance:	$535.00

Encounter Form

Provider Information

Name:	Goodman Pathology Medical Group
Address:	P.O. Box 9999

City:	Long Beach	State:	CA	Zip Code:	90810

Telephone #:		Fax #:	

Medicare ID#:		UPIN #:	W00005

Tax ID #:	94-4679921	Accepts Medicare Assignment:	☒

Provider's Signature: _Paul Provider, MD_   Date: _8/16/CCYY_

Appointment Information

Appointment Date:		Time:	
Next Appt. Date:		Time:	
Date of First Visit:		Date of Injury:	
Referring Physician:	Gary Gephart, M.D.		

Guarantor Information

Name:	Greg Green			
Address:	160 Grain Avenue			
City:	Pasadena	State:	CA	Zip Code:	91114
Insurance ID #:	11-1111 ABC			
Insurance Name:	Winter Insurance Company			
Insurance Group #:	36928			
Employer Name:	ABC Corporation			

Patient Information

Name:	Gina Green
Address:	160 Grain Avenue

City:	Pasadena	State:	CA	Zip Code:	91114

Telephone #:	(626) 555-9111	Account #:	10013

Date of Birth:	04/16/CCYY-49	Gender:	Female

Marital Status:	Married	Relationship to Guarantor:	Spouse

Student Status:	☐ Full-time	☐ Part-time

Insurance Type: ☒ Pvt ☐ M/care ☐ M/caid ☐ WC ☐ Other _____

Hospitalization Date:	
Hospital Information:	

Authorization

☒ Authorization to Release Information
☒ Authorization for Assignment of Benefits
☐ Authorization for Consent for Treatment
☐ My insurance will be billed but there may be a balance due.

Signature: _Gina Green_   Date: _5/16/CCYY_

Clinical Information

	DOS	POS	CPT® /HCPCS Description	ICD-9-CM (*Indicates diagnosis for all lines)	Amount
1	05/14/CCYY	Office	Bld ct/smear, micro exam w/h manual diff/ WBC ct	*Unknown cause of mortality	$ 11.00
2	05/14/CCYY	Office	Creatine kinase; total	*	$ 56.00
3	05/15/CCYY	Office	Amylase	*	$ 19.00
4	05/15/CCYY	Office	Basic metabolic panel	*	$ 30.00
5	05/16/CCYY	Office	Lactate dehydrogenase	*	$ 16.00
6					

Remarks:	Services performed by Paul Provider, M.D. UPIN #: E45678			Referring Physician: Gary Gephart, M.D. UPIN #: F98654	
Previous Balance:		Payment:		Copay:		Adjustment:	
Total Fee:	$132.00	Cash ☐ Check ☐ Credit ☐		Cash ☐ Check ☐ Credit ☐		Remarks:	New Balance:	$132.00

Encounter Form

Provider Information

Name:	Gary Gephart, M.D.
Address:	1123 Geerly Blvd

City:	Glendora	State:	CA	Zip Code:	91110
Telephone #:		Fax #:			
Medicare ID#:		UPIN #:	F98654		
Tax ID #:	444-56-9801	Accepts Medicare Assignment:	☒		
Provider's Signature:	Gary Gephart, MD	Date: 2/8/CCYY			

Appointment Information

Appointment Date:		Time:	
Next Appt. Date:		Time:	
Date of First Visit:	12/16/CCPY	Date of Injury:	
Referring Physician:			

Guarantor Information

Name:	Greg Green
Address:	160 Grain Avenue

City:	Pasadena	State:	CA	Zip Code:	91114
Insurance ID #:	11-1111 ABC				
Insurance Name:	Winter Insurance Company				
Insurance Group #:	36928				
Employer Name:	ABC Corporation				

Patient Information

Name:	Greta Green
Address:	160 Grain Avenue

City:	Pasadena	State:	CA	Zip Code:	91114
Telephone #:	(626) 555-9111	Account #:	10014		
Date of Birth:	10/16/CCYY-18	Gender:	Female		
Marital Status:	Single	Relationship to Guarantor:	Child		
Student Status:	☒ Full-time	☐ Part-time			
Insurance Type:	☒ Pvt ☐ M/care ☐ M/caid ☐ WC ☐ Other _____				
Hospitalization Date:					
Hospital Information:					

Authorization

☒ Authorization to Release Information
☒ Authorization for Assignment of Benefits
☐ Authorization for Consent for Treatment
☐ My insurance will be billed but there may be a balance due.

Signature: Greg Green   Date: 2/8/CCYY

Clinical Information

	DOS	POS	CPT® /HCPCS Description	ICD-9-CM (*Indicates diagnosis for all lines)	Amount
1	02/08/CCYY	Office	Mammography, bilateral	*1	$250.00
2	02/08/CCYY	Office	Ultrasound, pelvic; B-scan,w/ image doc, complete	*	$250.00
3	02/08/CCYY	Office	X-ray sinuses, paranasal exam, less than three views	*2	$106.00
4	02/08/CCYY	Office	Collection of venous blood by venipuncture	*1	$ 22.00
5	02/08/CCYY	Office	Est pt, comprehensive hist & exam, high complexity	*Diffuse cystic mastopathy, *1Pelvic Pain,	$150.00
6				*2Acute URI	
Remarks:					

Previous Balance:		Payment:	$350.00	Copay:		Adjustment:			
Total Fee:	$778.00	Cash ☐ Check ☐ Credit ☒		Cash ☐ Check ☐ Credit ☐		Reason:		New Balance:	$428.00

Encounter Form

Provider Information

Name:	Glen Gardner, M.D.
Address:	113 Gatton Way

City:	Los Angeles	State:	CA	Zip Code:	90010
Telephone #:		Fax #:			
Medicare ID#:		UPIN #:	G55884		
Tax ID #:	33-2446123	Accepts Medicare Assignment:	☒		
Provider's Signature:	Glen Gardner, MD	Date: 6/10/CCYY			

Appointment Information

Appointment Date:		Time:	
Next Appt. Date:		Time:	
Date of First Visit:	06/10/CCYY	Date of Injury:	06/05/CCYY
Referring Physician:			

Guarantor Information

Name:	Greg Green
Address:	160 Grain Avenue

City:	Pasadena	State:	CA	Zip Code:	91114
Insurance ID #:	11-1111 ABC				
Insurance Name:	Winter Insurance Company				
Insurance Group #:	36928				
Employer Name:	ABC Corporation				

Patient Information

Name:	George Green
Address:	160 Grain Avenue

City:	Pasadena	State:	CA	Zip Code:	91114
Telephone #:	(626) 555-9111	Account #:	10011		
Date of Birth:	01/24/CCYY-17	Gender:	Male		
Marital Status:	Single	Relationship to Guarantor:	Child		
Student Status:	☒ Full-time	☐ Part-time			
Insurance Type:	☒ Pvt ☐ M/care ☐ M/caid ☐ WC ☐ Other _____				
Hospitalization Date:					
Hospital Information:					

Authorization

☒ Authorization to Release Information
☐ Authorization for Assignment of Benefits
☐ Authorization for Consent for Treatment
☐ My insurance will be billed but there may be a balance due.

Signature: Greg Green   Date: 6/10/CCYY

Clinical Information

	DOS	POS	CPT® /HCPCS Description	ICD-9-CM (*Indicates diagnosis for all lines)	Amount
1	06/10/CCYY	Office	Est pt, expanded prob foc hist & exam, low comp	*Open wound of index finger	$ 90.00
2	06/10/CCYY	Office	Radiological exam, finger(s), 2 views	*	$ 50.00
3	06/10/CCYY	Office	Supplies and materials	*	$ 50.00
4					
5					
6					
Remarks:	Parents stated that patient cut finger while slicing apple on 6/05/CCYY.				

Previous Balance:	$155.00	Payment:		Copay:		Adjustment:			
Total Fee:	$190.00	Cash ☐ Check ☐ Credit ☐		Cash ☐ Check ☐ Credit ☐		Reason:		New Balance:	$345.00

DXL Claims Beginning Financials
FRANCISCO FAMILY

Insurance Plan	Rover Insurers, Inc.—Ninja Enterprises				
Patient:	**FRANK**	**FELICIA**	**FRED**	**FREDA**	
C/O DEDUCTIBLE	0.00	0.00	0.00	0.00	
DEDUCTIBLE	0.00	100.00	125.00	75.00	
COINSURANCE	0.00	0.00	0.00	0.00	
ACCIDENT BENEFIT					
LIFETIME MAXIMUM	750.00	1,154.20	679.50	2,037.96	
M/N OFFICE VISITS					
OFFICE VISITS					
HOSPITAL VISITS					
DXL					
SURGERY					
ASSISTANT SURGERY					
ANESTHESIA					

Encounter Form

Provider Information

Name:	Foster Farmingham, M.D.
Address:	113 Fetter Blvd.
City:	Los Angeles · State: CA · Zip Code: 90020
Telephone #:	Fax #:
Medicare ID#:	UPIN #: H64458
Tax ID #:	95-2461234 · Accepts Medicare Assignment: ☒
Provider's Signature:	*Foster Farmingham., MD* · Date: 5/2/CCYY

Appointment Information

Appointment Date:	Time:
Next Appt. Date:	Time:
Date of First Visit: 05/02/CCYY	Date of Injury:
Referring Physician:	

Guarantor Information

Name:	Frank Francisco
Address:	1540 Farquat Avenue
City: N. Hollywood · State: CA · Zip Code: 91000	
Insurance ID #:	22-2222 NIN
Insurance Name:	Rover Insurers, Inc.
Insurance Group #:	21088
Employer Name:	Ninja Enterprises

Patient Information

Name:	Frank Francisco
Address:	1540 Farquat Avenue
City:	N. Hollywood · State: CA · Zip Code: 91000
Telephone #:	(818) 555-9100 · Account #: 10015
Date of Birth:	10/04/CCYY-45 · Gender: Male
Marital Status:	Married · Relationship to Guarantor: Self
Student Status:	☐ Full-time ☐ Part-time
Insurance Type:	☒ Pvt ☐ M/care ☐ M/caid ☐ WC ☐ Other
Hospitalization Date:	
Hospital Information:	

Authorization
☒ Authorization to Release Information
☒ Authorization for Assignment of Benefits
☐ Authorization for Consent for Treatment
☐ My insurance will be billed but there may be a balance due.

Signature: *Frank Francisco* Date: 5/2/CCYY

Clinical Information

	DOS	POS	CPT® /HCPCS Description	ICD-9-CM (*Indicates diagnosis for all lines)	Amount
1	05/02/CCYY	Office	New pt, expanded hist & exam, straightforward	Hemoptysis; *1Chest Pain	$150.00
2	05/02/CCYY	Office	Electrocardiogram; with interpretation and report	*1	$120.00
3	05/02/CCYY	Office	Spirometry incl graph record, total w/ max vol vent	*1	$150.00
4					
5					
6					

Remarks:			
Previous Balance:	Payment:	Copay:	Adjustment:
Total Fee: $420.00	Cash ☐ Check ☐ Credit ☐	Cash ☐ Check ☐ Credit ☐	Reason: · New Balance: $420.00

Encounter Form

Provider Information

Name:	Foster Farley, M.D.
Address:	101 Fetter Blvd.
City:	Montebello — State: CA — Zip Code: 90640
Telephone #:	Fax #:
Medicare ID#:	UPIN #: I42384
Tax ID #:	95-2433444 — Accepts Medicare Assignment: ☒
Provider's Signature:	Foster Farley, MD — Date: 10/2/CCYY

Appointment Information

Appointment Date:	Time:
Next Appt. Date:	Time:
Date of First Visit:	Date of Injury:
Referring Physician:	

Guarantor Information

Name:	Frank Francisco
Address:	1540 Farquat Blvd.
City: N. Hollywood	State: CA — Zip Code: 91000
Insurance ID #:	22-2222 NIN
Insurance Name:	Rover Insurers, Inc.
Insurance Group #:	21088
Employer Name:	Ninja Enterprises

Patient Information

Name:	Felicia Francisco
Address:	1540 Farquat Blvd.
City:	N. Hollywood — State: CA — Zip Code: 91000
Telephone #:	(818) 555-9100 — Account #: 10016
Date of Birth:	11/14/CCYY-44 — Gender: Female
Marital Status:	Married — Relationship to Guarantor: Spouse
Student Status:	☐ Full-time ☐ Part-time
Insurance Type:	☒ Pvt ☐ M/care ☐ M/caid ☐ WC ☐ Other _____
Hospitalization Date:	
Hospital Information:	

Authorization

☒ Authorization to Release Information
☐ Authorization for Assignment of Benefits
☐ Authorization for Consent for Treatment
☐ My insurance will be billed but there may be a balance due.

Signature: Felicia Francisco — Date: 10/2/CCYY

Clinical Information

	DOS	POS	CPT® /HCPCS Description	ICD-9-CM (*Indicates diagnosis for all lines)	Amount
1	10/02/CCYY	Office	Est pt, expanded prob foc hist & exam, low complexity	*Diabetes mellitus	$100.00
2	10/02/CCYY	Office	Glucose, blood, reagent strip	*	$ 40.00
3					
4					
5					
6					

Remarks:

Previous Balance:		Payment:		Copay:		Adjustment:		
Total Fee:	$140.00	Cash ☐ Check ☐ Credit ☐		Cash ☐ Check ☐ Credit ☐		Reason:	New Balance:	$140.00

Encounter Form

Provider Information

Name:	Farnilla Fah, M.D.
Address:	6315 Feltern Avenue
City:	Bell Gardens — State: CA — Zip Code: 90202
Telephone #:	Fax #:
Medicare ID#:	UPIN #: J45224
Tax ID #:	94-3390193 — Accepts Medicare Assignment: ☒
Provider's Signature:	Farnilla Fah, MD — Date: 9/12/CCYY

Appointment Information

Appointment Date:	Time:
Next Appt. Date:	Time:
Date of First Visit:	07/25/CCYY — Date of Injury:
Referring Physician:	

Guarantor Information

Name:	Frank Francisco
Address:	1540 Farquat Avenue
City: N. Hollywood	State: CA — Zip Code: 91000
Insurance ID #:	22-2222 NIN
Insurance Name:	Rover Insurers, Inc.
Insurance Group #:	21088
Employer Name:	Ninja Enterprises

Patient Information

Name:	Fred Francisco
Address:	1540 Farquat Avenue
City:	N. Hollywood — State: CA — Zip Code: 91000
Telephone #:	(818) 555-9100 — Account #: 10017
Date of Birth:	11/14/CCYY-18 — Gender: Male
Marital Status:	Single — Relationship to Guarantor: Child
Student Status:	☒ Full-time ☐ Part-time
Insurance Type:	☒ Pvt ☐ M/care ☐ M/caid ☐ WC ☐ Other _____
Hospitalization Date:	
Hospital Information:	

Authorization

☒ Authorization to Release Information
☒ Authorization for Assignment of Benefits
☐ Authorization for Consent for Treatment
☐ My insurance will be billed but there may be a balance due.

Signature: Frank Francisco — Date: 9/12/CCYY

Clinical Information

	DOS	POS	CPT® /HCPCS Description	ICD-9-CM (*Indicates diagnosis for all lines)	Amount
1	09/12/CCYY	Office	Est pt, detailed hist & exam, moderate complexity	*Anemia	$150.00
2	09/12/CCYY	Office	Intramuscular Therapeutic injection of B-complex	*	$ 25.00
3	09/12/CCYY	Office	Iron	*	$125.00
4	09/12/CCYY	Office	Blood count/smear, micro exam w/ different WBC ct	*	$ 45.00
5					
6					

Remarks:

Previous Balance:		Payment:		Copay:		Adjustment:		
Total Fee:	$345.00	Cash ☐ Check ☐ Credit ☐		Cash ☐ Check ☐ Credit ☐		Reason:	New Balance:	$345.00

Encounter Form

DOCUMENT 35

Provider Information

Name:	Felicia Freeze, M.D.
Address:	P.O. Box 2339
City:	Beverly Hills	State:	CA	Zip Code:	90200
Telephone #:		Fax #:
Medicare ID#:		UPIN #:	K11115
Tax ID #:	33-4060446	Accepts Medicare Assignment: ☒
Provider's Signature:	*Felicia Freeze, MD*	Date: *11/2/CCYY*

Patient Information

Name:	Felicia Francisco
Address:	1540 Farquat Blvd.
City:	N. Hollywood	State:	CA	Zip Code:	91000
Telephone #:	(818) 555-9100	Account #:	10016
Date of Birth:	11/14/CCYY-44	Gender:	Female
Marital Status:	Married	Relationship to Guarantor:	Spouse
Student Status:	☐ Full-time	☐ Part-time
Insurance Type:	☒ Pvt ☐ M/care ☐ M/caid ☐ WC ☐ Other _____
Hospitalization Date:	
Hospital Information:	

Appointment Information

Appointment Date:		Time:	
Next Appt. Date:		Time:	
Date of First Visit:		Date of Injury:	
Referring Physician:			

Guarantor Information

Name:	Frank Francisco
Address:	1540 Farquat Blvd.
City:	N. Hollywood	State:	CA	Zip Code:	91000
Insurance ID #:	22-2222 NIN
Insurance Name:	Rover Insurers, Inc.
Insurance Group #:	21088
Employer Name:	Ninja Enterprises

Authorization

☒ Authorization to Release Information
☒ Authorization for Assignment of Benefits
☐ Authorization for Consent for Treatment
☐ My insurance will be billed but there may be a balance due.

Signature: *Felicia Francisco*　　　　Date: *11/2/CCYY*

Clinical Information

	DOS	POS	CPT® /HCPCS Description	ICD-9-CM (*Indicates diagnosis for all lines)	Amount
1	11/02/CCYY	Office	Basic metabolic panel	Venous (peripheral) insufficiency	$ 142.00
2	11/02/CCYY	Office	Cholesterol, serum or whole blood, total	*	$ 25.00
3					
4					
5					
6					

Remarks:					
Previous Balance:	$140.00	Payment:	$45.00	Copay:		Adjustment:		
Total Fee:	$167.00	Cash ☒ Check ☐ Credit ☐	Cash ☐ Check ☐ Credit ☐	Reason:	New Balance: $262.00

Encounter Form

DOCUMENT 36

Provider Information

Name:	Francis Frame, M.D.
Address:	9100 Florence Avenue
City:	Huntington Beach	State:	CA	Zip Code:	90322
Telephone #:		Fax #:
Medicare ID#:		UPIN #:	L87777
Tax ID #:	93-0128391	Accepts Medicare Assignment: ☒
Provider's Signature:	*Francis Frame, MD*	Date: *9/14/CCYY*

Patient Information

Name:	Freda Francisco
Address:	1540 Farquat Avenue
City:	N. Hollywood	State:	CA	Zip Code:	91000
Telephone #:	(818) 555-9100	Account #:	10018
Date of Birth:	08/25/CCYY-17	Gender:	Female
Marital Status:	Single	Relationship to Guarantor:	Child
Student Status:	☒ Full-time	☐ Part-time
Insurance Type:	☒ Pvt ☐ M/care ☐ M/caid ☐ WC ☐ Other _____
Hospitalization Date:	
Hospital Information:	

Appointment Information

Appointment Date:		Time:	
Next Appt. Date:		Time:	
Date of First Visit:	09/14/CCYY	Date of Injury:	
Referring Physician:			

Guarantor Information

Name:	Frank Francisco
Address:	1540 Farquat Avenue
City:	N. Hollywood	State:	CA	Zip Code:	91000
Insurance ID #:	22-2222 NIN
Insurance Name:	Rover Insurers, Inc.
Insurance Group #:	21088
Employer Name:	Ninja Enterprises

Authorization

☒ Authorization to Release Information
☒ Authorization for Assignment of Benefits
☐ Authorization for Consent for Treatment
☐ My insurance will be billed but there may be a balance due.

Signature: *Frank Francisco*　　　　Date: *9/14/CCYY*

Clinical Information

	DOS	POS	CPT® /HCPCS Description	ICD-9-CM (*Indicates diagnosis for all lines)	Amount
1	09/14/CCYY	Office	Abdominal ultrasound, B-scan, complete	Abdominal pain	$350.00
2	09/14/CCYY	Office	X-ray, gastrointestinal tract w/ film and KUB	*Urinary tract infection	$275.00
3	09/14/CCYY	Office	Lab - surgical pathology, gross and microscopic exam	*1Secondary syphilis of mucous membranes	$225.00
4	09/14/CCYY	Office	New pt, comprehensive hist & exam, high complexity	*, *1	$225.00
5					
6					

Remarks:					
Previous Balance:		Payment:	$550.00	Copay:		Adjustment:		
Total Fee:	$1075.00	Cash ☐ Check ☒ Credit ☐	Cash ☐ Check ☐ Credit ☐	Reason:	New Balance: $525.00

DXL Claims Beginning Financials
HERNANDEZ FAMILY

Insurance Plan	Ball Insurance Carriers—XYZ Corporation				
Patient:	**HENRIQUEZ**	**HORTENCIA**	**HECTOR**		
C/O DEDUCTIBLE					
DEDUCTIBLE	125.00	50.00	75.00		
COINSURANCE	365.15	0.00	0.00		
ACCIDENT BENEFIT	0.00	45.00	105.00		
LIFETIME MAXIMUM	2,781.50	45.00	1,200.00		
M/N LIFETIME					
M/N OFFICE VISITS					
OFFICE VISITS	0.00	0.00	50.00		
HOSPITAL VISITS					
DXL	0.00	0.00	93.60		
SURGERY					
ASSISTANT SURGERY					
ANESTHESIA					

Encounter Form

Provider Information

Name:	Hapsheth Urgent Care
Address:	P.O. Box 1998
City:	Montebello State: CA Zip Code: 90640
Telephone #:	Fax #:
Medicare ID#:	UPIN #: W00006
Tax ID #:	33-4212790 Accepts Medicare Assignment: ☒
Provider's Signature:	Harry Hapsheth, MD Date: 12/15/CCYY

Appointment Information

Appointment Date:	Time:
Next Appt. Date:	Time:
Date of First Visit:	12/15/CCYY Date of Injury: 12/15/CCY
Referring Physician:	

Guarantor Information

Name:	Henriquez Hernandez
Address:	7931 Harbor Avenue
City:	Harbor State: CA Zip Code: 90202
Insurance ID #:	44-4444 XYZ
Insurance Name:	Ball Insurance Carriers
Insurance Group #:	62958
Employer Name:	XYZ Corporation

Patient Information

Name:	Hector Hernandez
Address:	7931 Harbor Avenue
City:	Harbor State: CA Zip Code: 90202
Telephone #:	(310) 555-9020 Account #: 10019
Date of Birth:	05/02/CCYY-17 Gender: Male
Marital Status:	Single Relationship to Guarantor: Child
Student Status:	☒ Full-time ☐ Part-time
Insurance Type:	☒ Pvt ☐ M/care ☐ M/caid ☐ WC ☐ Other _____
Hospitalization Date:	
Hospital Information:	

Authorization

☒ Authorization to Release Information
☐ Authorization for Assignment of Benefits
☐ Authorization for Consent for Treatment
☐ My insurance will be billed but there may be a balance due.

Signature: Henriquez Hernandez Date: 12/15/CCYY

Clinical Information

	DOS	POS	CPT® /HCPCS Description	ICD-9-CM (*Indicates diagnosis for all lines)	Amount
1	12/15/CCYY	Office	New pt, comprehensive hist & exam, low complexity	*Headache, *1Epistaxis, *2Head Injury	$100.00
2	12/15/CCYY	Office	X-ray, skull, complete, 4 views	*	$150.00
3	12/15/CCYY	Office	X-ray, spine, 2 views, comp, incl oblique and flexion	*2	$150.00
4					
5					
6					

Remarks:	Services performed by Harry Hapsheth, M.D. UPIN #: M98666 Parents stated that patient tripped at home and hit his head on driveway.
Previous Balance:	Payment: Copay: Adjustment:
Total Fee:	$400.00 Cash ☐ Check ☐ Credit ☐ Cash ☐ Check ☐ Credit ☐ Reason: New Balance: $400.00

Encounter Form

Provider Information

Name:	La Hiero Medical Center
Address:	1877 La Hiero Drive
City:	Hacienda Heights State: CA Zip Code: 91740
Telephone #:	Fax #:
Medicare ID#:	UPIN #: W00007
Tax ID #:	95-3405565 Accepts Medicare Assignment: ☒
Provider's Signature:	Henry Harrison, MD Date: 9/1/CCYY

Appointment Information

Appointment Date:	Time:
Next Appt. Date:	Time:
Date of First Visit:	08/30/CCYY Date of Injury:
Referring Physician:	

Guarantor Information

Name:	Henriquez Hernandez
Address:	7931 Harbor Avenue
City: Harbor	State: CA Zip Code: 90202
Insurance ID #:	44-4444 XYZ
Insurance Name:	Ball Insurance Carriers
Insurance Group #:	62958
Employer Name:	XYZ Corporation

Patient Information

Name:	Hortencia Hernandez
Address:	7931 Harbor Avenue
City:	Harbor State: CA Zip Code: 90202
Telephone #:	(310) 555-9020 Account #: 10020
Date of Birth:	10/17/CCYY-45 Gender: Female
Marital Status:	Married Relationship to Guarantor: Spouse
Student Status:	☐ Full-time ☐ Part-time
Insurance Type:	☒ Pvt ☐ M/care ☐ M/caid ☐ WC ☐ Other _____
Hospitalization Date:	
Hospital Information:	

Authorization

☒ Authorization to Release Information
☒ Authorization for Assignment of Benefits
☐ Authorization for Consent for Treatment
☐ My insurance will be billed but there may be a balance due.

Signature: Hortencia Hernandez Date: 9/1/CCYY

Clinical Information

	DOS	POS	CPT® /HCPCS Description	ICD-9-CM (*Indicates diagnosis for all lines)	Amount
1	09/01/CCYY	Office	Est pt, problem foc hist & exam, straightforward	*Chronic bronchitis, *1Asbestosis	$ 80.00
2	09/01/CCYY	Office	X-ray, chest, two views	*, *1	$ 98.00
3					
4					
5					
6					

Remarks:	Services performed by Henry Harrison, M.D. UPIN #: A45667
Previous Balance:	Payment: $60.00 Copay: Adjustment:
Total Fee: $178.00	Cash ☐ Check ☒ Credit ☐ Cash ☐ Check ☐ Credit ☐ Reason: New Balance: $118.00

Encounter Form

Provider Information

Name:	Happy Health Clinic
Address:	3175 E. Helming Drive
City:	Southgate State: CA Zip Code: 90280
Telephone #:	Fax #:
Medicare ID#:	UPIN #: W00008
Tax ID #:	33-0144402 Accepts Medicare Assignment: ☒
Provider's Signature:	Hugo Huxtable, MD Date: 12/27/CCYY

Appointment Information

Appointment Date:	Time:
Next Appt. Date:	Time:
Date of First Visit:	Date of Injury:
Referring Physician:	

Guarantor Information

Name:	Henriquez Hernandez
Address:	7931 Harbor Avenue
City: Harbor	State: CA Zip Code: 90202
Insurance ID #:	44-4444 XYZ
Insurance Name:	Ball Insurance Carriers
Insurance Group #:	62958
Employer Name:	XYZ Corporation

Patient Information

Name:	Hector Hernandez
Address:	7931 Harbor Avenue
City:	Harbor State: CA Zip Code: 90202
Telephone #:	(310) 555-9020 Account #: 10019
Date of Birth:	05/02/CCYY-17 Gender: Male
Marital Status:	Single Relationship to Guarantor: Child
Student Status:	☒ Full-time ☐ Part-time
Insurance Type:	☒ Pvt ☐ M/care ☐ M/caid ☐ WC ☐ Other _____
Hospitalization Date:	
Hospital Information:	

Authorization

☒ Authorization to Release Information
☒ Authorization for Assignment of Benefits
☐ Authorization for Consent for Treatment
☐ My insurance will be billed but there may be a balance due.

Signature: Henriquez Hernandez Date: 12/27/CCYY

Clinical Information

	DOS	POS	CPT® /HCPCS Description	ICD-9-CM (*Indicates diagnosis for all lines)	Amount
1	12/27/CCYY	Office	Throat culture with sensitivity	*Streptococcal Pharyngitis	$ 80.00
2	12/27/CCYY	Office	Basic metabolic panel	*	$ 75.00
3					
4					
5					
6					

Remarks:	Services performed by Hugo Huxtable, M.D. UPIN #: B87765
Previous Balance: $400.00	Payment: Copay: Adjustment:
Total Fee: $155.00	Cash ☐ Check ☐ Credit ☐ Cash ☐ Check ☐ Credit ☐ Reason: New Balance: $555.00

Encounter Form

Provider Information

Name:	Hispanic Medical Group
Address:	2256 Hooks Blvd.
City:	Los Angeles **State:** CA **Zip Code:** 90020
Telephone #:	**Fax #:**
Medicare ID#:	**UPIN #:** W00009
Tax ID #:	95-2743311 **Accepts Medicare Assignment:** ☒
Provider's Signature:	Hin Harry, MD **Date:** 9/17/CCYY

Appointment Information

Appointment Date:		Time:
Next Appt. Date:		Time:
Date of First Visit:	09/17/CCYY	Date of Injury:
Referring Physician:		

Guarantor Information

Name:	Henriquez Hernandez
Address:	7931 Harbor Avenue
City:	Harbor **State:** CA **Zip Code:** 90202
Insurance ID #:	44-4444 XYZ
Insurance Name:	Ball Insurance Carriers
Insurance Group #:	62958
Employer Name:	XYZ Corporation

Patient Information

Name:	Hortencia Hernandez
Address:	7931 Harbor Avenue
City:	Harbor **State:** CA **Zip Code:** 90202
Telephone #:	(310) 555-9020 **Account #:** 10020
Date of Birth:	10/17/CCYY-45 **Gender:** Female
Marital Status:	Married **Relationship to Guarantor:** Spouse
Student Status:	☐ Full-time ☐ Part-time
Insurance Type:	☒ Pvt ☐ M/care ☐ M/caid ☐ WC ☐ Other _____
Hospitalization Date:	
Hospital Information:	

Authorization

☒ Authorization to Release Information
☒ Authorization for Assignment of Benefits
☐ Authorization for Consent for Treatment
☐ My insurance will be billed but there may be a balance due.

Signature: _Hortencia Hernandez_ Date: 9/17/CCYY

Clinical Information

	DOS	POS	CPT® /HCPCS Description	ICD-9-CM (*Indicates diagnosis for all lines)	Amount
1	09/17/CCYY	Office	New pt, comprehensive hist & exam, high complexity	*Fibrocystic Breast Disease; *1Vaginitis	$300.00
2	09/17/CCYY	Office	Basic metabolic panel	*	$160.00
3	09/17/CCYY	Office	Cytpoathology, vaginal; manual screening	*1	$ 40.00
4	09/17/CCYY	Office	Cytopahtology, slides , vaginal, hormonal evaluation	*1	$ 65.00
5	09/17/CCYY	Office	Thyroxine; total	*	$130.00
6					

Remarks:	Services performed by Hin Harry, M.D. UPIN #: C45456		
Previous Balance: $118.00	Payment:	Copay:	Adjustment:	
Total Fee: $695.00	Cash ☐ Check ☐ Credit ☐	Cash ☐ Check ☐ Credit ☐	Reason:	New Balance: $813.00

Encounter Form

Provider Information

Name:	Henry Higgs, M.D.
Address:	300 N. Hildegarde
City:	Los Angeles **State:** CA **Zip Code:** 90023
Telephone #:	**Fax #:**
Medicare ID#:	**UPIN #:** D98985
Tax ID #:	57-1471339 **Accepts Medicare Assignment:** ☒
Provider's Signature:	Henry Higgins, MD **Date:** 5/18/CCYY

Appointment Information

Appointment Date:		Time:
Next Appt. Date:		Time:
Date of First Visit:		Date of Injury:
Referring Physician:		

Guarantor Information

Name:	Henriquez Hernandez
Address:	7931 Harbor Avenue
City:	Harbor **State:** CA **Zip Code:** 90202
Insurance ID #:	44-4444 XYZ
Insurance Name:	Ball Insurance Carriers
Insurance Group #:	62958
Employer Name:	XYZ Corporation

Patient Information

Name:	Henriquez Hernandez
Address:	7931 Harbor Avenue
City:	Harbor **State:** CA **Zip Code:** 90202
Telephone #:	(310) 555-9020 **Account #:** 10021
Date of Birth:	05/16/CCYY-47 **Gender:** Male
Marital Status:	Married **Relationship to Guarantor:** Self
Student Status:	☐ Full-time ☐ Part-time
Insurance Type:	☒ Pvt ☐ M/care ☐ M/caid ☐ WC ☐ Other _____
Hospitalization Date:	
Hospital Information:	

Authorization

☒ Authorization to Release Information
☒ Authorization for Assignment of Benefits
☐ Authorization for Consent for Treatment
☐ My insurance will be billed but there may be a balance due.

Signature: _Henriquez Hernandez_ Date: 5/18/CCYY

Clinical Information

	DOS	POS	CPT® /HCPCS Description	ICD-9-CM (*Indicates diagnosis for all lines)	Amount
1	05/18/CCYY	Office	Est pt, detailed hist & exam, moderate complexity	*Acute Bronchiolitis, *1Bacterial Pneumonia	$250.00
2	05/18/CCYY	Office	CBC, automated, differential WBC count	*, *1	$ 25.00
3	05/18/CCYY	Office	Breathing response to CO2	*, *1	$ 65.00
4	05/18/CCYY	Office	Collection of venous blood by venipuncture	*, *1	$ 25.00
5					
6					

Remarks:			
Previous Balance:	Payment:	Copay:	Adjustment:	
Total Fee: $365.00	Cash ☐ Check ☐ Credit ☐	Cash ☐ Check ☐ Credit ☐	Reason:	New Balance: $365.00

Health Claims Examining Exercises

(**Instructor's Note:** Medical Billing exercises in the entire text should be completed prior to students starting Health Claims Examining Exercise 3–A. New files should be set up for the Health Claims Examining exercises.)

Exercise **3-A**

Directions: Complete an Insurance Coverage Form (located in the **Forms** chapter) and set up Family Files for all families in this chapter. Refer to the Family Data Tables (**Documents 22–24**) located in the beginning of this chapter, and the Contracts located in the **Contracts, UCR Conversion Factor Report, and Relative Value Study** chapter.

Exercise **3-B**

Directions: Complete a Payment Worksheet (located in the **Forms** chapter) for CMS-1500 claims (**Documents 26–30, 32–36, and 38–42**) using the guidelines contained in the **Introduction** chapter and using the UCR Conversion Factor Report, Relative Value Study, and Contracts located in the **Contracts, UCR Conversion Factor Report, and Relative Value Study** chapter.

When processing claims, the Beginning Financials (**Documents 25, 31, and 37**) should be incorporated as payment history and claim calculations should be adjusted accordingly. Any carryover deductible listed should be included in the current year deductible for that individual. Therefore, in figuring current year deductible, students should be instructed to subtract the carryover deductible from the current year's amount.

Upon completion of each claim complete or update the Family Benefits Tracking Sheet (located in the **Forms** chapter) by compiling all of the claims payment data for the family.

4
Surgery Services

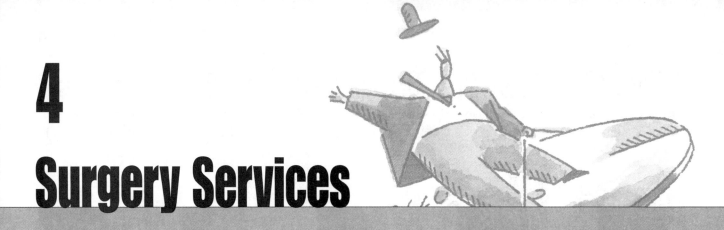

Medical Billing Exercises

Exercise 4-1

Directions: Complete Patient Information Sheets (leave **Assigned Provider** field blank), Ledger Cards, and Insurance Coverage Forms and set up patient charts for the following families using copies of the forms in the **Forms** chapter. Refer to the Family Data Tables (**Documents 43–45**) for information. Individual folders with dividers may be used to store information for each family. One Patient Information Sheet and Insurance Coverage Form should be filled out for the entire family.

DOCUMENT 43

FAMILY DATA TABLE

GATES FAMILY	INSURED'S INFORMATION	SPOUSE'S INFORMATION	CHILD #1	CHILD #2	CHILD #3
Name	**Guadalupe Gates**	**Guillermo Gates**	**Gloria Gates**		
Address	1428 E. Guest Avenue Gardena, CA 91114	1428 E. Guest Avenue Gardena, CA 91114	1428 E. Guest Avenue Gardena, CA 91114		
Email Address	guadalupeg@gates.com				
TELEPHONE #					
Home:	(310) 555-9114	(310) 555-9114	(310) 555-9114		
Work:	(310) 555-9115				
Cell:	(310) 555-9116				
Date of Birth	12/27/CCYY-35	08/12/CCYY-35	01/24/CCYY-12		
Social Security #	555-55-5555	555-55-5556	555-55-5557		
Marital Status/Gender	Married/Female	Married/Male	Single/Female		
Student Status			Full-time		
Patient Account #	10022	10024	10023		
Allergies/Medical Conditions	None	None	None		
PRIMARY INSURANCE CARRIER					
Name Address	Winter Insurance Company 9763 Western Way Whittier, CO 82963	Winter Insurance Company 9763 Western Way Whittier, CO 82963	Winter Insurance Company 9763 Western Way Whittier, CO 82963		
Effective Date	01/01/CCPY	01/01/CCPY	01/01/CCPY		
Member's ID #	55-5555 ABC	55-5555 ABC	55-5555 ABC		
Group Policy #	36928	36928	36928		
Policy/Employer	ABC Corporation 1234 Whitaker Lane Colter, CO 81222				
OTHER INSURANCE CARRIER					
Name Address					
Effective Date					
Member's ID #					
Group Policy #					
Policy/Employer					
Responsible Party	Self	Self	Insured		
EMERGENCY CONTACT					
Name	Gada Gately	Gada Gately	Gada Gately		
Telephone #	(310) 555-9117	(310) 555-9117	(310) 555-9117		
Address	8241 E. Guest Avenue Gardena, CA 91114	8241 E. Guest Avenue Gardena, CA 91114	8241 E. Guest Avenue Gardena, CA 91114		

DOCUMENT 44

FAMILY DATA TABLE

BUTLER FAMILY	INSURED'S INFORMATION	SPOUSE'S INFORMATION	CHILD #1	CHILD #2	CHILD #3
Name	Branford Butler	Barbara Butler	Brielle Butler		
Address	1111 E. Birmingham Blvd. Bayport, CA 90020	1111 E. Birmingham Blvd. Bayport, CA 90020	1111 E. Birmingham Blvd. Bayport, CA 90020		
Email Address	branfordb@butler.com				
TELEPHONE #					
Home:	(906) 555-9004	(906) 555-9004	(906) 555-9004		
Work:	(906) 555-9005				
Cell:	(906) 555-9006				
Date of Birth	03/12/CCYY-52	05/15/CCYY-50	04/02/CCYY-18		
Social Security #	000-00-0000	000-00-0001	000-00-0002		
Marital Status/Gender	Married/Male	Married/Female	Single/Female		
Student Status			Full-time		
Patient Account #	10026	10025	10027		
Allergies/Medical Conditions	None	None	None		
PRIMARY INSURANCE CARRIER					
Name	Ball Insurance Carriers	Ball Insurance Carriers	Ball Insurance Carriers		
Address	3895 Bubble Blvd. Ste. 283 Boxwood, CO 85926	3895 Bubble Blvd. Ste. 283 Boxwood, CO 85926	3895 Bubble Blvd. Ste. 283 Boxwood, CO 85926		
Effective Date	01/01/CCPY	01/01/CCPY	01/01/CCPY		
Member's ID #	00-0000 XYZ	00-0000 XYZ	00-0000 XYZ		
Group Policy #	62958	62958	62958		
Policy/Employer	XYZ Corporation 9817 Bobcat Blvd. Bastion, CO 81319				
OTHER INSURANCE CARRIER					
Name					
Address					
Effective Date					
Member's ID #					
Group Policy #					
Policy/Employer					
Responsible Party	Self	Self	Insured		
EMERGENCY CONTACT					
Name	Brian Bately	Brian Bately	Brian Bately		
Telephone #	(906) 555-9007	(906) 555-9007	(906) 555-9007		
Address	2222 E. Birmingham Blvd. Bayport, CA 90020	2222 E. Birmingham Blvd. Bayport, CA 90020	2222 E. Birmingham Blvd. Bayport, CA 90020		

FAMILY DATA TABLE

DOCUMENT 45

SMITH FAMILY	INSURED'S INFORMATION	SPOUSE'S INFORMATION	CHILD #1	CHILD #2	CHILD #3
Name	Sheryl Smith	Shawn Smith	Shane Smith		
Address	444 Slemons Street So. Sorrie, CA 29003	444 Slemons Street So. Sorrie, CA 29003	444 Slemons Street So. Sorrie, CA 29003		
Email Address	sheryls@smith.com				
TELEPHONE #					
Home:	(803) 555-2900	(803) 555-2900	(803) 555-2900		
Work:	(803) 555-2901				
Cell:	(803) 555-2902				
Date of Birth	05/22/CCYY-56	11/22/CCYY-58	09/12/CCYY-16		
Social Security #	121-21-2121	121-21-2122	121-22-2123		
Marital Status/Gender	Married/Female	Married/Male	Single/Male		
Student Status			Full-time		
Patient Account #	10028	10030	10029		
Allergies/Medical Conditions	None	None	None		
PRIMARY INSURNCE CARRIER					
Name	Rover Insurers, Inc.	Rover Insurers, Inc.	Rover Insurers, Inc.		
Address	5931 Rolling Road Ronson, CO 81369	5931 Rolling Road Ronson, CO 81369	5931 Rolling Road Ronson, CO 81369		
Effective Date	01/01/CCPY	01/01/CCPY	01/01/CCPY		
Member's ID #	21-2121 NIN	21-2121 NIN	21-2121 NIN		
Group Policy #	21088	21088	21088		
Policy/Employer	Ninja Enterprises 1234 Nockout Road Newton, NM 88012				
OTHER INSURANCE CARRIER					
Name					
Address					
Effective Date					
Member's ID #					
Group Policy #					
Policy/Employer					
Responsible Party	Self	Self	Insured		
EMERGENCY CONTACT					
Name	Sarah Sawyer	Sarah Sawyer	Sarah Sawyer		
Telephone #	(803) 555-2903	(803) 555-2903	(803) 555-2903		
Address	555 Slemons Street So. Sorrie, CA 29003	555 Slemons Street So. Sorrie, CA 29003	555 Slemons Street So. Sorrie, CA 29003		

Exercise 4-2

Directions: Complete a CMS-1500 for each of the Encounter Forms **(Documents 47–51, 53–57, and 59–63)** in this chapter. CMS-1500 forms may be provided by your instructor or purchased from a stationery store.

   After completion of each CMS-1500 form, complete a Patient Receipt (if a payment was made), and post the transaction(s) to the patient Ledger Card/Statement of Account previously created.

Exercise 4-3

Directions: Upon completion of all of the activities in Exercise 4–2, complete a Bank Deposit Slip/Ticket (located in the **Forms** chapter) for all payments made on the patient's account in this chapter.

Exercise 4-4

Directions: Using an Insurance Claims Register (located in the **Forms** chapter) list all claims that have been fully prepared and are ready for submission to the insurance carrier for payment. Enter the date that you created the CMS-1500 in the **Date Claim Filed** column.

Exercise 4-5

Directions: Using the stationery or Request for Additional Information Form (located in the **Forms** chapter), write a letter or request information for the following scenario. In each case, you are the medical biller working for Any Billing Services. Addresses and personal information are contained in the patient files that were previously set up. Also, refer to the Family Data Table **(Document 44)** for required information.

1. Create a correspondence for Branford Butler requesting the amount of $8,000 due on their account.

Surgery Claims Beginning Financials
GATES FAMILY

Insurance Plan	Winter Insurance Company—ABC Corporation				
Patient:	**GUADALUPE**	**GUILLERMO**	**GLORIA**		
C/O DEDUCTIBLE	0.00	0.00	0.00		
DEDUCTIBLE	15.70	25.25	65.00		
COINSURANCE	0.00	0.00	0.00		
ACCIDENT BENEFIT					
LIFETIME MAXIMUM	5,413.94	753.89	14,935.10		
M/N OFFICE VISITS					
OFFICE VISITS					
HOSPITAL VISITS					
DXL					
SURGERY					
ASSISTANT SURGERY					
ANESTHESIA					

Encounter Form

Provider Information

Name:	Gateway Medical Group
Address:	1567 Gampete Parkway
City:	Gardena State: CA Zip Code: 91115
Telephone #:	Fax #:
Medicare ID#:	UPIN #: W00010
Tax ID #:	33-1471339 Accepts Medicare Assignment: ☒
Provider's Signature:	*Gina Gelch, MD* Date: *8/14/CCYY*

Appointment Information

Appointment Date:		Time:
Next Appt. Date:		Time:
Date of First Visit:	07/28/CCYY	Date of Injury:
Referring Physician:	Arnold Aspen, M.D.	

Guarantor Information

Name:	Guadalupe Gates
Address:	1428 E. Guest Avenue
City: Gardena	State: CA Zip Code: 91114
Insurance ID #:	55-5555 ABC
Insurance Name:	Winter Insurance Company
Insurance Group #:	36928
Employer Name:	ABC Corporation

Patient Information

Name:	Guadalupe Gates
Address:	1428 E. Guest Avenue
City:	Gardena State: CA Zip Code: 91114
Telephone #:	(310) 555-9114 Account #: 10022
Date of Birth:	12/27/CCYY-35 Gender: Female
Marital Status:	Married Relationship to Guarantor: Self
Student Status:	☐ Full-time ☐ Part-time
Insurance Type:	☒ Pvt ☐ M/care ☐ M/caid ☐ WC ☐ Other
Hospitalization Date:	From: 07/27/CCYY To: 08/16/CCYY
Hospital Information:	Gateway Medical Center, P.O. Box 6677, Gardena, CA 91115

Authorization

☒ Authorization to Release Information
☒ Authorization for Assignment of Benefits
☐ Authorization for Consent for Treatment
☐ My insurance will be billed but there may be a balance due.

Signature: *Guadalupe Gates*   Date: *8/14/CCYY*

Clinical Information

	DOS	POS	CPT® /HCPCS Description	ICD-9-CM (*Indicates diagnosis for all lines)	Amount
1	07/28/CCYY	Inpt Hosp	Consult, comprehensive hist & exam, high complexity	*Chronic Cystitis	$300.00
2	07/29/CCYY	Inpt Hosp	Subhosp care expand prob foc hist & exam, moderate	*	$ 70.00
3	08/14/CCYY	Inpt Hosp	Cystourethroscopy w/ incision of cogen post ureth val	*	$900.00
4					
5					
6					

Remarks:	Services performed by Gina Gelch, M.D. UPIN #: E35354	Referring Physician Arnold Aspen, M.D. UPIN #: F88456	
Previous Balance:	Payment: $450.00 Copay:	Adjustment:	
Total Fee: $1270.00	Cash ☐ Check ☒ Credit ☐ Cash ☐ Check ☐ Credit ☐	Reason:	New Balance: $820.00

Encounter Form *DOCUMENT 48*

Provider Information

Name:	Arnold Aspen, M.D.
Address:	146 Arrow Highway
City:	Altadena State: CA Zip Code: 91124
Telephone #:	Fax #:
Medicare ID#:	UPIN #: F88456
Tax ID #:	95-5671779 Accepts Medicare Assignment: ☐
Provider's Signature:	*Arnold Aspen, MD* Date: *10/12/CCYY*

Appointment Information

Appointment Date:		Time:	
Next Appt. Date:		Time:	
Date of First Visit:		Date of Injury:	
Referring Physician:			

Guarantor Information

Name:	Guadalupe Gates
Address:	1428 E. Guest Avenue
City:	Gardena State: CA Zip Code: 91114
Insurance ID #:	55-5555 ABC
Insurance Name:	Winter Insurance Company
Insurance Group #:	36928
Employer Name:	ABC Corporation

Patient Information

Name:	Guadalupe Gates
Address:	1428 E. Guest Avenue
City:	Gardena State: CA Zip Code: 91114
Telephone #:	(310) 555-9114 Account #: 10022
Date of Birth:	12/27/CCYY-35 Gender: Female
Marital Status:	Married Relationship to Guarantor: Self
Student Status:	☐ Full-time ☐ Part-time
Insurance Type:	☒ Pvt ☐ M/care ☐ M/caid ☐ WC ☐ Other _____
Hospitalization Date:	
Hospital Information:	

Authorization

☒ Authorization to Release Information
☐ Authorization for Assignment of Benefits
☐ Authorization for Consent for Treatment
☐ My insurance will be billed but there may be a balance due.

Signature: *Guadalupe Gates* Date: *10/12/CCYY*

Clinical Information

	DOS	POS	CPT® /HCPCS Description	ICD-9-CM (*Indicates diagnosis for all lines)	Amount
1	09/28/CCYY	Office	Anoscopy; with collection of specimen by brushing	*Hemorrhoids	$ 95.00
2	10/12/CCYY	Office	Protosigmoidoscopy, rigid w/ removal of single	*	$350.00
3			polyp by hot forceps		
4					
5					
6					

Remarks:							
Previous Balance:	$820.00	Payment:	$50.00	Copay:		Adjustment:	
Total Fee:	$445.00	Cash ☒ Check ☐ Credit ☐		Cash ☐ Check ☐ Credit ☐		Reason:	New Balance: $1215.00

Encounter Form *DOCUMENT 49*

Provider Information

Name:	George Guemon, M.D.
Address:	1225 Great Goose Way
City:	Glendora State: CA Zip Code: 91120
Telephone #:	Fax #:
Medicare ID#:	UPIN #: G54327
Tax ID #:	94-4678909 Accepts Medicare Assignment: ☐
Provider's Signature:	*George Guemon, MD* Date: *9/14/CCYY*

Appointment Information

Appointment Date:		Time:	
Next Appt. Date:		Time:	
Date of First Visit:	09/07/CCYY	Date of Injury:	
Referring Physician:			

Guarantor Information

Name:	Guadalupe Gates
Address:	1428 E. Guest Avenue
City:	Gardena State: CA Zip Code: 91114
Insurance ID #:	55-5555 ABC
Insurance Name:	Winter Insurance Company
Insurance Group #:	36928
Employer Name:	ABC Corporation

Patient Information

Name:	Gloria Gates
Address:	1428 E. Guest Avenue
City:	Gardena State: CA Zip Code: 91114
Telephone #:	(310) 555-9114 Account #: 10023
Date of Birth:	01/24/CCYY-12 Gender: Female
Marital Status:	Single Relationship to Guarantor: Child
Student Status:	☒ Full-time ☐ Part-time
Insurance Type:	☒ Pvt ☐ M/care ☐ M/caid ☐ WC ☐ Other _____
Hospitalization Date:	9/10/CCYY
Hospital Information:	Gateway Medical Center, P.O. Box 6677, Gardena, CA 91115

Authorization

☒ Authorization to Release Information
☒ Authorization for Assignment of Benefits
☐ Authorization for Consent for Treatment
☐ My insurance will be billed but there may be a balance due.

Signature: *Guadalupe Gates* Date: *9/14/CCYY*

Clinical Information

	DOS	POS	CPT® /HCPCS Description	ICD-9-CM (*Indicates diagnosis for all lines)	Amount
1	09/07/CCYY	Office	New pt, comprehensive hist & exam, high complexity	*Cysts of Eyelid	$270.00
2	09/10/CCYY	Inpt Hosp	Excisional biopsy of lesion of eyelid w/flap reconstruct	*	$575.00
3	09/14/CCYY	Office	Supplies and material	*	$ 50.00
4					
5					
6					

Remarks:							
Previous Balance:		Payment:		Copay:		Adjustment:	
Total Fee:	$895.00	Cash ☐ Check ☐ Credit ☐		Cash ☐ Check ☐ Credit ☐		Reason:	New Balance: $895.00

Encounter Form   DOCUMENT 50

Provider Information

Name:	Garner Dermatology Medical Group				
Address:	4912 Gorin Avenue				
City:	San Fernando	State:	CA	Zip Code:	91130
Telephone #:		Fax #:			
Medicare ID#:		UPIN #:	W00011		
Tax ID #:	95-6783421	Accepts Medicare Assignment: ☐			
Provider's Signature:	_Gilbert Garcia, MD_	Date: _10/1/CCYY_			

Appointment Information

Appointment Date:		Time:	
Next Appt. Date:		Time:	
Date of First Visit:		Date of Injury:	
Referring Physician:			

Guarantor Information

Name:	Guadalupe Gates				
Address:	1428 E. Guest Avenue				
City:	Gardena	State:	CA	Zip Code:	91114
Insurance ID #:	55-5555 ABC				
Insurance Name:	Winter Insurance Company				
Insurance Group #:	36928				
Employer Name:	ABC Corporation				

Patient Information

Name:	Guillermo Gates				
Address:	1428 E. Guest Avenue				
City:	Gardena	State:	CA	Zip Code:	91114
Telephone #:	(310) 555-9114	Account #:	10024		
Date of Birth:	08/12/CCYY-35	Gender:	Male		
Marital Status:	Married	Relationship to Guarantor:		Spouse	
Student Status:	☐ Full-time	☐ Part-time			
Insurance Type:	☒ Pvt ☐ M/care ☐ M/caid ☐ WC ☐ Other _____				
Hospitalization Date:					
Hospital Information:					

Authorization

☒ Authorization to Release Information
☒ Authorization for Assignment of Benefits
☐ Authorization for Consent for Treatment
☐ My insurance will be billed but there may be a balance due.

Signature: _Guillermo Gates_   Date: _10/1/CCYY_

Clinical Information

	DOS	POS	CPT® /HCPCS Description	ICD-9-CM (*Indicates diagnosis for all lines)	Amount
1	10/01/CCYY	Office	Complex repair of 5.1 cm lesion of neck	Dermatosis	$950.00
2					
3					
4					
5					
6					

Remarks:	Services performed by Gilbert Garcia, M.D. UPIN #: H85564				
Previous Balance:		Payment:		Copay:	Adjustment:
Total Fee:	$950.00	Cash ☐ Check ☐ Credit ☐	Cash ☐ Check ☐ Credit ☐	Reason:	New Balance: $950.00

Encounter Form   DOCUMENT 51

Provider Information

Name:	Gavner Orthopedic Medical Group				
Address:	5900 Gathic Avenue				
City:	Huntington Park	State:	CA	Zip Code:	91311
Telephone #:		Fax #:			
Medicare ID#:		UPIN #:	W00012		
Tax ID #:	95-1442899	Accepts Medicare Assignment: ☐			
Provider's Signature:	_George Gilroy, MD_	Date: _12/15/CCYY_			

Appointment Information

Appointment Date:		Time:	
Next Appt. Date:		Time:	
Date of First Visit:		Date of Injury:	
Referring Physician:			

Guarantor Information

Name:	Guadalupe Gates				
Address:	1428 E. Guest Avenue				
City:	Gardena	State:	CA	Zip Code:	91114
Insurance ID #:	55-5555 ABC				
Insurance Name:	Winter Insurance Company				
Insurance Group #:	36928				
Employer Name:	ABC Corporation				

Patient Information

Name:	Guillermo Gates				
Address:	1428 E. Guest Avenue				
City:	Gardena	State:	CA	Zip Code:	91114
Telephone #:	(310) 555-9114	Account #:	10024		
Date of Birth:	08/12/CCYY-35	Gender:	Male		
Marital Status:	Married	Relationship to Guarantor:		Spouse	
Student Status:	☐ Full-time	☐ Part-time			
Insurance Type:	☒ Pvt ☐ M/care ☐ M/caid ☐ WC ☐ Other _____				
Hospitalization Date:					
Hospital Information:					

Authorization

☒ Authorization to Release Information
☒ Authorization for Assignment of Benefits
☐ Authorization for Consent for Treatment
☐ My insurance will be billed but there may be a balance due.

Signature: _Guillermo Gates_   Date: _12/15/CCYY_

Clinical Information

	DOS	POS	CPT® /HCPCS Description	ICD-9-CM (*Indicates diagnosis for all lines)	Amount
1	11/16/CCYY	Office	Injection of single tendon sheath	*Neuralgia; *1Costochondritis	$120.00
2	12/15/CCYY	Office	Arthrocentesis of the elbow	*; *1	$150.00
3					
4					
5					
6					

Remarks:	Services performed by George Gilroy, M.D. UPIN #: I85564				
Previous Balance:	$950.00	Payment:		Copay:	Adjustment:
Total Fee:	$270.00	Cash ☐ Check ☐ Credit ☐	Cash ☐ Check ☐ Credit ☐	Reason:	New Balance: $1220.00

Surgery Claims Beginning Financials

BUTLER FAMILY

Insurance Plan	Ball Insurance Carriers—XYZ Corporation				
Patient:	BRANFORD	BARBARA	BRIELLE		
C/O DEDUCTIBLE	0.00	0.00	0.00		
DEDUCTIBLE	75.50	125.00	5.00		
COINSURANCE	0.00	325.59	0.00		
ACCIDENT BENEFIT					
LIFETIME MAXIMUM	6,753.89	54,322.94	935.10		
M/N OFFICE VISITS					
OFFICE VISITS	25.00	160.00	0.00		
HOSPITAL VISITS					
DXL	125.00	75.00	0.00		
SURGERY	225.00	1,375.00	0.00		
ASSISTANT SURGERY					
ANESTHESIA					

Encounter Form

Provider Information

Name:	Babies R Us Medical Group
Address:	4440 Bobsey Way
City:	Backdoor State: CA Zip Code: 90120
Telephone #:	Fax #:
Medicare ID#:	UPIN #: W00013
Tax ID #:	33-1557669 Accepts Medicare Assignment: ☐
Provider's Signature:	Brian Brown, MD Date: 10/21/CCYY

Appointment Information

Appointment Date:	Time:
Next Appt. Date:	Time:
Date of First Visit:	03/15/CCYY Date of Injury:
Referring Physician:	

Guarantor Information

Name:	Branford Butler
Address:	1111 E. Birmingham Blvd.
City:	Bayport State: CA Zip Code: 90020
Insurance ID #:	00-0000 XYZ
Insurance Name:	Ball Insurance Carriers
Insurance Group #:	62958
Employer Name:	XYZ Corporation

Patient Information

Name:	Barbara Butler
Address:	1111 E. Birmingham Blvd.
City:	Bayport State: CA Zip Code: 90020
Telephone #:	(906) 555-9004 Account #: 10025
Date of Birth:	05/15/CCYY-50 Gender: Female
Marital Status:	Married Relationship to Guarantor: Spouse
Student Status:	☐ Full-time ☐ Part-time
Insurance Type:	☒ Pvt ☐ M/care ☐ M/caid ☐ WC ☐ Other _____
Hospitalization Date:	From: 10/21/CCYY To: 10/23/CCYY
Hospital Information:	Bayport Hospital, P.O. Box 7890, Backdoor, CA 90120

Authorization

☒ Authorization to Release Information
☒ Authorization for Assignment of Benefits
☐ Authorization for Consent for Treatment
☐ My insurance will be billed but there may be a balance due.

Signature: Barbara Butler Date: 10/21/CCYY

Clinical Information

	DOS	POS	CPT® /HCPCS Description	ICD-9-CM (*Indicates diagnosis for all lines)	Amount
1	09/20/CCYY	Office	Urinalysis, dip stick, with microscopic	*Pregnant state; *1Normal delivery	$ 10.00
2	10/21/CCYY	Inpt Hosp	Routine obstetric care, vaginal delivery	*; *1	$2720.00
3					
4					
5					
6					

Remarks:	Services performed by Brian Brown, M.D. UPIN#: J72816				
Previous Balance:	Payment: $1500.00	Copay:		Adjustment:	
Total Fee: $2730.00	Cash ☐ Check ☐ Credit ☒	Cash ☐ Check ☐ Credit ☐	Reason:	New Balance: $1230.00	

Encounter Form   DOCUMENT 54

Provider Information

Name:	Ben Beeve, M.D.				
Address:	1220 Bark Way				
City:	Bayport	State:	CA	Zip Code:	91120
Telephone #:		Fax #:			
Medicare ID#:		UPIN #:	K76453		
Tax ID #:	94-2224096	Accepts Medicare Assignment:	☐		
Provider's Signature:	_Ben Beeve, MD_		Date: _05/21/CCYY_		

Appointment Information

Appointment Date:		Time:	
Next Appt. Date:		Time:	
Date of First Visit:		Date of Injury:	
Referring Physician:			

Guarantor Information

Name:	Branford Butler				
Address:	1111 E. Birmingham Blvd.				
City:	Bayport	State:	CA	Zip Code:	90020
Insurance ID #:	00-0000 XYZ				
Insurance Name:	Ball Insurance Carriers				
Insurance Group #:	62958				
Employer Name:	XYZ Corporation				

Patient Information

Name:	Branford Butler				
Address:	1111 E. Birmingham Blvd.				
City:	Bayport	State:	CA	Zip Code:	90020
Telephone #:	(906) 555-9004	Account #:	10026		
Date of Birth:	03/12/CCYY-52	Gender:	Male		
Marital Status:	Married	Relationship to Guarantor:	Self		
Student Status:	☐ Full-time	☐ Part-time			
Insurance Type:	☒ Pvt ☐ M/care ☐ M/caid ☐ WC ☐ Other _____				
Hospitalization Date:	From: 04/26/CCYY To: 04/29/CCYY				
Hospital Information:	Bayport Hospital, P.O. Box 7890, Backdoor, CA 90120				

Authorization

☒ Authorization to Release Information
☒ Authorization for Assignment of Benefits
☐ Authorization for Consent for Treatment
☐ My insurance will be billed but there may be a balance due.

Signature: _Branford Butler_   Date: _05/21/CCYY_

Clinical Information

	DOS	POS	CPT® /HCPCS Description	ICD-9-CM (*Indicates diagnosis for all lines)	Amount
1	04/26/CCYY	Inpt Hosp	Cholecystectomy with exploration of common duct	*Chronic Cholecystitis	$2950.00
2	05/21/CCYY	Office	Expanded problem focused exam, low	*; Diabetes Mellitus	$ 50.00
3					
4					
5					
6					
Remarks:					
Previous Balance:		Payment:		Copay:		Adjustment:		
Total Fee:	$3000.00	Cash ☐ Check ☐ Credit ☐	Cash ☐ Check ☐ Credit ☐	Reason:	New Balance: $3000.00

Encounter Form   DOCUMENT 55

Provider Information

Name:	Bob Buam, M.D.				
Address:	220 Buyer Drive				
City:	Bridle	State:	CA	Zip Code:	92221
Telephone #:		Fax #:			
Medicare ID#:		UPIN #:	L15975		
Tax ID #:	34-3221239	Accepts Medicare Assignment:	☐		
Provider's Signature:	_Bob Buam, MD_		Date: _5/6/CCYY_		

Appointment Information

Appointment Date:		Time:	
Next Appt. Date:		Time:	
Date of First Visit:		Date of Injury:	
Referring Physician:			

Guarantor Information

Name:	Branford Butler				
Address:	1111 E. Birmingham Blvd.				
City:	Bayport	State:	CA	Zip Code:	90020
Insurance ID #:	00-0000 XYZ				
Insurance Name:	Ball Insurance Carriers				
Insurance Group #:	62958				
Employer Name:	XYZ Corporation				

Patient Information

Name:	Brielle Butler				
Address:	1111 E. Birmingham Blvd.				
City:	Bayport	State:	CA	Zip Code:	90020
Telephone #:	(906) 555-9004	Account #:	10027		
Date of Birth:	04/02/CCYY-18	Gender:	Female		
Marital Status:	Single	Relationship to Guarantor:	Child		
Student Status:	☒ Full-time	☐ Part-time			
Insurance Type:	☒ Pvt ☐ M/care ☐ M/caid ☐ WC ☐ Other _____				
Hospitalization Date:					
Hospital Information:	Bridle Medical Facility, P.O. Box 111, Bridle, CA 92221				

Authorization

☒ Authorization to Release Information
☐ Authorization for Assignment of Benefits
☐ Authorization for Consent for Treatment
☐ My insurance will be billed but there may be a balance due.

Signature: _Branford Butler_   Date: _5/6/CCYY_

Clinical Information

	DOS	POS	CPT® /HCPCS Description	ICD-9-CM (*Indicates diagnosis for all lines)	Amount
1	05/06/CCYY	Otpt Hosp	Excision of pilonidal cyst; simple	Pilondial Cyst	$1300.00
2					
3					
4					
5					
6					
Remarks:					
Previous Balance:		Payment:		Copay:		Adjustment:		
Total Fee:	$1300.00	Cash ☐ Check ☐ Credit ☐	Cash ☐ Check ☐ Credit ☐	Reason:	New Balance: $1300.00

Encounter Form   DOCUMENT 56

Provider Information

Name:	Emergency Medical Group				
Address:	1232 Boston Blvd.				
City:	Brighton	State:	CA	Zip Code:	90129
Telephone #:		Fax #:			
Medicare ID#:		UPIN #:	W00014		
Tax ID #:	94-4446749	Accepts Medicare Assignment:	☐		
Provider's Signature:	_Barbara Boxer, MD_		Date: _6/30/CCYY_		

Appointment Information

Appointment Date:		Time:	
Next Appt. Date:		Time:	
Date of First Visit:	06/30/CCYY	Date of Injury:	06/30/CCYY
Referring Physician:			

Patient Information

Name:	Brielle Butler				
Address:	1111 E. Birmingham Blvd.				
City:	Bayport	State:	CA	Zip Code:	90020
Telephone #:	(906) 555-9004	Account #:	10027		
Date of Birth:	04/02/CCYY-18	Gender:	Female		
Marital Status:	Single	Relationship to Guarantor:	Child		
Student Status:	☒ Full-time	☐ Part-time			
Insurance Type:	☒ Pvt ☐ M/care ☐ M/caid ☐ WC ☐ Other _____				
Hospitalization Date:					
Hospital Information:	Brighton Medical Facility, P.O. Box 2400, Brighton, CA 90129				

Guarantor Information

Name:	Branford Butler			
Address:	1111 E. Birmingham Blvd.			
City:	Bayport	State:	CA	Zip Code: 90020
Insurance ID #:	00-0000 XYZ			
Insurance Name:	Ball Insurance Carriers			
Insurance Group #:	62958			
Employer Name:	XYZ Corporation			

Authorization

☒ Authorization to Release Information
☒ Authorization for Assignment of Benefits
☐ Authorization for Consent for Treatment
☐ My insurance will be billed but there may be a balance due.
Signature: _Branford Butler_   Date: _6/30/CCYY_

Clinical Information

	DOS	POS	CPT® /HCPCS Description	ICD-9-CM (*Indicates diagnosis for all lines)	Amount
1	06/30/CCYY	Outpt Hosp	Open treatment of distal radius, internal fixation	Fractures of distal end of radius	$2500.00
2					
3					
4					
5					
6					
Remarks:	Services provided by Barbara Boxer, M.D. UPIN #: M35715			Parents state that patient fell from a horse today.	
Previous Balance:	$1300.00	Payment:		Copay:	Adjustment:	
Total Fee:	$2500.00	Cash ☐ Check ☐ Credit ☐	Cash ☐ Check ☐ Credit ☐	Reason:	New Balance: $3800.00

Encounter Form   DOCUMENT 57

Provider Information

Name:	Sight for Sore Eyes Medical Group				
Address:	1501 Bass Drive				
City:	Brighton	State:	CA	Zip Code:	90132
Telephone #:		Fax #:			
Medicare ID#:		UPIN #:	W00015		
Tax ID #:	95-4336712	Accepts Medicare Assignment:	☐		
Provider's Signature:	_Bobby Brown, M.D._		Date: _7/30/CCYY_		

Appointment Information

Appointment Date:		Time:	
Next Appt. Date:		Time:	
Date of First Visit:		Date of Injury:	
Referring Physician:			

Patient Information

Name:	Branford Butler				
Address:	1111 E. Birmingham Blvd.				
City:	Bayport	State:	CA	Zip Code:	90020
Telephone #:	(906) 555-9004	Account #:	10026		
Date of Birth:	03/12/CCYY-52	Gender:	Male		
Marital Status:	Married	Relationship to Guarantor:	Self		
Student Status:	☐ Full-time	☐ Part-time			
Insurance Type:	☒ Pvt ☐ M/care ☐ M/caid ☐ WC ☐ Other _____				
Hospitalization Date:					
Hospital Information:	Brighton Medical Facility, P.O. Box 2400, Brighton, CA 90129				

Guarantor Information

Name:	Branford Butler			
Address:	1111 E. Birmingham Blvd.			
City:	Bayport	State:	CA	Zip Code: 90020
Insurance ID #:	00-0000 XYZ			
Insurance Name:	Ball Insurance Carriers			
Insurance Group #:	62958			
Employer Name:	XYZ Corporation			

Authorization

☒ Authorization to Release Information
☐ Authorization for Assignment of Benefits
☐ Authorization for Consent for Treatment
☐ My insurance will be billed but there may be a balance due.
Signature: _Branford Butler_   Date: _7/30/CCYY_

Clinical Information

	DOS	POS	CPT® /HCPCS Description	ICD-9-CM (*Indicates diagnosis for all lines)	Amount
1	06/30/CCYY	Otpt Hosp	Removal of lens; intracapsular	*Cataract; *1Retinal Detachment	$2500.00
2	07/30/CCYY	Otpt Hosp	Repair of retinal detachment, cryotherapy, w/ drainage	*; *1	$5500.00
3			photocoagulation, right eye		
4					
5					
6					
Remarks:	Services performed by Bobby Brown, M.D. UPIN #: A98513				
Previous Balance:	$3000.00	Payment:		Copay:	Adjustment:	
Total Fee:	$8000.00	Cash ☐ Check ☐ Credit ☐	Cash ☐ Check ☐ Credit ☐	Reason:	New Balance: 11000.00

Surgery Claims Beginning Financials

SMITH FAMILY

Insurance Plan	Rover Insurers, Inc.—Ninja Enterprises				
Patient:	SHERYL	SHAWN	SHANE		
C/O DEDUCTIBLE	0.00	0.00	0.00		
DEDUCTIBLE	0.00	5.00	75.15		
COINSURANCE	0.00	0.00	0.00		
ACCIDENT BENEFIT					
LIFETIME MAXIMUM	0.00	0.00	0.00		
M/N OFFICE VISITS					
OFFICE VISITS					
HOSPITAL VISITS					
DXL					
SURGERY					
ASSISTANT SURGERY					
ANESTHESIA					

Encounter Form

Provider Information

Name:	Gateway Medical Group				
Address:	1567 Gampete Parkway				
City:	Gardena	State:	CA	Zip Code:	91115
Telephone #:		Fax #:			
Medicare ID#:		UPIN #:	W00010		
Tax ID #:	33-1471339	Accepts Medicare Assignment:	☒		
Provider's Signature:	*Gina Gelch, MD*		Date: *8/14/CCYY*		

Appointment Information

Appointment Date:		Time:	
Next Appt. Date:		Time:	
Date of First Visit:	07/28/CCYY	Date of Injury:	
Referring Physician:	Arnold Aspen, M.D.		

Guarantor Information

Name:	Guadalupe Gates				
Address:	1428 E. Guest Avenue				
City:	Gardena	State:	CA	Zip Code:	91114
Insurance ID #:	55-5555 ABC				
Insurance Name:	Winter Insurance Company				
Insurance Group #:	36928				
Employer Name:	ABC Corporation				

Patient Information

Name:	Guadalupe Gates				
Address:	1428 E. Guest Avenue				
City:	Gardena	State:	CA	Zip Code:	91114
Telephone #:	(310) 555-9114	Account #:	10022		
Date of Birth:	12/27/CCYY-35	Gender:	Female		
Marital Status:	Married	Relationship to Guarantor:	Self		
Student Status:	☐ Full-time	☐ Part-time			
Insurance Type:	☒ Pvt ☐ M/care ☐ M/caid ☐ WC ☐ Other _____				
Hospitalization Date:	From: 07/27/CCYY	To: 08/16/CCYY			
Hospital Information:	Gateway Medical Center, P.O. Box 6677, Gardena, CA 91115				

Authorization

☒ Authorization to Release Information
☒ Authorization for Assignment of Benefits
☐ Authorization for Consent for Treatment
☐ My insurance will be billed but there may be a balance due.
Signature: *Guadalupe Gates*   Date: *8/14/CCYY*

Clinical Information

	DOS	POS	CPT® /HCPCS Description	ICD-9-CM (*Indicates diagnosis for all lines)	Amount
1	07/28/CCYY	Inpt Hosp	Consult, comprehensive hist & exam, high complexity	*Chronic Cystitis	$300.00
2	07/29/CCYY	Inpt Hosp	Subhosp care expand prob foc hist & exam, moderate	*	$ 70.00
3	08/14/CCYY	Inpt Hosp	Cystourethroscopy w/ incision of cogen post ureth val	*	$900.00
4					
5					
6					
Remarks:	Services performed by Gina Gelch, M.D. UPIN #: E35354			Referring Physician Arnold Aspen, M.D. UPIN #: F88456	
Previous Balance:		Payment:	$450.00	Copay:		Adjustment:		
Total Fee:	$1270.00	Cash ☐ Check ☒ Credit ☐		Cash ☐ Check ☐ Credit ☐	Reason:		New Balance:	$820.00

Encounter Form

Provider Information

Name:	Sarmiento Medical Group
Address:	555 North Sill Avenue
City: Charlotte	State: NC Zip Code: 28201
Telephone #:	Fax #:
Medicare ID#:	UPIN #: W00016
Tax ID #: 23-6781254	Accepts Medicare Assignment: ☒
Provider's Signature: _Shawn Sheen, MD_	Date: 8/23/CCYY

Patient Information

Name:	Shane Smith
Address:	444 S. Slemons St.
City: So. Sorrie	State: SC Zip Code: 29003
Telephone #: (803) 555-2900	Account #: 10029
Date of Birth: 09/12/CCYY-16	Gender: Male
Marital Status: Single	Relationship to Guarantor: Child
Student Status: ☒ Full-time ☐ Part-time	
Insurance Type: ☒ Pvt ☐ M/care ☐ M/caid ☐ WC ☐ Other _____	
Hospitalization Date:	
Hospital Information:	

Appointment Information

Appointment Date:	Time:
Next Appt. Date:	Time:
Date of First Visit: 08/23/CCYY	Date of Injury:
Referring Physician:	

Guarantor Information

Name:	Sheryl Smith
Address:	444 S. Slemons St.
City: So. Sorrie	State: SC Zip Code: 29003
Insurance ID #:	21-2121 NIN
Insurance Name:	Rover Insurers, Inc.
Insurance Group #:	21088
Employer Name:	Ninja Enterprises

Authorization

☒ Authorization to Release Information
☒ Authorization for Assignment of Benefits
☐ Authorization for Consent for Treatment
☐ My insurance will be billed but there may be a balance due.

Signature: _Sheryl Smith_ Date: 8/23/CCYY

Clinical Information

	DOS	POS	CPT® /HCPCS Description	ICD-9-CM (*Indicates diagnosis for all lines)	Amount
1	08/23/CCYY	Office	Excision of nail and nail matrix, complete	Ingrowing Nail	$400.00
2					
3					
4					
5					
6					

Remarks:	Services performed by Shawn Sheen, M.D. UPIN #: C98756				
Previous Balance:		Payment: $400.00	Copay:	Adjustment:	
Total Fee: $400.00	Cash ☐ Check ☐ Credit ☒	Cash ☐ Check ☐ Credit ☐	Reason:	New Balance: $0.00	

Encounter Form

Provider Information

Name:	Shinaya Shimfa, M.D.
Address:	4955 Siesta
City: Greensboro	State: NC Zip Code: 27502
Telephone #:	Fax #:
Medicare ID#:	UPIN #: D42215
Tax ID #: 13-3691221	Accepts Medicare Assignment: ☒
Provider's Signature: _Shinava Shimfa, MD_	Date: 5/11/CCYY

Patient Information

Name:	Shawn Smith
Address:	444 S. Slemons St
City: So. Sorrie	State: SC Zip Code: 29003
Telephone #: (803) 555-2900	Account #: 10030
Date of Birth: 11/22/CCYY-58	Gender: Male
Marital Status: Married	Relationship to Guarantor: Spouse
Student Status: ☐ Full-time ☐ Part-time	
Insurance Type: ☒ Pvt ☐ M/care ☐ M/caid ☐ WC ☐ Other _____	
Hospitalization Date: From: 05/10/CCYY To: 05/16/CCYY	
Hospital Information: Greensboro Singletarian Hospital, P.O. Box 432, Greensboro, NC 27502	

Appointment Information

Appointment Date:	Time:
Next Appt. Date:	Time:
Date of First Visit: 03/14/CCYY	Date of Injury: 03/14/CCYY
Referring Physician:	

Guarantor Information

Name:	Sheryl Smith
Address:	444 S. Slemons St.
City: So. Sorrie	State: SC Zip Code: 29003
Insurance ID #:	21-2121 NIN
Insurance Name:	Rover Insurers, Inc.
Insurance Group #:	21088
Employer Name:	Ninja Enterprises

Authorization

☒ Authorization to Release Information
☒ Authorization for Assignment of Benefits
☐ Authorization for Consent for Treatment
☐ My insurance will be billed but there may be a balance due.

Signature: _Shawn Smith_ Date: 5/11/CCYY

Clinical Information

	DOS	POS	CPT® /HCPCS Description	ICD-9-CM (*Indicates diagnosis for all lines)	Amount
1	05/11/CCYY	Inpt Hosp	Laminectomy with myelotomy	Displacement of intervertebral disc	$3000.00
2					
3					
4					
5					
6					

Remarks:	A second surgical opinion was performed by Sam Spade, M.D. UPIN #: F33352		Patient in car accident.		
Previous Balance:		Payment:	Copay:	Adjustment:	
Total Fee: $3000.00	Cash ☐ Check ☐ Credit ☐	Cash ☐ Check ☐ Credit ☐	Reason:	New Balance: $3000.00	

Encounter Form — DOCUMENT 62

Provider Information

Name:	Permanent Weight Loss Group
Address:	12450 Squirrel Avenue

City:	Sorrie	State:	SC	Zip Code:	29002

Telephone #:		Fax #:	

Medicare ID#:		UPIN #:	W00017

Tax ID #:	23-2573141	Accepts Medicare Assignment:	☒

Provider's Signature: _Sylvia Sweet, MD_   Date: _12/30/CCYY_

Appointment Information

Appointment Date:		Time:	
Next Appt. Date:		Time:	
Date of First Visit:	05/14/CCYY	Date of Injury:	
Referring Physician:			

Guarantor Information

Name:	Sheryl Smith
Address:	444 S. Slemons St.

City:	So. Sorrie	State:	SC	Zip Code:	29003

Insurance ID #:	21-2121 NIN
Insurance Name:	Rover Insurers, Inc.
Insurance Group #:	21088
Employer Name:	Ninja Enterprises

Patient Information

Name:	Sheryl Smith
Address:	444 S. Slemons St.

City:	So. Sorrie	State:	SC	Zip Code:	29003

Telephone #:	(803) 555-2900	Account #:	10028

Date of Birth:	05/22/CCYY-56	Gender:	Female

Marital Status:	Married	Relationship to Guarantor:	Self

Student Status:	☐ Full-time	☐ Part-time

Insurance Type: ☒ Pvt ☐ M/care ☐ M/caid ☐ WC ☐ Other _____

Hospitalization Date:	From: 12/30/CCYY	To: 01/04/CCNY

Hospital Information: Sorrie Medical Center, P.O. Box 333, Sorrie, SC 29002

Authorization

☒ Authorization to Release Information
☒ Authorization for Assignment of Benefits
☐ Authorization for Consent for Treatment
☐ My insurance will be billed but there may be a balance due.

Signature: _Sheryl Smith_   Date: _12/30/CCYY_

Clinical Information

	DOS	POS	CPT® /HCPCS Description	ICD-9-CM (*Indicates diagnosis for all lines)	Amount
1	12/30/CCYY	Inpt Hosp	Gastric stapling, w/out bypass, nonvertical-banded	Morbid obesity	$ 3505.00
2					
3					
4					
5					
6					

Remarks:	Services performed by Sylvia Sweet, M.D. UPIN #: E44444	Patient has history of morbid exogenous obesity.

Previous Balance:	$1050.00	Payment:		Copay:		Adjustment:		
Total Fee:	$3505.00	Cash ☐ Check ☐ Credit ☐		Cash ☐ Check ☐ Credit ☐		Reason:	New Balance:	$4555.00

Encounter Form — DOCUMENT 63

Provider Information

Name:	Sharon Stack, M.D.
Address:	321 S. 7th Street

City:	Raleigh	State:	NC	Zip Code:	27612

Telephone #:		Fax #:	

Medicare ID#:		UPIN #:	F55555

Tax ID #:	43-4461294	Accepts Medicare Assignment:	☒

Provider's Signature: _Sharon Stack, MD_   Date: _11/14/CCYY_

Appointment Information

Appointment Date:		Time:	
Next Appt. Date:		Time:	
Date of First Visit:	10/21/CCYY	Date of Injury:	
Referring Physician:			

Guarantor Information

Name:	Sheryl Smith
Address:	444 S. Slemons St.

City:	So. Sorrie	State:	SC	Zip Code:	29003

Insurance ID #:	21-2121 NIN
Insurance Name:	Rover Insurers, Inc.
Insurance Group #:	21088
Employer Name:	Ninja Enterprises

Patient Information

Name:	Shane Smith
Address:	444 S. Slemons St

City:	So. Sorrie	State:	SC	Zip Code:	29003

Telephone #:	(803) 555-2900	Account #:	10029

Date of Birth:	09/12/CCYY-16	Gender:	Male

Marital Status:	Single	Relationship to Guarantor:	Child

Student Status:	☒ Full-time	☐ Part-time

Insurance Type: ☒ Pvt ☐ M/care ☐ M/caid ☐ WC ☐ Other _____

Hospitalization Date:	
Hospital Information:	

Authorization

☒ Authorization to Release Information
☒ Authorization for Assignment of Benefits
☐ Authorization for Consent for Treatment
☐ My insurance will be billed but there may be a balance due.

Signature: _Sheryl Smith_   Date: _11/14/CCYY_

Clinical Information

	DOS	POS	CPT® /HCPCS Description	ICD-9-CM (*Indicates diagnosis for all lines)	Amount
1	10/21/CCYY	Office	Removal foreign body, intranasal	Foreign body in nose	$ 80.00
2	11/14/CCYY	Office	Removal impacted cerumen, both ears	Impacted cerumen	$ 75.00
3					
4					
5					
6					

Remarks:	Bean removed from patient's nose.

Previous Balance:		Payment:		Copay:		Adjustment:		
Total Fee:	$155.00	Cash ☐ Check ☐ Credit ☐		Cash ☐ Check ☐ Credit ☐		Reason:	New Balance:	$155.00

Health Claims Examining Exercises

(**Instructor's Note:** Medical Billing exercises in the entire text should be completed prior to students starting Health Claims Examining Exercise 4–A. New files should be set up for the Health Claims Examining exercises.)

Exercise **4-A**

Directions: Complete an Insurance Coverage Form (located in the **Forms** chapter) and set up Family Files for all families in this chapter. Refer to the Family Data Tables (**Documents 43–45**) located in the beginning of this chapter, and the Contracts located in the **Contracts, UCR Conversion Factor Report, and Relative Value Study** chapter.

Exercise **4-B**

Directions: Complete a Payment Worksheet (located in the **Forms** chapter) for CMS-1500 claims (**Documents 47–51, 53–57, and 59–63**) using the guidelines contained in the **Introduction** chapter and using the UCR Conversion Factor Report, Relative Value Study, and Contracts located in the **Contracts, UCR Conversion Factor Report, and Relative Value Study** chapter.

When processing claims, the Beginning Financials (**Documents 46, 52, 58**) should be incorporated as payment history and claim calculations should be adjusted accordingly. Any carryover deductible listed should be included in the current year deductible for that individual. Therefore, in figuring current year deductible, students should be instructed to subtract the carryover deductible from the current year's amount.

Upon completion of each claim complete or update the Family Benefits Tracking Sheet (located in the **Forms** chapter) by compiling all of the claims payment data for the family.

5
Multiple Surgery
Services

Medical Billing Exercises

Exercise 5-1

Directions: Complete Patient Information Sheets (leave **Assigned Provider** field blank), Ledger Cards, and Insurance Coverage Forms and set up patient charts for the following families using copies of the forms in the **Forms** chapter. Refer to the Family Data Tables **(Documents 64–65)** for information. Individual folders with dividers may be used to store information for each family. One Patient Information Sheet and Insurance Coverage Form should be filled out for the entire family.

FAMILY DATA TABLE

THOMPSON FAMILY	INSURED'S INFORMATION	SPOUSE'S INFORMATION	CHILD #1	CHILD #2	CHILD #3
Name	Tony Thompson	Terry Thompson	Traci Thompson	Tina Thompson	
Address	222 Tamarack Lane Tomahawk, TN 37308	222 Tamarack Lane Tomahawk, TN 37308	222 Tamarack Lane Tomahawk, TN 37308	222 Tamarack Lane Tomahawk, TN 37308	
Email Address	tonyt@thompson.com				
TELEPHONE #					
Home:	(903) 555-3730	(903) 555-3730	(903) 555-3730	(903) 555-3730	
Work:	(903) 555-3731				
Cell:	(903) 555-3732				
Date of Birth	07/10/CCYY-55	08/21/CCYY-51	03/11/CCYY-17	12/14/CCYY-18	
Social Security #	999-99-9999	999-99-9900	999-99-9901	999-99-9902	
Marital Status/Gender	Married/Male	Married/Female	Single/Female	Single/Female	
Student Status			Full-time	Full-time	
Patient Account #	10031	10032	10033	10034	
Allergies/Medical Conditions	None	None	None	None	
PRIMARY INSURANCE CARRIER					
Name Address	Ball Insurance Carriers 3895 Bubble Blvd. Ste. 283 Boxwood, CO 85926	Ball Insurance Carriers 3895 Bubble Blvd. Ste. 283 Boxwood, CO 85926	Ball Insurance Carriers 3895 Bubble Blvd. Ste. 283 Boxwood, CO 85926	Ball Insurance Carriers 3895 Bubble Blvd. Ste. 283 Boxwood, CO 85926	
Effective Date	01/01/CCPY	01/01/CCPY	01/01/CCPY	01/01/CCPY	
Member's ID #	99-9999 XYZ	99-9999 XYZ	99-9999 XYZ	99-9999 XYZ	
Group Policy #	62958	62958	62958	62958	
Policy/Employer	XYZ Corporation 9817 Bobcat Blvd. Bastion, CO 81319				
OTHER INSURANCE CARRIER					
Name Address					
Effective Date					
Member's ID #					
Group Policy #					
Policy/Employer					
Responsible Party	Self	Self	Insured	Insured	
EMERGENCY CONTACT					
Name	Tonya Timberlake	Tonya Timberlake	Tonya Timberlake	Tonya Timberlake	
Telephone #	(903) 555-3733	(903) 555-3733	(903) 555-3733	(903) 555-3733	
Address	333 Tamarack Lane Tomahawk, TN 37308	333 Tamarack Lane Tomahawk, TN 37308	333 Tamarack Lane Tomahawk, TN 37308	333 Tamarack Lane Tomahawk, TN 37308	

FAMILY DATA TABLE

MARTIN FAMILY	INSURED'S INFORMATION	SPOUSE'S INFORMATION	CHILD #1	CHILD #2	CHILD #3
Name	Mark Martin, Sr.	Maria Martin	Melissa Martin	Melody Martin	
Address	1238 Marvale Manor Rd. Many Meadows, ME 04168	1238 Marvale Manor Rd. Many Meadows, ME 04168	1238 Marvale Manor Rd. Many Meadows, ME 04168	1238 Marvale Manor Rd. Many Meadows, ME 04168	
Email Address	markm@martin.com				
TELEPHONE #					
Home: Work: Cell:	(410) 555-0416 (410) 555-0417 (410) 555-0418	(410) 555-0416	(410) 555-0416	(410) 555-0416	
Date of Birth	01/10/CCYY-56	06/23/CCYY-42	06/12/CCYY-17	06/12/CCYY-17	
Social Security #	999-99-9991	999-99-9903	999-99-9904	999-99-9905	
Marital Status/Gender	Married/Male	Married/Female	Single/Female	Single/Female	
Student Status			Full-time	Full-time	
Patient Account #	10035	10037	10036	10038	
Allergies/Medical Conditions	None	None	None	None	
PRIMARY INSURANCE CARRIER					
Name Address	Rover Insurers, Inc. 5931 Rolling Road Ronson, CO 81369	Rover Insurers, Inc. 5931 Rolling Road Ronson, CO 81369	Rover Insurers, Inc. 5931 Rolling Road Ronson, CO 81369	Rover Insurers, Inc. 5931 Rolling Road Ronson, CO 81369	
Effective Date	01/01/CCPY	01/01/CCPY	01/01/CCPY	01/01/CCPY	
Member's ID #	99-9991 NIN	99-9991 NIN	99-9991 NIN	99-9991 NIN	
Group Policy #	21088	21088	21088	21088	
Policy/Employer	Ninja Enterprises 1234 Nockout Road Newton, NM 88012				
OTHER INSURANCE CARRIER					
Name Address					
Effective Date					
Member's ID #					
Group Policy #					
Policy/Employer					
Responsible Party	Self	Self	Insured	Insured	
EMERGENCY CONTACT					
Name	Monica Martini	Monica Martini	Monica Martini	Monica Martini	
Telephone #	(410) 555-0419	(410) 555-0419	(410) 555-0419	(410) 555-0419	
Address	8321 Marvale Manor Rd. Many Meadows, ME 04168	8321 Marvale Manor Rd. Many Meadows, ME 04168	8321 Marvale Manor Rd. Many Meadows, ME 04168	8321 Marvale Manor Rd. Many Meadows, ME 04168	

Exercise 5-2

Directions: Complete a CMS-1500 for each of the Encounter Forms (**Documents 67–71, 73–77**) in this chapter. CMS-1500 forms may be provided by your instructor or purchased from a stationery store.

After completion of each CMS-1500 form, complete a Patient Receipt (if a payment was made), and post the transaction(s) to the patient Ledger Card/Statement of Account previously created.

Exercise 5-3

Directions: Upon completion of all of the activities in Exercise 5–2, complete a Bank Deposit Slip/Ticket (located in the **Forms** chapter) for all payments made on the patient's account in this chapter.

Exercise 5-4

Directions: Using an Insurance Claims Register (located in the **Forms** chapter) list all claims that have been fully prepared and are ready for submission to the insurance carrier for payment. Enter the date that you created the CMS-1500 in the **Date Claim Filed** column.

Exercise 5-5

Directions: Using the stationery or Request for Additional Information Form (located in the **Forms** chapter), write a letter or request information for the following scenario. In each case, you are the medical biller working for Any Billing Services. Addresses and personal information are contained in the patient files that were previously set up. Also, refer to the Family Data Table (**Document 65**) for required information.

1. Create a correspondence for Mark Martin, Sr. advising him to schedule appointments for his dependents Melissa Martin and Melody Martin for school or sports physical, as these appointments fill up early.

DOCUMENT 66

Multiple Surgery Claims Beginning Financials
THOMPSON FAMILY

Insurance Plan	Winter Insurance Company—ABC Corporation				
Patient:	**TONY**	**TERRY**	**TRACI**	**TINA**	
C/O DEDUCTIBLE					
DEDUCTIBLE	0.00	125.00	125.00	55.00	
COINSURANCE	0.00	0.00	122.46	0.00	
ACCIDENT BENEFIT					
LIFETIME MAXIMUM	51,200.00	15,555.00	2,021.77	4,658.92	
M/N OFFICE VISITS					
OFFICE VISITS	285.00	0.00	0.00	0.00	
HOSPITAL VISITS					
DXL					
SURGERY	625.00	0.00	0.00	0.00	
ASSISTANT SURGERY					
ANESTHESIA					

Encounter Form

DOCUMENT 67

Provider Information

Name:	Terrence Tew, M.D.
Address:	Tomahawk Memorial Hospital
City:	Tomahawk State: TN Zip Code: 37308
Telephone #:	Fax #:
Medicare ID#:	UPIN #: G21348
Tax ID #:	22-2222222 Accepts Medicare Assignment: ☒
Provider's Signature:	_Terrence Tew, MD_ Date: _7/9/CCYY_

Appointment Information

Appointment Date:		Time:	
Next Appt. Date:		Time:	
Date of First Visit:		Date of Injury:	
Referring Physician:	Tamara Teeson, M.D.		

Guarantor Information

Name:	Tony Thompson
Address:	222 Tamarack Lane
City: Tomahawk	State: TN Zip Code: 37308
Insurance ID #:	99-9999 XYZ
Insurance Name:	Ball Insurance Carriers
Insurance Group #:	62958
Employer Name:	XYZ Corporation

Patient Information

Name:	Tony Thompson
Address:	222 Tamarack Lane
City:	Tomahawk State: TN Zip Code: 37308
Telephone #:	(903) 555-3730 Account #: 10031
Date of Birth:	07/10/CCYY-55 Gender: Male
Marital Status:	Married Relationship to Guarantor: Self
Student Status:	☐ Full-time ☐ Part-time
Insurance Type:	☒ Pvt ☐ M/care ☐ M/caid ☐ WC ☐ Other _____
Hospitalization Date:	
Hospital Information:	Tomahawk Memorial Hospital, Tomahawk, TN 37308

Authorization

☒ Authorization to Release Information
☒ Authorization for Assignment of Benefits
☐ Authorization for Consent for Treatment
☐ My insurance will be billed but there may be a balance due.

Signature: _Tony Thompson_   Date: _7/9/CCYY_

Clinical Information

	DOS	POS	CPT® /HCPCS Description	ICD-9-CM (*Indicates diagnosis for all lines)	Amount
1	07/09/CCYY	Otpt Hosp	Excision, curettage of bone cyst, humerus	*Olecranon Bursitis	$1800.00
2	07/09/CCYY	Otpt Hosp	Excision, olecranon bursa	*	$ 500.00
3					
4					
5					
6					
Remarks:	Referring Physician: Tamara Teeson, M.D. UPIN #: H02315				

Previous Balance:		Payment:		Copay:		Adjustment:		
Total Fee:	$2300.00	Cash ☐ Check ☐ Credit ☐		Cash ☐ Check ☐ Credit ☐		Reason:	New Balance:	$2300.00

Encounter Form   DOCUMENT 68

Provider Information

Name:	Tamara Teeson, M.D.
Address:	Tomahawk Women's Clinic

City:	Tomahawk	State:	TN	Zip Code:	37308

Telephone #:		Fax #:	

Medicare ID#:		UPIN #:	H02315

Tax ID #:	22-2222238	Accepts Medicare Assignment:	☒

Provider's Signature:	*Tamara Teeson, MD*	Date: *7/21/CCYY*

Appointment Information

Appointment Date:		Time:	
Next Appt. Date:		Time:	
Date of First Visit:	04/28/CCYY	Date of Injury:	
Referring Physician:			

Guarantor Information

Name:	Tony Thompson
Address:	222 Tamarack Lane

City:	Tomahawk	State:	TN	Zip Code:	37308

Insurance ID #:	99-9999 XYZ
Insurance Name:	Ball Insurance Carriers
Insurance Group #:	62958
Employer Name:	XYZ Corporation

Patient Information

Name:	Terry Thompson
Address:	222 Tamarack Lane

City:	Tomahawk	State:	TN	Zip Code:	37308

Telephone #:	(903) 555-3730	Account #:	10032

Date of Birth:	08/21/CCYY-51	Gender:	Female

Marital Status:	Married	Relationship to Guarantor:	Spouse

Student Status:	☐ Full-time	☐ Part-time

Insurance Type:	☒ Pvt ☐ M/care ☐ M/caid ☐ WC ☐ Other _____

Hospitalization Date:	From: 07/21/CCYY To: 07/22/CCYY

Hospital Information:	Tomahawk Women's Hospital, P.O. Box 444, Tomahawk, TN 37308

Authorization

☒ Authorization to Release Information
☒ Authorization for Assignment of Benefits
☐ Authorization for Consent for Treatment
☐ My insurance will be billed but there may be a balance due.

Signature: *Terry Thompson*   Date: *7/21/CCYY*

Clinical Information

	DOS	POS	CPT® /HCPCS Description	ICD-9-CM (*Indicates diagnosis for all lines)	Amount
1	07/21/CCYY	Inpt Hosp	Laparoscopy; visual pelvis viscera; lysis of adhesions	*Excessive menstruation; *1 Pelvic Pain	$ 800.00
2	07/21/CCYY	Inpt Hosp	Dilation and curettage	*, *1	$ 150.00
3					
4					
5					
6					
Remarks:					

Previous Balance:		Payment:		Copay:		Adjustment:			
Total Fee:	$950.00	Cash ☐ Check ☐ Credit ☐		Cash ☐ Check ☐ Credit ☐		Reason:		New Balance:	$950.00

Encounter Form   DOCUMENT 69

Provider Information

Name:	Tory T. Tamer, M.D.
Address:	Tomahawk Surgi-Center

City:	Tomahawk	State:	TN	Zip Code:	37308

Telephone #:		Fax #:	

Medicare ID#:		UPIN #:	L22345

Tax ID #:	22-2222212	Accepts Medicare Assignment:	☒

Provider's Signature:	*Tory T. Tamer, MD*	Date: *6/11/CCYY*

Appointment Information

Appointment Date:		Time:	
Next Appt. Date:		Time:	
Date of First Visit:	04/24/CCYY	Date of Injury:	
Referring Physician:	Terrence Tew, M.D.		

Guarantor Information

Name:	Tony Thompson
Address:	222 Tamarack Lane

City:	Tomahawk	State:	TN	Zip Code:	37308

Insurance ID #:	99-9999 XYZ
Insurance Name:	Ball Insurance Carriers
Insurance Group #:	62958
Employer Name:	XYZ Corporation

Patient Information

Name:	Traci Thompson
Address:	222 Tamarack Lane

City:	Tomahawk	State:	TN	Zip Code:	37308

Telephone #:	(903) 555-3730	Account #:	10033

Date of Birth:	03/11/CCYY-17	Gender:	Female

Marital Status:	Single	Relationship to Guarantor:	Child

Student Status:	☒ Full-time	☐ Part-time

Insurance Type:	☒ Pvt ☐ M/care ☐ M/caid ☐ WC ☐ Other _____

Hospitalization Date:	

Hospital Information:	Tomahawk Surgi Center, Tomahawk, TN 33708

Authorization

☒ Authorization to Release Information
☒ Authorization for Assignment of Benefits
☐ Authorization for Consent for Treatment
☐ My insurance will be billed but there may be a balance due.

Signature: *Tony Thompson*   Date: *6/11/CCYY*

Clinical Information

	DOS	POS	CPT® /HCPCS Description	ICD-9-CM (*Indicates diagnosis for all lines)	Amount
1	05/11/CCYY	ASC	Rhinoplasty, primary; lateral cartilages, nasal tip, prior	Prior Fracture of Nasal Bones and Septum	$3125.00
2	06/11/CCYY	ASC	Ethmoidectomy; intranasal, anterior	Hemorrhagic Sinusitis	$ 500.00
3	06/11/CCYY	ASC	Submucous resection turbinate, partial	Hypertrophy of Nasal Turbinates	$ 350.00
4					
5					
6					
Remarks:	Referring Physician: Terrence Tew, M.D. UPIN #: G21348				

Previous Balance:		Payment:		Copay:		Adjustment:			
Total Fee:	$3975.00	Cash ☐ Check ☐ Credit ☐		Cash ☐ Check ☐ Credit ☐		Reason:		New Balance:	$3975.00

Encounter Form

Provider Information

Name:	Thomas Tom, D.P.M.
Address:	Tomahawk Surgi-Center

City:	Tomahawk	State:	TN	Zip Code:	37308

Telephone #:	Fax #:	
Medicare ID#:	UPIN #:	T12234
Tax ID #:	22-2222256	Accepts Medicare Assignment: ☒
Provider's Signature:	_Thomas Tom, DPM_	Date: _8/22/CCYY_

Patient Information

Name:	Tony Thompson
Address:	222 Tamarack Lane

City:	Tomahawk	State:	TN	Zip Code:	37308
Telephone #:	(903) 555-3730	Account #:	10031		
Date of Birth:	07/10/CCYY-55	Gender:	Male		
Marital Status:	Married	Relationship to Guarantor:		Self	

Student Status: ☐ Full-time   ☐ Part-time
Insurance Type: ☒ Pvt ☐ M/care ☐ M/caid ☐ WC ☐ Other _____

Hospitalization Date:	
Hospital Information:	Tomahawk Surgi Center, Tomahawk, TN 33708

Appointment Information

Appointment Date:		Time:	
Next Appt. Date:		Time:	
Date of First Visit:		Date of Injury:	
Referring Physician:			

Guarantor Information

Name:	Tony Thompson
Address:	222 Tamarack Lane

City:	Tomahawk	State:	TN	Zip Code:	37308
Insurance ID #:	99-9999 XYZ				
Insurance Name:	Ball Insurance Carriers				
Insurance Group #:	62958				
Employer Name:	XYZ Corporation				

Authorization

☒ Authorization to Release Information
☒ Authorization for Assignment of Benefits
☐ Authorization for Consent for Treatment
☐ My insurance will be billed but there may be a balance due.

Signature: _Tony Thompson_   Date: _8/22/CCYY_

Clinical Information

	DOS	POS	CPT® /HCPCS Description	ICD-9-CM (*Indicates diagnosis for all lines)	Amount
1	08/22/CCYY	ASC	Excision of nail and nail matrix, complete, right	*, *1	$ 600.00
2	08/22/CCYY	ASC	Excision of nail and nail matrix, complete, left	*, *1	$ 600.00
3	08/22/CCYY	ASC	Arthrocentesis; small joint and bursa	*, *1	$ 90.00
4	08/22/CCYY	ASC	Supplies and materials	*Calcaneal Heel Spur; *1 Plantar Fascial	$ 50.00
5				Fibromatosis	
6					

Remarks:							
Previous Balance:	$2300.00	Payment:		Copay:		Adjustment:	
Total Fee:	$1340.00	Cash ☐ Check ☐ Credit ☐		Cash ☐ Check ☐ Credit ☐		Reason:	New Balance: $3640.00

Encounter Form

Provider Information

Name:	Tamara Teeson, M.D.
Address:	Tomahawk Women's Clinic

City:	Tomahawk	State:	TN	Zip Code:	37308

Telephone #:	Fax #:	
Medicare ID#:	UPIN #:	H02315
Tax ID #:	22-2222238	Accepts Medicare Assignment: ☒
Provider's Signature:	_Tamara Teeson, MD_	Date: _6/15/CCYY_

Patient Information

Name:	Tina Thompson
Address:	222 Tamarack Lane

City:	Tomahawk	State:	TN	Zip Code:	37308
Telephone #:	(903) 555-3730	Account #:	10034		
Date of Birth:	12/14/CCYY-18	Gender:	Female		
Marital Status:	Single	Relationship to Guarantor:		Child	

Student Status: ☒ Full-time   ☐ Part-time
Insurance Type: ☒ Pvt ☐ M/care ☐ M/caid ☐ WC ☐ Other _____

Hospitalization Date:	
Hospital Information:	Tomahawk Women's Clinic, Tomahawk, TN 37308

Appointment Information

Appointment Date:		Time:	
Next Appt. Date:		Time:	
Date of First Visit:		Date of Injury:	
Referring Physician:			

Guarantor Information

Name:	Tony Thompson
Address:	222 Tamarack Lane

City:	Tomahawk	State:	TN	Zip Code:	37308
Insurance ID #:	99-9999 XYZ				
Insurance Name:	Ball Insurance Carriers				
Insurance Group #:	62958				
Employer Name:	XYZ Corporation				

Authorization

☒ Authorization to Release Information
☒ Authorization for Assignment of Benefits
☐ Authorization for Consent for Treatment
☐ My insurance will be billed but there may be a balance due.

Signature: _Tony Thompson_   Date: _6/15/CCYY_

Clinical Information

	DOS	POS	CPT® /HCPCS Description	ICD-9-CM (*Indicates diagnosis for all lines)	Amount
1	06/15/CCYY	Otpt Hosp	Laparoscopy; lysis of adhesions	*2	$1200.00
2	06/15/CCYY	Otpt Hosp	Combined anterioposterior colporrhaphy	*, *1, *2	$ 600.00
3	06/15/CCYY	Otpt Hosp	Dilation and curettage, diagnostic	*Ovarian Mass; *1 Pelvic Adhesions; *2 Severe	$ 775.00
4				Rectro-Cystocele	
5					
6					

Remarks:							
Previous Balance:	$2575.00	Payment:		Copay:		Adjustment:	
Total Fee:	$2575.00	Cash ☐ Check ☐ Credit ☐		Cash ☐ Check ☐ Credit ☐		Reason:	New Balance: $2575.00

Multiple Surgery Claims Beginning Financials
MARTIN FAMILY

Insurance Plan	Rover Insurers Inc.—Ninja Enterprises				
Patient:	**MARK SR.**	**MARIA**	**MELISSA**	**MELODY**	
C/O DEDUCTIBLE					
DEDUCTIBLE	55.00	0.00	4.83	0.00	
COINSURANCE	0.00	97.49	0.00	0.00	
ACCIDENT BENEFIT					
LIFETIME MAXIMUM	45.00	1,427.49	2,781.50	0.00	
M/N OFFICE VISITS					
OFFICE VISITS					
HOSPITAL VISITS					
DXL					
SURGERY					
ASSISTANT SURGERY					
ANESTHESIA					

Encounter Form

Provider Information

		Appointment Information		
Name:	Michelle Mann, M.D.	Appointment Date:		Time:
Address:	Many Meadows Memorial Hospital	Next Appt. Date:		Time:
City:	Many Meadows State: ME Zip Code: 04168	Date of First Visit:		Date of Injury:
Telephone #:	Fax #:	Referring Physician:	Matthew Mayhew, M.D.	

Guarantor Information

Medicare ID#:	UPIN #: L22345	
Tax ID #:	44-9999996 Accepts Medicare Assignment: ☒	Name: Mark Martin, Sr.
Provider's Signature:	*Michelle Mann, MD* Date: 1/2/CCYY	Address: 1238 Marvale Manor Road

City: Many Meadows State: ME Zip Code: 04168

Patient Information

Name:	Mark Martin, Sr.
Address:	1238 Marvale Manor Road
City:	Many Meadows State: ME Zip Code: 04168
Telephone #:	(410) 555-0416 Account #: 10035
Date of Birth:	01/10/CCYY-56 Gender: Male
Marital Status:	Married Relationship to Guarantor: Self
Student Status:	☐ Full-time ☐ Part-time
Insurance Type:	☒ Pvt ☐ M/care ☐ M/caid ☐ WC ☐ Other
Hospitalization Date:	From: 01/01/CCYY To: 01/05/CCYY
Hospital Information:	Many Meadows Memorial Hospital, Many Meadows, ME 04168

Insurance ID #:	99-9991 NIN
Insurance Name:	Rover Insurers, Inc.
Insurance Group #:	21088
Employer Name:	Ninja Enterprises

Authorization

☒ Authorization to Release Information
☒ Authorization for Assignment of Benefits
☐ Authorization for Consent for Treatment
☐ My insurance will be billed but there may be a balance due.

Signature: *Mark Martin* Date: 1/2/CCYY

Clinical Information

	DOS	POS	CPT® /HCPCS Description	ICD-9-CM (*Indicates diagnosis for all lines)	Amount
1	01/01/CCYY	Inpt Hosp	Comprehensive exam, high complexity	*Angina Unstable; *1 Coronary Artery Disease	$ 300.00
2	01/01/CCYY	Inpt Hosp	Left heart cathe; retrograde from brachial percutaneous	*, *1	$2600.00
3	01/02/CCYY	Inpt Hosp	Sub hosp care, detail exam, high complexity	*, *1	$ 115.00
4					
5					
6					

Remarks:	Referring Physician: Matthew Mayhem, M.D. UPIN#: A11223			
Previous Balance:	Payment:	Copay:	Adjustment:	
Total Fee: $3015.00	Cash ☐ Check ☐ Credit ☐	Cash ☐ Check ☐ Credit ☐	Reason:	New Balance: $3015.00

Encounter Form   DOCUMENT 74

Provider Information						Appointment Information			
Name:	Minnie Malorn, M.D.					Appointment Date:		Time:	
Address:	Many Meadows Centers					Next Appt. Date:		Time:	
City:	Many Meadows	State:	ME	Zip Code:	04160	Date of First Visit:		Date of Injury:	
Telephone #:		Fax #:				Referring Physician:	Marlene Matsen, M.D.		
Medicare ID#:		UPIN #:	M14410			**Guarantor Information**			
Tax ID #:	44-9999980	Accepts Medicare Assignment:		⊠		Name:	Mark Martin, Sr.		
Provider's Signature:	*Minnie Malorn, MD*		Date: *10/27/CCYY*			Address:	1238 Marvale Manor Road		

Patient Information						City:	Many Meadows	State:	ME	Zip Code:	04168
Name:	Melissa Martin					Insurance ID #:	99-9991 NIN				
Address:	1238 Marvale Manor Road					Insurance Name:	Rover Insurers, Inc.				
City:	Many Meadows	State:	ME	Zip Code:	04168	Insurance Group #:	21088				
Telephone #:	(410) 555-0416	Account #:	10036			Employer Name:	Ninja Enterprises				
Date of Birth:	06/12/CCYY-17	Gender:	Female			**Authorization**					

Marital Status: Single   Relationship to Guarantor: Child
Student Status: ⊠ Full-time   ☐ Part-time
Insurance Type: ⊠ Pvt ☐ M/care ☐ M/caid ☐ WC ☐ Other
Hospitalization Date: From: 10/25/CCYY   To: 10/28/CCYY
Hospital Information: Many Meadows Centers, Many Meadows, ME 04160

⊠ Authorization to Release Information
⊠ Authorization for Assignment of Benefits
☐ Authorization for Consent for Treatment
☐ My insurance will be billed but there may be a balance due.
Signature: *Mark Martin*   Date: *10/27/CCYY*

Clinical Information

	DOS	POS	CPT® /HCPCS Description	ICD-9-CM (*Indicates diagnosis for all lines)	Amount
1	10/25/CCYY	Inpt Hosp	Int consult, comp hist & exam high complexity	*Anemia,;*1 Peptic Ulcer Disease,	$250.00
2	10/25/CCYY	Inpt Hosp	Colonoscopy, proximal-splenic flexure, diag, brushing	*1	$777.00
3	10/25/CCYY	Inpt Hosp	Upper gastrointestinal endoscopy, simple prim exam	Gastroenteritis	$500.00
4	10/26/CCYY	Inpt Hosp	Sub hosp care, prob foc exam, straightforward	*, *1	$ 80.00
5	10/27/CCYY	Inpt Hosp	Sub hosp care, prob foc exam, straightforward	*, *1	$ 80.00
6					

Remarks:	Referring Physician: Marlene Matsen, M.D. UPIN #: B22334				
Previous Balance:		Payment:	Copay:	Adjustment:	
Total Fee:	$1687.00	Cash ☐ Check ☐ Credit ☐	Cash ☐ Check ☐ Credit ☐	Reason:	New Balance: $1687.00

Encounter Form   DOCUMENT 75

Provider Information						Appointment Information			
Name:	Michael Mitchell, M.D.					Appointment Date:		Time:	
Address:	Many Meadows Memorial Hospital					Next Appt. Date:		Time:	
City:	Many Meadows	State:	ME	Zip Code:	04160	Date of First Visit:		Date of Injury:	
Telephone #:		Fax #:				Referring Physician:			
Medicare ID#:		UPIN #:	A65459			**Guarantor Information**			
Tax ID #:	44-9999999	Accepts Medicare Assignment:		⊠		Name:	Mark Martin, Sr.		
Provider's Signature:	*Michelle Mitchell, MD*		Date: *4/2/CCYY*			Address:	1238 Marvale Manor Road		

Patient Information						City:	Many Meadows	State:	ME	Zip Code:	04168
Name:	Maria Martin					Insurance ID #:	99-9991 NIN				
Address:	1238 Marvale Manor Road					Insurance Name:	Rover Insurers, Inc.				
City:	Many Meadows	State:	ME	Zip Code:	04168	Insurance Group #:	21088				
Telephone #:	(410) 555-0416	Account #:	10037			Employer Name:	Ninja Enterprises				
Date of Birth:	06/23/CCYY-42	Gender:	Female			**Authorization**					

Marital Status: Married   Relationship to Guarantor: Spouse
Student Status: ☐ Full-time   ☐ Part-time
Insurance Type: ⊠ Pvt ☐ M/care ☐ M/caid ☐ WC ☐ Other
Hospitalization Date: From: 04/02/CCYY   To: 04/04/CCYY
Hospital Information: Many Meadows Memorial Hospital, Many Meadows, ME 04160

⊠ Authorization to Release Information
⊠ Authorization for Assignment of Benefits
☐ Authorization for Consent for Treatment
☐ My insurance will be billed but there may be a balance due.
Signature: *Maria Martin*   Date: *4/2/CCYY*

Clinical Information

	DOS	POS	CPT® /HCPCS Description	ICD-9-CM (*Indicates diagnosis for all lines)	Amount
1	04/02/CCYY	Inpt Hosp	Routine ob care,c-section, including ante & post care	*Previous Cesarean Section; *1 Multiparity	$3590.00
2	04/02CCYY	Inpt Hosp	Ligation or transaction of fallopian tube, cesarean	*, *1	$1000.00
3					
4					
5					
6					

Remarks:					
Previous Balance:		Payment:	Copay:	Adjustment:	
Total Fee:	$4590.00	Cash ☐ Check ☐ Credit ☐	Cash ☐ Check ☐ Credit ☐	Reason:	New Balance: $4590.00

Encounter Form

Provider Information

Name:	Moira Minton, D.P.M.
Address:	5678 Montana Road
City:	Many Meadows State: ME Zip Code: 04168
Telephone #:	Fax #:
Medicare ID#:	UPIN #: T44561
Tax ID #:	44-9999977 Accepts Medicare Assignment: ☒
Provider's Signature:	_Moira Minton, DPM_ Date: _10/26/CCYY_

Appointment Information

Appointment Date:		Time:	
Next Appt. Date:		Time:	
Date of First Visit:		Date of Injury:	
Referring Physician:			

Guarantor Information

Name:	Mark Martin, Sr.
Address:	1238 Marvale Manor Road
City:	Many Meadows State: ME Zip Code: 04168
Insurance ID #:	99-9991 NIN
Insurance Name:	Rover Insurers, Inc.
Insurance Group #:	21088
Employer Name:	Ninja Enterprises

Patient Information

Name:	Melody Martin
Address:	1238 Marvale Manor Road
City:	Many Meadows State: ME Zip Code: 04168
Telephone #:	(410) 555-0416 Account #: 10038
Date of Birth:	06/12/CCYY-17 Gender: Female
Marital Status:	Single Relationship to Guarantor: Child
Student Status:	☒ Full-time ☐ Part-time
Insurance Type:	☒ Pvt ☐ M/care ☐ M/caid ☐ WC ☐ Other _____
Hospitalization Date:	
Hospital Information:	

Authorization

☒ Authorization to Release Information
☒ Authorization for Assignment of Benefits
☐ Authorization for Consent for Treatment
☐ My insurance will be billed but there may be a balance due.

Signature: _Mark Martin_   Date: _10/26/CCYY_

Clinical Information

	DOS	POS	CPT® /HCPCS Description	ICD-9-CM (*Indicates diagnosis for all lines)	Amount
1	10/25/CCYY	Office	New pt, detailed hist & exam, low complexity	*Onychomycosis; *1 Atrophoderma	$ 75.00
2	10/25/CCYY	Office	Biopsy of skin; single lesion	*, *1	$ 45.00
3	10/25/CCYY	Office	Additional lesion	*, *1	$ 50.00
4	10/26/CCYY	Office	Excision of nail and nail matrix; left hallux	*, *1	$350.00
5	10/26/CCYY	Office	Excision of nail and nail matrix; right hallux	*, *1	$350.00
6	10/26/CCYY	Office	Supplies and materials	*, *1	$450.00

Remarks:

Previous Balance:		Payment:		Copay:		Adjustment:			
Total Fee:	$1320.00	Cash ☐ Check ☐ Credit ☐		Cash ☐ Check ☐ Credit ☐		Reason:		New Balance:	$1320.00

Encounter Form

Provider Information

Name:	Marsha Matsen, M.D.
Address:	Many Meadows Medical Center
City:	Many Meadows State: ME Zip Code: 04160
Telephone #:	Fax #:
Medicare ID#:	UPIN #: C11513
Tax ID #:	44-8888877 Accepts Medicare Assignment: ☒
Provider's Signature:	_Marsha Matsen, MD_ Date: _6/19/CCYY_

Appointment Information

Appointment Date:		Time:	
Next Appt. Date:		Time:	
Date of First Visit:		Date of Injury:	
Referring Physician:			

Guarantor Information

Name:	Mark Martin, Sr.
Address:	1238 Marvale Manor Road
City:	Many Meadows State: ME Zip Code: 04168
Insurance ID #:	99-9991 NIN
Insurance Name:	Rover Insurers, Inc.
Insurance Group #:	21088
Employer Name:	Ninja Enterprises

Patient Information

Name:	Maria Martin
Address:	1238 Marvale Manor Road
City:	Many Meadows State: ME Zip Code: 04168
Telephone #:	(410) 555-0416 Account #: 10037
Date of Birth:	06/23/CCYY-42 Gender: Female
Marital Status:	Married Relationship to Guarantor: Spouse
Student Status:	☐ Full-time ☐ Part-time
Insurance Type:	☒ Pvt ☐ M/care ☐ M/caid ☐ WC ☐ Other _____
Hospitalization Date:	From: 06/19/CCYY To: 06/22/CCYY
Hospital Information:	Many Meadows Medical Center, Many Meadows, ME 04160

Authorization

☒ Authorization to Release Information
☒ Authorization for Assignment of Benefits
☐ Authorization for Consent for Treatment
☐ My insurance will be billed but there may be a balance due.

Signature: _Maria Martin_   Date: _6/19/CCYY_

Clinical Information

	DOS	POS	CPT® /HCPCS Description	ICD-9-CM (*Indicates diagnosis for all lines)	Amount
1	06/19/CCYY	Intpt Hosp	Trachelectomy, amputation of cervix	*, *1, *2	$1300.00
2	06/19/CCYY	Inpt Hosp	Excision, benign lesion, genitalia, 1.0 cm	*Abnormal Uterine Bleeding; *1 Enlarged	$ 200.00
3				Fibroid Uterus; *2 Benign Neoplasm of Vulva	
4					
5					
6					

Remarks:

Previous Balance:	$4590.00	Payment:		Copay:		Adjustment:			
Total Fee:	$1500.00	Cash ☐ Check ☐ Credit ☐		Cash ☐ Check ☐ Credit ☐		Reason:		New Balance:	$6090.00

Health Claims Examining Exercises

(**Instructor's Note:** Medical Billing exercises in the entire text should be completed prior to students starting Health Claims Examining Exercise 5–A. New files should be set up for the Health Claims Examining exercises.)

Exercise **5-A**

Directions: Complete an Insurance Coverage Form (located in the **Forms** chapter) and set up Family Files for all families in this chapter. Refer to the Family Data Tables **(Documents 64–65)** located in the beginning of this chapter, and the Contracts located in the **Contracts, UCR Conversion Factor Report, and Relative Value Study** chapter.

Exercise **5-B**

Directions: Complete a Payment Worksheet (located in the **Forms** chapter) for CMS-1500 claims **(Documents 67–71, 73–77)** using the guidelines contained in the **Introduction** chapter and using the UCR Conversion Factor Report, Relative Value Study, and Contracts located in the **Contracts, UCR Conversion Factor Report, and Relative Value Study** chapter.

When processing claims, the Beginning Financials **(Documents 66 and 72)** should be incorporated as payment history and claim calculations should be adjusted accordingly. Any carryover deductible listed should be included in the current year deductible for that individual. Therefore, in figuring current year deductible, students should be instructed to subtract the carryover deductible from the current year's amount.

Upon completion of each claim complete or update the Family Benefits Tracking Sheet (located in the **Forms** chapter) by compiling all of the claims payment data for the family.

6

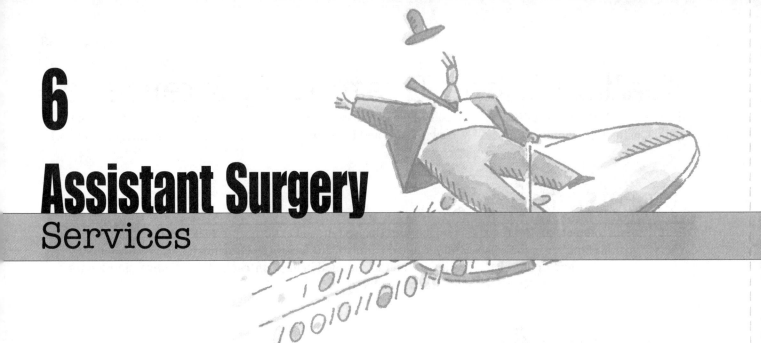

Assistant Surgery
Services

Medical Billing Exercises

Exercise 6-1

Directions: Complete Patient Information Sheets (leave **Assigned Provider** field blank), Ledger Cards, and Insurance Coverage Forms and set up patient charts for the following families using copies of the forms in the **Forms** chapter. Refer to the following Family Data Tables **(Documents 78–80)** for information.

    Individual folders with dividers may be used to store information for each family. One Patient Information Sheet and Insurance Coverage Form should be filled out for the entire family.

DOCUMENT 78

FAMILY DATA TABLE

DODSON FAMILY	INSURED'S INFORMATION	SPOUSE'S INFORMATION	CHILD #1	CHILD #2	CHILD #3
Name	Doris Dodson		Debbie Dodson	Daniel Dodson	Deedee Dodson
Address	6789 Duchesne Drive Durham, ND 58163		6789 Duchesne Drive Durham, ND 58163	6789 Duchesne Drive Durham, ND 58163	6789 Duchesne Drive Durham, ND 58163
Email Address	dorisd@dodson.com				
TELEPHONE #					
Home: Work: Cell:	(701) 555-5816 (701) 555-5817 (701) 555-5818		(701) 555-5816	(701) 555-5816	(701) 555-5816
Date of Birth	05/12/CCYY-47		08/15/CCYY-18	12/24/CCYY-17	12/24/CCYY-17
Social Security #	999-99-9992		999-99-9906	999-99-9907	999-99-9908
Marital Status/Gender	Single/Female		Single/Female	Single/Male	Single/Female
Student Status			Full-time	Full-time	Full-time
Patient Account #	10039		10040	10041	10052
Allergies/Medical Conditions	None		None	None	None
PRIMARY INSURANCE CARRIER					
Name Address	Winter Insurance Company 9763 Western Way Whittier, CO 82963		Winter Insurance Company 9763 Western Way Whittier, CO 82963	Winter Insurance Company 9763 Western Way Whittier, CO 82963	Winter Insurance Company 9763 Western Way Whittier, CO 82963
Effective Date	01/01/CCPY		01/01/CCPY	01/01/CCPY	01/01/CCPY
Member's ID #	99-9992 ABC		99-9992 ABC	99-9992 ABC	99-9992 ABC
Group Policy #	36928		36928	36928	36928
Policy/Employer	ABC Corporation 1234 Whitaker Lane Colter, CO 81222				
OTHER INSURANCE CARRIER					
Name Address					
Effective Date					
Member's ID #					
Group Policy #					
Policy/Employer					
Responsible Party	Self		Insured	Insured	Insured
EMERGENCY CONTACT					
Name Telephone # Address	David Dawson (710) 555-5816 9876 Duchesne Drive Durham, ND 58163		David Dawson (710) 555-5816 9876 Duchesne Drive Durham, ND 58163	David Dawson (701) 555-5816 9876 Duchesne Drive Durham, ND 58163	David Dawson (701) 555-5816 9876 Duchesne Drive Durham, ND 58163

FAMILY DATA TABLE

WESTIN FAMILY	Insured's Information	Spouse's Information	Child #1	Child #2	Child #3
Name	William Westin	Wilma Westin	Wendy Westin	Wally Westin	
Address	Route 1 Box 83 Walla Walla, WA 98977	Route 1 Box 83 Walla Walla, WA 98977	Route 1 Box 83 Walla Walla, WA 98977	Route 1 Box 83 Walla Walla, WA 98977	
Email Address	williamw@westin.com				
TELEPHONE #					
Home: Work: Cell:	(206) 555-9897 (206) 555-9898 (206) 555-9899	(206) 555-9897	(206) 555-9897	(206) 555-9897	
Date of Birth	04/03/CCYY-33	03/23/CCYY-31	06/28/CCYY-10	10/16/CCYY-11	
Social Security #	777-77-7777	777-77-7778	777-77-7779	777-77-7770	
Marital Status/Gender	Married/Male	Married/Female	Single/Female	Single/Male	
Student Status			Full-time	Full-time	
Patient Account #	10042	10043	10044	10053	
Allergies/Medical Conditions	None	None	None	None	
PRIMARY INSURANCE CARRIER					
Name Address	Ball Insurance Carriers 3895 Bubble Blvd. Ste. 283 Boxwood, CO 85926	Ball Insurance Carriers 3895 Bubble Blvd. Ste. 283 Boxwood, CO 85926	Ball Insurance Carriers 3895 Bubble Blvd. Ste. 283 Boxwood, CO 85926	Ball Insurance Carriers 3895 Bubble Blvd. Ste. 283 Boxwood, CO 85926	
Effective Date	01/01/CCPY	01/01/CCPY	01/01/CCPY	01/01/CCPY	
Member's ID #	77-7777 XYZ	77-7777 XYZ	77-7777 XYZ	77-7777 XYZ	
Group Policy #	62958	62958	62958	62958	
Policy/Employer	XYZ Corporation 9817 Bobcat Blvd. Bastion, CO 81319				
OTHER INSURANCE CARRIER					
Name Address					
Effective Date					
Member's ID #					
Group Policy #					
Policy/Employer					
Responsible Party	Self	Self	Insured	Insured	
EMERGENCY CONTACT					
Name Telephone # Address	Waldo Woods (206) 555-9890 Route 83 Box 1 Walla Walla, WA 98977	Waldo Woods (206) 555-9890 Route 83 Box 1 Walla Walla, WA 98977	Waldo Woods (206) 555-9890 Route 83 Box 1 Walla Walla, WA 98977	Waldo Woods (206) 555-9890 Route 83 Box 1 Walla Walla, WA 98977	

DOCUMENT 80

FAMILY DATA TABLE

SMITH FAMILY	INSURED'S INFORMATION	SPOUSE'S INFORMATION	CHILD #1	CHILD #2	CHILD #3
Name	**Sherry Smith**	**Sherman Smith**	**Sean Smith**		
Address	6767 Sampson Square Silent Shores, SC 29608	6767 Sampson Square Silent Shores, SC 29608	6767 Sampson Square Silent Shores, SC 29608		
Email Address	sherrys@smith.com				
TELEPHONE #					
Home: Work: Cell:	(864) 555-2960 (864) 555-2961 (864) 555-2962	(864) 555-2960	(864) 555-2960		
Date of Birth	12/08/CCYY-39	10/16/CCYY-39	02/03/CCYY-15		
Social Security #	888-99-7777	888-99-7778	888-99-7779		
Marital Status/Gender	Married/Female	Married/Male	Single/Male		
Student Status			Full-time		
Patient Account #	10046	10045	10047		
Allergies/Medical Conditions	None	None	None		
PRIMARY INSURANCE CARRIER					
Name Address	Rover Insurers, Inc. 5931 Rolling Road Ronson, CO 81369	Rover Insurers, Inc. 5931 Rolling Road Ronson, CO 81369	Rover Insurers, Inc. 5931 Rolling Road Ronson, CO 81369		
Effective Date	01/01/CCPY	01/01/CCPY	01/01/CCPY		
Member's ID #	99-7777 NIN	99-7777 NIN	99-7777 NIN		
Group Policy #	21088	21088	21088		
Policy/Employer	Ninja Enterprises 1234 Nockout Road Newton, NM 88012				
OTHER INSURANCE CARRIER					
Name Address					
Effective Date					
Member's ID #					
Group Policy #					
Policy/Employer					
Responsible Party	Self	Self	Insured		
EMERGENCY CONTACT					
Name Telephone # Address	Sandra Soriano (864) 555-2963 7676 Sampson Square Silent Shores, SC 29608	Sandra Soriano (864) 555-2963 7676 Sampson Square Silent Shores, SC 29608	Sandra Soriano (864) 555-2963 7676 Sampson Square Silent Shores, SC 29608		

Exercise 6-2

Directions: Complete a CMS-1500 for each of the Encounter Forms (**Documents 82–86, 88–92, and 94–98**) in this chapter. CMS-1500 forms may be provided by your instructor or purchased from a stationery store.

After completion of each CMS-1500 form, complete a Patient Receipt (if a payment was made), and post the transaction(s) to the patient Ledger Card/Statement of Account previously created.

Exercise 6-3

Directions: Upon completion of all of the activities in Exercise 6–2, complete a Bank Deposit Slip/Ticket (located in the **Forms** chapter) for all payments made on the patient's account in this chapter.

Exercise 6-4

Directions: Using an Insurance Claims Register (located in the **Forms** chapter) list all claims that have been fully prepared and are ready for submission to the insurance carrier for payment. Enter the date that you created the CMS-1500 in the **Date Claim Filed** column.

Exercise 6-5

Directions: Complete an Insurance Tracer Form (located in the **Forms** Chapter) for the following claim. For additional information refer to the Family Data Table (**Document 1**), completed claim form, or the Encounter Form.

Patient	Date Billed	Date of Service	Date of Illness	Diagnosis	Claim #
Evan Espinosa	08/31/CCYY	08/11/CCYY	08/11/CCYY	574.10	Document 9

Assistant Surgery Claims Beginning Financials
DODSON FAMILY

Insurance Plan	Winter Insurance Company—ABC Corporation				
Patient:	**DORIS**	**DEBBIE**	**DANIEL**	**DEEDEE**	
C/O DEDUCTIBLE	0.00	0.00	0.00	0.00	
DEDUCTIBLE	15.00	55.00	0.00	0.00	
COINSURANCE	0.00	0.00	0.00	0.00	
ACCIDENT BENEFIT					
LIFETIME MAXIMUM	54,000.00	5,674.45	4,444.77	332.56	
M/N OFFICE VISITS					
OFFICE VISITS					
HOSPITAL VISITS					
DXL					
SURGERY					
ASSISTANT SURGERY					
ANESTHESIA					

Encounter Form

Provider Information

Name:	David Dorton, M.D.				
Address:	1111 Durry Drive				
City:	Durham	State:	ND	Zip Code:	58163
Telephone #:		Fax #:			
Medicare ID#:		UPIN #:	D66666		
Tax ID #:	55-6666666	Accepts Medicare Assignment:	☒		
Provider's Signature:	David Dorton, MD		Date: 2/16/CCYY		

Patient Information

Name:	Doris Dodson				
Address:	6789 Duchesne Drive				
City:	Durham	State:	ND	Zip Code:	58163
Telephone #:	(701) 555-5816	Account #:	10039		
Date of Birth:	05/12/CCYY-47	Gender:	Female		
Marital Status:	Single	Relationship to Guarantor:	Self		
Student Status:	☐ Full-time	☐ Part-time			
Insurance Type:	☒ Pvt ☐ M/care ☐ M/caid ☐ WC ☐ Other				
Hospitalization Date:	From: 02/15/CCYY	To: 02/18/CCYY			
Hospital Information:	Durham Medical Center, P.O. Box 001, Durham, ND 58163				

Appointment Information

Appointment Date:		Time:	
Next Appt. Date:		Time:	
Date of First Visit:		Date of Injury:	
Referring Physician:	Butch M. N. Hackim, M.D.		

Guarantor Information

Name:	Doris Dodson			
Address:	6789 Duchesne Drive			
City:	Durham	State:	ND	Zip Code: 58163
Insurance ID #:	99-9992 ABC			
Insurance Name:	Winter Insurance Company			
Insurance Group #:	36928			
Employer Name:	ABC Corporation			

Authorization

☒ Authorization to Release Information
☒ Authorization for Assignment of Benefits
☐ Authorization for Consent for Treatment
☐ My insurance will be billed but there may be a balance due.

Signature: Doris Dodson   Date: 2/16/CCYY

Clinical Information

	DOS	POS	CPT® /HCPCS Description	ICD-9-CM (*Indicates diagnosis for all lines)	Amount
1	02/16/CCYY	Inpt Hosp	Cystoplasty, operation on bladder, w/ resection	Hydronephrosis; Calculus of kidney	$500.00
2					
3					
4					
5					
6					
Remarks:	David Dorton, M.D. was the Assistant Surgeon for Butch M. N. Hackim, M.D. UPIN #: M42781				
Previous Balance:		Payment:		Copay:		Adjustment:	
Total Fee:	$500.00	Cash ☐ Check ☐ Credit ☐	Cash ☐ Check ☐ Credit ☐	Remarks:	New Balance: $500.00

Encounter Form

Provider Information

Name:	Doreen Davis, M.D.
Address:	2222 Durry Drive
City:	Durham	State: ND	Zip Code: 58163
Telephone #:		Fax #:
Medicare ID#:		UPIN #: E46480
Tax ID #:	55-6666655	Accepts Medicare Assignment: ☒
Provider's Signature:	Doreen Davis, MD	Date: 2/15/CCYY

Patient Information

Name:	Debbie Dodson
Address:	6789 Duchesne Drive
City:	Durham	State: ND	Zip Code: 58163
Telephone #:	(701) 555-5816	Account #: 10040
Date of Birth:	08/15/CCYY-18	Gender: Female
Marital Status:	Single	Relationship to Guarantor: Child
Student Status:	☒ Full-time	☐ Part-time
Insurance Type:	☒ Pvt ☐ M/care ☐ M/caid ☐ WC ☐ Other _____
Hospitalization Date:	
Hospital Information:	Durham Medical Center, P.O. Box 001, Durham, ND 58163

Appointment Information

Appointment Date:		Time:	
Next Appt. Date:		Time:	
Date of First Visit:		Date of Injury:	
Referring Physician:	Butch M. N. Hackim, M.D.		

Guarantor Information

Name:	Doris Dodson
Address:	6789 Duchesne Drive
City: Durham	State: ND	Zip Code: 58163
Insurance ID #:	99-9992 ABC
Insurance Name:	Winter Insurance Company
Insurance Group #:	36928
Employer Name:	ABC Corporation

Authorization

☒ Authorization to Release Information
☒ Authorization for Assignment of Benefits
☐ Authorization for Consent for Treatment
☐ My insurance will be billed but there may be a balance due.
Signature: Doris Dodson   Date: 2/15/CCYY

Clinical Information

	DOS	POS	CPT® /HCPCS Description	ICD-9-CM (*Indicates diagnosis for all lines)	Amount
1	02/15/CCYY	Otpt Hosp	Missed abortion, second trimester	Missed abortion	$750.00
2					
3					
4					
5					
6					
Remarks:	Doreen Davis, M.D. was the Assistant Surgeon for Butch M. N. Hackim, M.D. UPIN #: M42781				
Previous Balance:		Payment:		Copay:	Adjustment:	
Total Fee:	$750.00	Cash ☐ Check ☐ Credit ☐	Cash ☐ Check ☐ Credit ☐	Remarks:	New Balance: $750.00

Encounter Form

Provider Information

Name:	Donald Dapeter, M.D.
Address:	4444 Dugoak Drive
City:	Durham	State: ND	Zip Code: 58163
Telephone #:		Fax #:
Medicare ID#:		UPIN #: F44456
Tax ID #:	55-6666677	Accepts Medicare Assignment: ☒
Provider's Signature:	Donald Dapeter, MD	Date: 8/15/CCYY

Patient Information

Name:	Daniel Dodson
Address:	6789 Duchesne Drive
City:	Durham	State: ND	Zip Code: 58163
Telephone #:	(701) 555-5816	Account #: 10041
Date of Birth:	12/24/CCYY-17	Gender: Male
Marital Status:	Single	Relationship to Guarantor: Child
Student Status:	☒ Full-time	☐ Part-time
Insurance Type:	☒ Pvt ☐ M/care ☐ M/caid ☐ WC ☐ Other _____
Hospitalization Date:	From: 8/15/CCYY To: 8/20/CCYY
Hospital Information:	Durham Medical Center, P.O. Box 001, Durham, ND 58163

Appointment Information

Appointment Date:		Time:	
Next Appt. Date:		Time:	
Date of First Visit:		Date of Injury:	
Referring Physician:	Butch M. N. Hackim, M.D.		

Guarantor Information

Name:	Doris Dodson
Address:	6789 Duchesne Drive
City: Durham	State: ND	Zip Code: 58163
Insurance ID #:	99-9992 ABC
Insurance Name:	Winter Insurance Company
Insurance Group #:	36928
Employer Name:	ABC Corporation

Authorization

☒ Authorization to Release Information
☒ Authorization for Assignment of Benefits
☐ Authorization for Consent for Treatment
☐ My insurance will be billed but there may be a balance due.
Signature: Doris Dodson   Date: 8/15/CCYY

Clinical Information

	DOS	POS	CPT® /HCPCS Description	ICD-9-CM (*Indicates diagnosis for all lines)	Amount
1	08/15/CCYY	Inpt Hosp	Surgery of simple intracranial aneurysm,intracra aprch	Intracranial hemorrhage;	$1000.00
2				Subarachnoid hemorrhage	
3					
4					
5					
6					
Remarks:	Donald Dapeter, M.D. was the Assistant Surgeon for Butch M. N. Hackim, M.D. UPIN #: M42781				
Previous Balance:		Payment:		Copay:	Adjustment:	
Total Fee:	$1000.00	Cash ☐ Check ☐ Credit ☐	Cash ☐ Check ☐ Credit ☐	Remarks:	New Balance: $1000.00

Encounter Form

Provider Information

Name:	Douglas Donns, M.D.
Address:	4444 Durry Drive
City:	Shapney State: ND Zip Code: 57762
Telephone #:	Fax #:
Medicare ID#:	UPIN #: G42215
Tax ID #:	55-6666000 Accepts Medicare Assignment: ☒
Provider's Signature:	*Douglas Donns, MD* Date: 1/18/CCYY

Appointment Information

Appointment Date:	Time:
Next Appt. Date:	Time:
Date of First Visit:	Date of Injury:
Referring Physician:	Butch M. N. Hackim, M.D.

Guarantor Information

Name:	Doris Dodson
Address:	6789 Duchesne Drive
City:	Durham State: ND Zip Code: 58163
Insurance ID #:	99-9992 ABC
Insurance Name:	Winter Insurance Company
Insurance Group #:	36928
Employer Name:	ABC Corporation

Patient Information

Name:	Deedee Dodson
Address:	6789 Duchesne Drive
City:	Durham State: ND Zip Code: 58163
Telephone #:	(701) 555-5816 Account #: 10052
Date of Birth:	12/24/CCYY-17 Gender: Female
Marital Status:	Single Relationship to Guarantor: Child
Student Status:	☒ Full-time ☐ Part-time
Insurance Type:	☒ Pvt ☐ M/care ☐ M/caid ☐ WC ☐ Other
Hospitalization Date:	From: 01/17/CCYY To: 01/22/CCYY
Hospital Information:	Shapney Medical Center, P.O. Box 100, Shapney, ND 57762

Authorization

☒ Authorization to Release Information
☒ Authorization for Assignment of Benefits
☐ Authorization for Consent for Treatment
☐ My insurance will be billed but there may be a balance due.
Signature: *Doris Dodson* Date: 1/18/CCYY

Clinical Information

	DOS	POS	CPT® /HCPCS Description	ICD-9-CM (*Indicates diagnosis for all lines)	Amount
1	01/18/CCYY	Inpt Hosp	Repair initial ventral hernia; reducible	Ventral Hernia	$575.00
2					
3					
4					
5					
6					
Remarks:	Douglas Donns, M.D. was the Assistant Surgeon for Butch M. N. Hackim, M.D. UPIN #: M42781				
Previous Balance:		Payment:		Copay:	Adjustment:
Total Fee:	$575.00	Cash ☐ Check ☐ Credit ☐		Cash ☐ Check ☐ Credit ☐	Remarks:	New Balance: $575.00

Encounter Form

Provider Information

Name:	Doug Duncan, M.D.
Address:	7384 Dogwood Drive
City:	Durham State: ND Zip Code: 58163
Telephone #:	Fax #:
Medicare ID#:	UPIN #: H46485
Tax ID #:	55-6666333 Accepts Medicare Assignment: ☒
Provider's Signature:	*Doug Duncan, MD* Date: 12/16/CCYY

Appointment Information

Appointment Date:	Time:
Next Appt. Date:	Time:
Date of First Visit:	08/14/CCYY Date of Injury:
Referring Physician:	Butch M. N. Hackim, M.D.

Guarantor Information

Name:	Doris Dodson
Address:	6789 Duchesne Drive
City:	Durham State: ND Zip Code: 58163
Insurance ID #:	99-9992 ABC
Insurance Name:	Winter Insurance Company
Insurance Group #:	36928
Employer Name:	ABC Corporation

Patient Information

Name:	Daniel Dodson
Address:	6789 Duchesne Drive
City:	Durham State: ND Zip Code: 58163
Telephone #:	(701) 555-5816 Account #: 10041
Date of Birth:	12/24/CCYY-17 Gender: Male
Marital Status:	Single Relationship to Guarantor: Child
Student Status:	☒ Full-time ☐ Part-time
Insurance Type:	☒ Pvt ☐ M/care ☐ M/caid ☐ WC ☐ Other
Hospitalization Date:	
Hospital Information:	Durham Medical Center, P.O. Box 001, Durham, ND 58163

Authorization

☒ Authorization to Release Information
☒ Authorization for Assignment of Benefits
☐ Authorization for Consent for Treatment
☐ My insurance will be billed but there may be a balance due.
Signature: *Doris Dodson* Date: 12/16/CCYY

Clinical Information

	DOS	POS	CPT® /HCPCS Description	ICD-9-CM (*Indicates diagnosis for all lines)	Amount
1	12/16/CCYY	Otpt Hosp	Tympanoplasty w/out mastoidectomy & ossicular	Chronic Suppurative Otitis Media;	$600.00
2				Perforation of Ear Drum	
3					
4					
5					
6					
Remarks:	Doug Duncan, M.D. was the Assistant Surgeon for Butch M. N. Hackim, M.D. UPIN #: M42781				
Previous Balance:	$1000.00	Payment:		Copay:	Adjustment:
Total Fee:	$600.00	Cash ☐ Check ☐ Credit ☐		Cash ☐ Check ☐ Credit ☐	Remarks:	New Balance: $1600.00

Assistant Surgery Claims Beginning Financials

WESTIN FAMILY

Insurance Plan	Ball Insurance Carriers—XYZ Corporation				
Patient:	**WILLIAM**	**WILMA**	**WENDY**		
C/O DEDUCTIBLE	0.00	0.00	0.00		
DEDUCTIBLE	65.00	25.00	49.93		
COINSURANCE	0.00	0.00	0.00		
ACCIDENT BENEFIT					
LIFETIME MAXIMUM	961.20	5,000.00	6,771.50		
M/N OFFICE VISITS					
OFFICE VISITS	40.00	16.00	40.00		
HOSPITAL VISITS					
DXL	0.00	0.00	0.00		
SURGERY	0.00	0.00	0.00		
ASSISTANT SURGERY	0.00	0.00	175.00		
ANESTHESIA					

Encounter Form

Provider Information

Name:	Walter Wind, M.D.
Address:	4242 West Winter
City:	Walla Walla State: WA Zip Code: 98977
Telephone #:	Fax #:
Medicare ID#:	UPIN #: M45777
Tax ID #:	77-3445689 Accepts Medicare Assignment: ☒
Provider's Signature:	*Walter Wind, MD* Date: *1/1/CCYY*

Appointment Information

Appointment Date:	Time:
Next Appt. Date:	Time:
Date of First Visit:	Date of Injury:
Referring Physician:	Butch M. N. Hackim, M.D.

Guarantor Information

Name:	William Westin
Address:	Route 1 Box 83
City: Walla Walla State: WA Zip Code: 98977
Insurance ID #:	77-7777 XYZ
Insurance Name:	Ball Insurance Carriers
Insurance Group #:	62958
Employer Name:	XYZ Corporation

Patient Information

Name:	William Westin
Address:	Route 1 Box 83
City:	Walla Walla State: WA Zip Code: 98977
Telephone #:	(206) 555-9897 Account #: 10042
Date of Birth:	04/03/CCYY-33 Gender: Male
Marital Status:	Married Relationship to Guarantor: Self
Student Status:	☐ Full-time ☐ Part-time
Insurance Type:	☒ Pvt ☐ M/care ☐ M/caid ☐ WC ☐ Other _____
Hospitalization Date:	From: 01/09/CCYY To: 01/12/CCYY
Hospital Information:	White Memorial Center, P.O. Box 600 Walla Walla, WA 98977

Authorization

☒ Authorization to Release Information
☒ Authorization for Assignment of Benefits
☐ Authorization for Consent for Treatment
☐ My insurance will be billed but there may be a balance due.

Signature: *William Westin*   Date: *1/1/CCYY*

Clinical Information

	DOS	POS	CPT® /HCPCS Description	ICD-9-CM (*Indicates diagnosis for all lines)	Amount
1	01/10/CCYY	Inpt Hosp	Repair lung hernia through chest wall	Hernia of Mediastinum	$2000.00
2					
3					
4					
5					
6					
Remarks:	Walter Wind, M.D. was the Assistant Surgeon for Butch M. N. Hackim, M.D. UPIN #: M42781				
Previous Balance:		Payment:		Copay:	Adjustment:
Total Fee:	$2000.00	Cash ☐ Check ☐ Credit ☐	Cash ☐ Check ☐ Credit ☐	Remarks:	New Balance: $2000.00

Encounter Form
DOCUMENT 89

Provider Information

Name:	Wanda Whister, M.D.
Address:	2600 Whitney Way
City:	Walla Walla State: WA Zip Code: 98977
Telephone #:	Fax #:
Medicare ID#:	UPIN #: J54688
Tax ID #:	77-3445690 Accepts Medicare Assignment: ☒
Provider's Signature:	*Wanda Whister, MD* Date: *1/16/CCYY*

Appointment Information

Appointment Date:	Time:
Next Appt. Date:	Time:
Date of First Visit:	Date of Injury:
Referring Physician:	Butch M. N. Hackim, M.D.

Guarantor Information

Name:	William Westin
Address:	Route 1 Box 83
City: Walla Walla	State: WA Zip Code: 98977
Insurance ID #:	77-7777 XYZ
Insurance Name:	Ball Insurance Carriers
Insurance Group #:	62958
Employer Name:	XYZ Corporation

Patient Information

Name:	Wilma Westin
Address:	Route 1 Box 83
City:	Walla Walla State: WA Zip Code: 98977
Telephone #:	(206) 555-9897 Account #: 10043
Date of Birth:	03/23/CCYY-31 Gender: Female
Marital Status:	Married Relationship to Guarantor: Spouse
Student Status:	☐ Full-time ☐ Part-time
Insurance Type:	☒ Pvt ☐ M/care ☐ M/caid ☐ WC ☐ Other _____
Hospitalization Date:	From: 01/16/CCYY To: 01/22/CCYY
Hospital Information:	White Memorial Center, P.O. Box 600, Walla Walla, WA 98977

Authorization

☒ Authorization to Release Information
☒ Authorization for Assignment of Benefits
☐ Authorization for Consent for Treatment
☐ My insurance will be billed but there may be a balance due.

Signature: *Wilma Westin*   Date: *1/16/CCYY*

Clinical Information

	DOS	POS	CPT® /HCPCS Description	ICD-9-CM (*Indicates diagnosis for all lines)	Amount
1	01/16/CCYY	Inpt Hosp	Revision of arteriovebous fistula with thrombectomy;	Chronic Renal Failure	$1000.00
2			autogenous graft		
3					
4					
5					
6					

Remarks:	Wanda Whister, M.D. was the Assistant Surgeon for Butch M. N. Hackim, M.D. UPIN #: M42781
Previous Balance:	Payment: Copay: Adjustment:
Total Fee: $1000.00	Cash ☐ Check ☐ Credit ☐ Cash ☐ Check ☐ Credit ☐ Remarks: New Balance: $1000.00

Encounter Form
DOCUMENT 90

Provider Information

Name:	Wanda Whister, M.D.
Address:	2600 Whitney Way
City:	Walla Walla State: WA Zip Code: 98977
Telephone #:	Fax #:
Medicare ID#:	UPIN #: J54688
Tax ID #:	77-3445690 Accepts Medicare Assignment: ☒
Provider's Signature:	*Wanda Whister, MD* Date: *3/15/CCYY*

Appointment Information

Appointment Date:	Time:
Next Appt. Date:	Time:
Date of First Visit:	Date of Injury:
Referring Physician:	Butch M. N. Hackim, M. D.

Guarantor Information

Name:	William Westin
Address:	Route 1 Box 83
City: Walla Walla	State: WA Zip Code: 98977
Insurance ID #:	77-7777 XYZ
Insurance Name:	Ball Insurance Carriers
Insurance Group #:	62958
Employer Name:	XYZ Corporation

Patient Information

Name:	Wilma Westin
Address:	Route 1 Box 83
City:	Walla Walla State: WA Zip Code: 98977
Telephone #:	(206) 555-9897 Account #: 10043
Date of Birth:	03/23/CCYY-31 Gender: Female
Marital Status:	Married Relationship to Guarantor: Spouse
Student Status:	☐ Full-time ☐ Part-time
Insurance Type:	☒ Pvt ☐ M/care ☐ M/caid ☐ WC ☐ Other _____
Hospitalization Date:	From: 03/14/CCYY To: 03/16/CCYY
Hospital Information:	White Memorial Center, P.O. Box 600, Walla Walla, WA 98977

Authorization

☒ Authorization to Release Information
☒ Authorization for Assignment of Benefits
☐ Authorization for Consent for Treatment
☐ My insurance will be billed but there may be a balance due.

Signature: *Wilma Westin*   Date: *3/15/CCYY*

Clinical Information

	DOS	POS	CPT® /HCPCS Description	ICD-9-CM (*Indicates diagnosis for all lines)	Amount
1	03/15/CCYY	Inpt Hosp	Laparoscopy; with lysis of adhesions	*Ovarian Mass; *1Pelvic Peritoneal Adhesions	$100.00
2	03/15/CCYY	Inpt Hosp	Saplingo-oophorectomy	*; *1	$600.00
3					
4					
5					
6					

Remarks:	Wanda Whister, M.D. was the Assistant Surgeon for Butch M. N. Hackim, M.D. UPIN #: M42781
Previous Balance: $1000.00	Payment: Copay: Adjustment:
Total Fee: $700.00	Cash ☐ Check ☐ Credit ☐ Cash ☐ Check ☐ Credit ☐ Remarks: New Balance: $1700.00

Encounter Form
DOCUMENT 91

Provider Information					Appointment Information		
Name:	Wade Wallace, M.D.				Appointment Date:		Time:
Address:	1000 Willow Way				Next Appt. Date:		Time:
City:	Walla Walla	State:	WA	Zip Code: 98977	Date of First Visit:		Date of Injury:
Telephone #:		Fax #:			Referring Physician:	Butch M. N. Hackim, M.D.	
Medicare ID#:		UPIN #:	L66851		**Guarantor Information**		
Tax ID #:	77-3445777	Accepts Medicare Assignment: ☒			Name:	William Westin	
Provider's Signature:	Wade Wallace, MD	Date: 1/25/CCYY			Address:	Route 1 Box 83	

Patient Information				
City:	Walla Walla	State: WA	Zip Code:	98977

Patient Information					
Name:	Wendy Westin			Insurance ID #:	77-7777 XYZ
Address:	Route 1 Box 83			Insurance Name:	Ball Insurance Carriers
City:	Walla Walla	State: WA	Zip Code: 98977	Insurance Group #:	62958
Telephone #:	(206) 555-9897	Account #:	10044	Employer Name:	XYZ Corporation
Date of Birth:	06/28/CCYY-10	Gender:	Female	**Authorization**	
Marital Status:	Single	Relationship to Guarantor:	Child	☒ Authorization to Release Information	
Student Status:	☒ Full-time	☐ Part-time		☒ Authorization for Assignment of Benefits	
Insurance Type:	☒ Pvt ☐ M/care ☐ M/caid ☐ WC ☐ Other ____			☐ Authorization for Consent for Treatment	
Hospitalization Date:				☐ My insurance will be billed but there may be a balance due.	
Hospital Information:	White Memorial Center, P.O. Box 600, Walla Walla, WA 98977			Signature: William Westin Date: 1/25/CCYY	

Clinical Information				
	DOS	POS	CPT® /HCPCS Description	ICD-9-CM (*Indicates diagnosis for all lines)	Amount
1	01/25/CCYY	Otpt Hosp	Excision, trochanteric pressure ulcer, w/ primary suture	Dermatosis	$800.00
2					
3					
4					
5					
6					
Remarks:	Wade Wallace, M.D. was the Assistant Surgeon for Butch M. N. Hackim, M.D. UPIN #: M42781				
Previous Balance:		Payment:		Copay:	Adjustment:	
Total Fee:	$800.00	Cash ☐ Check ☐ Credit ☐	Cash ☐ Check ☐ Credit ☐	Remarks:	New Balance: $800.00

Encounter Form
DOCUMENT 92

Provider Information					Appointment Information		
Name:	Wayne Winters, M.D.				Appointment Date:		Time:
Address:	4747 Willow Way				Next Appt. Date:		Time:
City:	Walla Walla	State:	WA	Zip Code: 98977	Date of First Visit:		Date of Injury:
Telephone #:		Fax #:			Referring Physician:	Butch M. N. Hackim, M.D.	
Medicare ID#:		UPIN #:	I88884		**Guarantor Information**		
Tax ID #:	77-3445555	Accepts Medicare Assignment: ☒			Name:	William Westin	
Provider's Signature:	Wayne Winters, MD	Date: 12/9/CCYY			Address:	Route 1 Box 83	

Patient Information				
City:	Walla Walla	State: WA	Zip Code:	98977

Patient Information					
Name:	William Westin			Insurance ID #:	77-7777 XYZ
Address:	Route 1 Box 83			Insurance Name:	Ball Insurance Carriers
City:	Walla Walla	State: WA	Zip Code: 98977	Insurance Group #:	62958
Telephone #:	(206) 555-9897	Account #:	10042	Employer Name:	XYZ Corporation
Date of Birth:	04/03/CCYY-33	Gender:	Male	**Authorization**	
Marital Status:	Married	Relationship to Guarantor:	Self	☒ Authorization to Release Information	
Student Status:	☐ Full-time	☐ Part-time		☒ Authorization for Assignment of Benefits	
Insurance Type:	☒ Pvt ☐ M/care ☐ M/caid ☐ WC ☐ Other ____			☐ Authorization for Consent for Treatment	
Hospitalization Date:				☐ My insurance will be billed but there may be a balance due.	
Hospital Information:	White Memorial Center, P.O. Box 600, Walla Walla, WA 98977			Signature: William Westin Date: 12/9/CCYY	

Clinical Information				
	DOS	POS	CPT® /HCPCS Description	ICD-9-CM (*Indicates diagnosis for all lines)	Amount
1	12/09/CCYY	Otpt Hosp	Excision of bone cyst; humerus	*Olecranon Bursitis; *1Lateral Epicondylitis	$500.00
2	12/09/CCYY	Otpt Hosp	Excision, olecranon bursa	*; *1	$150.00
3					
4					
5					
6					
Remarks:	Wayne Winters, M.D. was the Assistant Surgeon for Butch M. N. Hackim, M.D. UPIN #: M42781				
Previous Balance:	$2000.00	Payment:		Copay:	Adjustment:	
Total Fee:	$650.00	Cash ☐ Check ☐ Credit ☐	Cash ☐ Check ☐ Credit ☐	Remarks:	New Balance: $2650.00

Assistant Surgery Claims Beginning Financials
SMITH FAMILY

Insurance Plan	Rover Insurers, Inc.—Ninja Enterprises				
Patient:	**SHERRY**	**SHERMAN**	**SEAN**		
C/O DEDUCTIBLE	0.00	0.00	0.00		
DEDUCTIBLE	75.15	100.00	0.00		
COINSURANCE	0.00	0.00	0.00		
ACCIDENT BENEFIT	0.00	0.00	0.00		
LIFETIME MAXIMUM	140.00	600.33	0.00		
M/N OFFICE VISITS					
OFFICE VISITS					
HOSPITAL VISITS					
DXL					
SURGERY					
ASSISTANT SURGERY					
ANESTHESIA					
Family Coverage Effective 4/1/CCYY					

Encounter Form

Provider Information

Name:	Steve Sorby, M.D.
Address:	2444 Silver Lane
City:	Silent Shores State: SC Zip Code: 29608
Telephone #:	Fax #:
Medicare ID#:	UPIN #: A89666
Tax ID #:	11-7814784 Accepts Medicare Assignment: ☒
Provider's Signature:	*Steve Sorby, MD* Date: *10/12/CCYY*

Appointment Information

Appointment Date:	Time:
Next Appt. Date:	Time:
Date of First Visit:	Date of Injury:
Referring Physician:	Butch M. N. Hackim, M.D.

Patient Information

Name:	Sherman Smith
Address:	6767 Sampson Square
City:	Silent Shores State: SC Zip Code: 29608
Telephone #:	(864) 555-2960 Account #: 10045
Date of Birth:	10/16/CCYY-39 Gender: Male
Marital Status:	Married Relationship to Guarantor: Spouse
Student Status:	☐ Full-time ☐ Part-time
Insurance Type:	☒ Pvt ☐ M/care ☐ M/caid ☐ WC ☐ Other _____
Hospitalization Date:	From: 10/12/CCYY To: 10/14/CCYY
Hospital Information:	Silent Shores Medical Center, P.O. Box 600, Silent Shores, SC 29608

Guarantor Information

Name:	Sherry Smith
Address:	6767 Sampson Square
City:	Silent Shores State: SC Zip Code: 29608
Insurance ID #:	99-7777 NIN
Insurance Name:	Rover Insurers, Inc.
Insurance Group #:	21088
Employer Name:	Ninja Enterprises

Authorization

☒ Authorization to Release Information
☒ Authorization for Assignment of Benefits
☐ Authorization for Consent for Treatment
☐ My insurance will be billed but there may be a balance due.
Signature: *Sherman Smith*   Date: *10/12/CCYY*

Clinical Information

	DOS	POS	CPT®/HCPCS Description	ICD-9-CM (*Indicates diagnosis for all lines)	Amount
1	10/12/CCYY	Inpt Hosp	Drainage perineal urinary extravasation; complicated	Malignant Neoplasm of Prostate	$1900.00
2					
3					
4					
5					
6					
Remarks:	Steve Sorby, M.D. was the Assistant Surgeon for Butch M. N. Hackim, M.D. UPIN #: M42781				
Previous Balance:		Payment:	Copay:	Adjustment:	
Total Fee:	$1900.00	Cash ☐ Check ☐ Credit ☐	Cash ☐ Check ☐ Credit ☐	Remarks:	New Balance: $1900.00

Encounter Form

Provider Information

Name:	Samuel Stone, M.D.
Address:	4000 Silent Shores

City:	Silent Shores	State:	SC	Zip Code:	29608

		Fax #:	
Telephone #:		Fax #:	

Medicare ID#:		UPIN #:	B77778

Tax ID #:	11-7833334	Accepts Medicare Assignment:	☒

Provider's Signature:	Samuel Stone, MD	Date: 1/11/CCYY

Appointment Information

Appointment Date:		Time:	
Next Appt. Date:		Time:	
Date of First Visit:		Date of Injury:	06/11/CCYY
Referring Physician:	Butch M. N. Hackim, M.D.		

Guarantor Information

Name:	Sherry Smith
Address:	6767 Sampson Square

City:	Silent Shores	State:	SC	Zip Code:	29608

Insurance ID #:	99-7777 NIN
Insurance Name:	Rover Insurers, Inc.
Insurance Group #:	21088
Employer Name:	Ninja Enterprises

Patient Information

Name:	Sherry Smith
Address:	6767 Sampson Square

City:	Silent Shores	State:	SC	Zip Code:	29608

Telephone #:	(864) 555-2960	Account #:	10046
Date of Birth:	12/08/CCYY-39	Gender:	Female

Marital Status:	Married	Relationship to Guarantor:	Self
Student Status:	☐ Full-time	☐ Part-time	
Insurance Type:	☒ Pvt ☐ M/care ☐ M/caid ☐ WC ☐ Other _____		
Hospitalization Date:	From: 01/11/CCYY	To: 01/13/CCYY	
Hospital Information:	Silent Shores Medical Center, P.O. Box 600, Silent Shores, SC 29608		

Authorization

☒ Authorization to Release Information
☒ Authorization for Assignment of Benefits
☐ Authorization for Consent for Treatment
☐ My insurance will be billed but there may be a balance due.

Signature:	Sherry Smith	Date: 1/11/CCYY

Clinical Information

	DOS	POS	CPT® /HCPCS Description	ICD-9-CM (*Indicates diagnosis for all lines)	Amount
1	01/11/CCYY	Inpt Hosp	Septal dermatoplasty	Fracture of Nasal Bones	$900.00
2	01/11/CCYY	Inpt Hosp	Septoplasty, w/ cartilage scoring	Acute Sinusitis	$200.00
3	01/11/CCYY	Inpt Hosp	Excision turbinate, partial	Hypertrophy of Nasal Turbinates	$150.00
4					
5					
Remarks:	Patient's nose was fractured when hit by a baseball on June 11, CCYY, while playing at home.				
	Samuel Stone, M.D. was the Assistant Surgeon for Butch M. N. Hackim, M.D. UPIN #: M42781				

Previous Balance:		Payment:		Copay:		Adjustment:		
Total Fee:	$1250.00	Cash ☐ Check ☐ Credit ☐		Cash ☐ Check ☐ Credit ☐		Remarks:	New Balance:	$1250.00

Encounter Form

Provider Information

Name:	Sarah Shaw, M.D.
Address:	2222 South Silver

City:	Silent Shore	State:	SC	Zip Code:	29608

Telephone #:		Fax #:	

Medicare ID#:		UPIN #:	C54456

Tax ID #:	11-7833666	Accepts Medicare Assignment:	☒

Provider's Signature:	Sarah Shaw, MD	Date: 9/3/CCYY

Appointment Information

Appointment Date:		Time:	
Next Appt. Date:		Time:	
Date of First Visit:		Date of Injury:	
Referring Physician:	Butch M. N. Hackim, M.D.		

Guarantor Information

Name:	Sherry Smith
Address:	6767 Sampson Square

City:	Silent Shore	State:	SC	Zip Code:	29608

Insurance ID #:	99-7777 NIN
Insurance Name:	Rover Insurers, Inc.
Insurance Group #:	21088
Employer Name:	Ninja Enterprises

Patient Information

Name:	Sherry Smith
Address:	6767 Sampson Square

City:	Silent Shores	State:	SC	Zip Code:	29608

Telephone #:	(864) 555-2960	Account #:	10046
Date of Birth:	12/08/CCYY-39	Gender:	Female

Marital Status:	Married	Relationship to Guarantor:	Self
Student Status:	☐ Full-time	☐ Part-time	
Insurance Type:	☒ Pvt ☐ M/care ☐ M/caid ☐ WC ☐ Other _____		
Hospitalization Date:	From: 09/03/CCYY	To: 09/05/CCYY	
Hospital Information:	Silent Shores Medical Center, P.O. Box 600, Silent Shores, SC 29608		

Authorization

☒ Authorization to Release Information
☒ Authorization for Assignment of Benefits
☐ Authorization for Consent for Treatment
☐ My insurance will be billed but there may be a balance due.

Signature:	Sherry Smith	Date: 9/3/CCYY

Clinical Information

	DOS	POS	CPT® /HCPCS Description	ICD-9-CM (*Indicates diagnosis for all lines)	Amount
1	09/03/CCYY	Inpt Hosp	Cesarean delivery only	Cesarean delivery; Pregnant State	$500.00
2					
3					
4					
5					
6					
Remarks:	Sarah Shaw, M.D. was the Assistant Surgeon for Butch M. N. Hackim, M.D. UPIN #: M42781				

Previous Balance:	$1250.00	Payment:		Copay:		Adjustment:		
Total Fee:	$500.00	Cash ☐ Check ☐ Credit ☐		Cash ☐ Check ☐ Credit ☐		Remarks:	New Balance:	$1750.00

Encounter Form

Provider Information

Name:	Shay Share, M.D.
Address:	322 S. Shorne Street

City:	Raleigh	State:	NC	Zip Code:	27512

Telephone #:		Fax #:	
Medicare ID#:		UPIN #:	D78932
Tax ID #:	13-5567902	Accepts Medicare Assignment:	☐
Provider's Signature:	Shay Share, MD	Date:	9/3/CCYY

Patient Information

Name:	Sean Smith
Address:	6767 Sampson Square

City:	Silent Shores	State:	SC	Zip Code:	29608

Telephone #:	(864) 555-2960	Account #:	10047
Date of Birth:	02/03/CCYY-15	Gender:	Male
Marital Status:	Single	Relationship to Guarantor:	Child
Student Status:	☒ Full-time	☐ Part-time	
Insurance Type:	☒ Pvt ☐ M/care ☐ M/caid ☐ WC ☐ Other		
Hospitalization Date:	From: 09/02/CCYY To: 09/05/CCYY		
Hospital Information:	Silent Shores Medical Center, P.O. Box 600, Silent Shores, SC 29608		

Appointment Information

Appointment Date:		Time:	
Next Appt. Date:		Time:	
Date of First Visit:		Date of Injury:	
Referring Physician:	Butch M. N. Hackim, M.D.		

Guarantor Information

Name:	Sherry Smith
Address:	6767 Sampson Square

City:	Silent Shores	State:	SC	Zip Code:	29608

Insurance ID #:	99-7777 NIN
Insurance Name:	Rover Insurers, Inc.
Insurance Group #:	21088
Employer Name:	Ninja Enterprises

Authorization

☒ Authorization to Release Information
☒ Authorization for Assignment of Benefits
☐ Authorization for Consent for Treatment
☐ My insurance will be billed but there may be a balance due.

Signature: Sherry Smith   Date: 9/3/CCYY

Clinical Information

	DOS	POS	CPT® /HCPCS Description	ICD-9-CM (*Indicates diagnosis for all lines)	Amount
1	09/03/CCYY	Inpt Hosp	Repair, diaphragmatic hernia; transthoacic	Anomalies of Diaphragm; Ventral Hernia	$775.00
2					
3					
4					
5					
Remarks:	Shay Share, M.D. was the Assistant Surgeon for Butch M. N. Hackim, M.D. UPIN #: M42781.				
	Hospitalization Pre-Certified Auth #: 12574612				

Previous Balance:		Payment:		Copay:		Adjustment:			
Total Fee:	$775.00	Cash ☐ Check ☐ Credit ☐		Cash ☐ Check ☐ Credit ☐		Remarks:		New Balance:	$775.00

Encounter Form

Provider Information

Name:	Shirley Sott, M.D.
Address:	1436 S. Scott Street

City:	Raleigh	State:	NC	Zip Code:	27512

Telephone #:		Fax #:	
Medicare ID#:		UPIN #:	E45876
Tax ID #:	13-4567112	Accepts Medicare Assignment:	☐
Provider's Signature:	Shirley Sott, MD	Date:	11/15/CCYY

Patient Information

Name:	Sherman Smith
Address:	6767 Sampson Square

City:	Silver Shores	State:	SC	Zip Code:	29608

Telephone #:	(864) 555-2960	Account #:	10045
Date of Birth:	10/16/CCYY-39	Gender:	Male
Marital Status:	Married	Relationship to Guarantor:	Spouse
Student Status:	☐ Full-time	☐ Part-time	
Insurance Type:	☒ Pvt ☐ M/care ☐ M/caid ☐ WC ☐ Other		
Hospitalization Date:	From: 11/14/CCYY To: 11/20/CCYY		
Hospital Information:	Silent Shores Medical Center, P.O. Box 600, Silent Shores, SC 29608		

Appointment Information

Appointment Date:		Time:	
Next Appt. Date:		Time:	
Date of First Visit:		Date of Injury:	
Referring Physician:	Butch M. N. Hackim, M.D.		

Guarantor Information

Name:	Sherry Smith
Address:	6767 Sampson Square

City:	Silver Shore	State:	SC	Zip Code:	29608

Insurance ID #:	99-7777 NIN
Insurance Name:	Rover Insurers, Inc.
Insurance Group #:	21088
Employer Name:	Ninja Enterprises

Authorization

☒ Authorization to Release Information
☒ Authorization for Assignment of Benefits
☐ Authorization for Consent for Treatment
☐ My insurance will be billed but there may be a balance due.

Signature: Sherman Smith   Date: 11/15/CCYY

Clinical Information

	DOS	POS	CPT® /HCPCS Description	ICD-9-CM (*Indicates diagnosis for all lines)	Amount
1	11/15/CCYY	Inpt Hosp	Gastrojejunostomy, with vagotomy	Antral Ulcer; Gastritis	$800.00
2					
3					
4					
5					
Remarks:	Shirley Sott, M.D. was the Assistant Surgeon for Butch M. N. Hackim, M.D. UPIN #: M42781.				
	Hospitalization Pre-Certified Auth#: 363712926				

Previous Balance:	$1900.00	Payment:		Copay:		Adjustment:			
Total Fee:	$800.00	Cash ☐ Check ☐ Credit ☐		Cash ☐ Check ☐ Credit ☐		Remarks:		New Balance:	$2700.00

Health Claims Examining Exercises

(**Instructor's Note:** Medical Billing exercises in the entire text should be completed prior to students starting Health Claims Examining Exercise 6–A. New files should be set up for the Health Claims Examining exercises.)

Exercise **6–A**

Directions: Complete an Insurance Coverage Form (located in the **Forms** chapter) and set up Family Files for all families in this chapter. Refer to the Family Data Tables (**Documents 78–80**) located in the beginning of this chapter, and the Contracts located in the **Contracts, UCR Conversion Factor Report, and Relative Value Study** chapter.

Exercise **6–B**

Directions: Complete a Payment Worksheet (located in the **Forms** chapter) for CMS-1500 claims (**Documents 82–86, 88–92, and 94–98**) using the guidelines contained in the **Introduction** chapter and using the UCR Conversion Factor Report, Relative Value Study, and Contracts located in the **Contracts, UCR Conversion Factor Report, and Relative Value Study** chapter.

When processing claims, the Beginning Financials (**Documents 81, 87, and 93**) should be incorporated as payment history and claim calculations should be adjusted accordingly. Any carryover deductible listed should be included in the current year deductible for that individual. Therefore, in figuring current year deductible, students should be instructed to subtract the carryover deductible from the current year's amount.

Upon completion of each claim complete or update the Family Benefits Tracking Sheet (located in the **Forms** chapter) by compiling all of the claims payment data for the family.

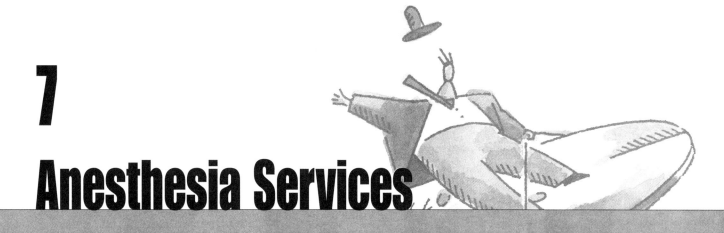

7
Anesthesia Services

Medical Billing Exercises

Exercise 7-1

Directions: Complete Patient Information Sheets (leave **Assigned Provider** field blank), Ledger Cards, and Insurance Coverage Forms and set up patient charts for the following families using copies of the forms in the **Forms** chapter. Refer to the Family Data Table **(Document 99)** for information. Refer to Chapter 6 for the Family Data Table **(Document 79)** for the Westin family.

Individual folders with dividers may be used to store information for each family. One Patient Information Sheet and Insurance Coverage Form should be filled out for the entire family.

FAMILY DATA TABLE

DOCUMENT 99

NORTON FAMILY	INSURED'S INFORMATION	SPOUSE'S INFORMATION	CHILD #1	CHILD #2	CHILD #3
Name	Ned Norton	Nancy Norton	Neil Norton	Nina Norton	
Address	34578 Navaho Lane Nampa, NV 89462	34578 Navaho Lane Nampa, NV 89462	34578 Navaho Lane Nampa, NV 89462	34578 Navaho Lane Nampa, NV 89462	
Email Address	nedn@norton.com				
TELEPHONE #					
Home: **Work:** **Cell:**	(702) 555-8946 (702) 555-8947 (702) 555-8948	(702) 555-8946	(702) 555-8946	(702) 555-8946	
Date of Birth	05/05/CCYY-50	06/10/CCYY-49	12/02/CCYY-17	09/01/CCYY-18	
Social Security #	777-44-3333	777-44-3334	777-44-3335	777-44-3336	
Marital Status/Gender	Married/Male	Married/Female	Single/Male	Single/Female	
Student Status			Full-time	Full-time	
Patient Account #	10048	10049	10050	10051	
Allergies/Medical Conditions	None	None	None	None	
PRIMARY INSURANCE CARRIER					
Name **Address**	Winter Insurance Company 9763 Western Way Whittier, CO 82963	Winter Insurance Company 9763 Western Way Whittier, CO 82963	Winter Insurance Company 9763 Western Way Whittier, CO 82963	Winter Insurance Company 9763 Western Way Whittier, CO 82963	
Effective Date	01/01/CCPY	01/01/CCPY	01/01/CCPY	01/01/CCPY	
Member's ID #	44-3333 ABC	44-3333 ABC	44-3333 ABC	44-3333 ABC	
Group Policy #	36928	36928	36928	36928	
Policy/Employer	ABC Corporation 1234 Whitaker Lane Colter, CO 81222				
OTHER INSURANCE CARRIER					
Name **Address**					
Effective Date					
Member's ID #					
Group Policy #					
Policy/Employer					
Responsible Party	Self	Self	Insured	Insured	
EMERGENCY CONTACT					
Name	Nick Noon	Nick Noon	Nick Noon	Nick Noon	
Telephone #	(702) 555-8949	(702) 555-8949	(702) 555-8949	(702) 555-8949	
Address	87543 Navaho Lane Nampa, NV 89462	87543 Navaho Lane Nampa, NV 89462	87543 Navaho Lane Nampa, NV 89462	87543 Navaho Lane Nampa, NV 89462	

Exercise 7-2

Directions: Complete a CMS-1500 for each of the Encounter Forms **(Documents 101–105** and **107–111)** in this chapter. CMS-1500 forms may be provided by your instructor or purchased from a stationery store. After completion of each CMS-1500 form complete a Patient Receipt (if a payment was made), and post the transaction(s) to the patient Ledger Card/Statement of Account previously created.

Exercise 7-3

Directions: Upon completion of all of the activities in Exercise 7–2 complete a Bank Deposit Slip/Ticket (located in the **Forms** chapter) for all payments made on the patient's account in this chapter.

Exercise 7-4

Directions: Using an Insurance Claims Register (located in the **Forms** chapter) list all claims that have been fully prepared and are ready for submission to the insurance carrier for payment. Enter the date that you created the CMS-1500 in the **Date Claim Filed** column.

Exercise 7-5

Directions: Complete an Insurance Tracer Form (located in the **Forms** Chapter) for the following claim. For additional information refer to the Family Data Table **(Document 2)**, completed claim form, or the Encounter Form.

Patient	Date Billed	Date of Service	Date of Illness	Diagnosis	Claim #
Sharon Smith	11/31/CCYY	11/19/CCYY	11/19/CCYY	574.20	Document 15

Anesthesia Claims Beginning Financials

NORTON FAMILY

Insurance Plan	Winter Insurance Company—ABC Corporation				
Patient:	**NED**	**NANCY**	**NEIL**	**NINA**	
C/O DEDUCTIBLE	0.00	0.00	0.00	0.00	
DEDUCTIBLE	31.00	5.00	9.93	12.48	
COINSURANCE	55.00	0.00	0.00	0.00	
ACCIDENT BENEFIT					
LIFETIME MAXIMUM	25,000.00	8,961.20	6,771.50	4,500.00	
M/N OFFICE VISITS					
OFFICE VISITS					
HOSPITAL VISITS					
DXL					
SURGERY					
ASSISTANT SURGERY					
ANESTHESIA					

Encounter Form

Provider Information

Name:	Nathan Navarro, M.D.
Address:	1234 Nampa Avenue
City:	Nampa State: NV Zip Code: 89462
Telephone #:	Fax #:
Medicare ID#:	UPIN #: F32105
Tax ID #:	88-8754489 Accepts Medicare Assignment: ☒
Provider's Signature:	*Nathan Navarro, MD* Date: *5/5/CCYY*

Appointment Information

Appointment Date:	Time:
Next Appt. Date:	Time:
Date of First Visit:	Date of Injury:
Referring Physician:	Butch M. N. Hackim, M.D.

Guarantor Information

Name:	Ned Norton
Address:	34578 Navaho Lane
City: Nampa	State: NV Zip Code: 89462
Insurance ID #:	44-3333 ABC
Insurance Name:	Winter Insurance Company
Insurance Group #:	36928
Employer Name:	ABC Corporation

Patient Information

Name:	Ned Norton
Address:	34578 Navaho Lane
City:	Nampa State: NV Zip Code: 89462
Telephone #:	(702) 555-8946 Account #: 10048
Date of Birth:	05/05/CCYY-50 Gender: Male
Marital Status:	Married Relationship to Guarantor: Self
Student Status:	☐ Full-time ☐ Part-time
Insurance Type:	☒ Pvt ☐ M/care ☐ M/caid ☐ WC ☐ Other _____
Hospitalization Date:	
Hospital Information:	Nampa Medical Center, P.O. Box 500, Nampa, NV 89462

Authorization

☒ Authorization to Release Information
☒ Authorization for Assignment of Benefits
☐ Authorization for Consent for Treatment
☐ My insurance will be billed but there may be a balance due.

Signature: *Ned Norton* Date: *5/5/CCYY*

Clinical Information

	DOS	POS	CPT® /HCPCS Description	ICD-9-CM (*Indicates diagnosis for all lines)	Amount
1	05/05/CCYY	Outpt Hosp	Colonoscopy with biopsy beyond splenic flexure	Flatulence	$350.00
2					
3					
4					
5					
6					

Remarks:	Anesthesia Time: Start – 8:40am, Stop – 9:20am Surgeon: Butch M. N. Hackim, M.D. UPIN #: M42781					
Previous Balance:		Payment:		Copay:	Adjustment:	
Total Fee:	$350.00	Cash ☐ Check ☐ Credit ☐	Cash ☐ Check ☐ Credit ☐	Remarks:		New Balance: $350.00

Encounter Form   *DOCUMENT 102*

Provider Information

Name:	Norma Nelson, M.D.
Address:	475 Nancy Lane

City:	Nampa	State:	NV	Zip Code:	89462

Telephone #:	Fax #:	
Medicare ID#:	UPIN #:	G05548
Tax ID #:	88-8778493	Accepts Medicare Assignment: ☒

Provider's Signature: _Norma Nelson, MD_   Date: _10/28/CCYY_

Appointment Information

Appointment Date:		Time:	
Next Appt. Date:		Time:	
Date of First Visit:		Date of Injury:	
Referring Physician:	Butch M. N. Hackim, M.D.		

Guarantor Information

Name:	Ned Norton
Address:	34578 Navaho Lane

City:	Nampa	State:	NV	Zip Code:	89462

Insurance ID #:	44-3333 ABC
Insurance Name:	Winter Insurance Company
Insurance Group #:	36928
Employer Name:	ABC Corporation

Patient Information

Name:	Nancy Norton
Address:	34578 Navaho Lane

City:	Nampa	State:	NV	Zip Code:	89462

Telephone #:	(702) 555-8946	Account #:	10049
Date of Birth:	06/10/CCYY-49	Gender:	Female
Marital Status:	Married	Relationship to Guarantor:	Spouse
Student Status:	☐ Full-time	☐ Part-time	
Insurance Type:	☒ Pvt ☐ M/care ☐ M/caid ☐ WC ☐ Other _____		
Hospitalization Date:	From: 10/28/CCYY	To: 10/31/CCYY	
Hospital Information:	Nampa Medical Center, P.O. Box 500, Nampa, NV 89462		

Authorization

☒ Authorization to Release Information
☒ Authorization for Assignment of Benefits
☐ Authorization for Consent for Treatment
☐ My insurance will be billed but there may be a balance due.

Signature: _Nancy Norton_   Date: _10/28/CCYY_

Clinical Information

	DOS	POS	CPT® /HCPCS Description	ICD-9-CM (*Indicates diagnosis for all lines)	Amount
1	10/28/CCYY	Inpt Hosp	Continuous epidural labor and delivery; lumbar, sacral	Normal delivery; Pregnant State	$1950.00
2					
3					
4					
5					
6					

Remarks:	Anesthesia Time: Start – 12:00pm, Stop – 7:00pm Surgeon: Butch M. N. Hackim, M.D. UPIN # M42781

Previous Balance:		Payment:		Copay:		Adjustment:		
Total Fee:	$1950.00	Cash ☐ Check ☐ Credit ☐		Cash ☐ Check ☐ Credit ☐		Remarks:	New Balance:	$1950.00

Encounter Form   *DOCUMENT 103*

Provider Information

Name:	Nicholas Nolan, M.D.
Address:	4742 Nathan Avenue

City:	Nathan	State:	NV	Zip Code:	89162

Telephone #:	Fax #:	
Medicare ID#:	UPIN #:	H04456
Tax ID #:	88-8778493	Accepts Medicare Assignment: ☒

Provider's Signature: _Nicholas Nolan, MD_   Date: _11/10/CCYY_

Appointment Information

Appointment Date:		Time:	
Next Appt. Date:		Time:	
Date of First Visit:		Date of Injury:	
Referring Physician:	Butch M. N. Hackim, M.D.		

Guarantor Information

Name:	Ned Norton
Address:	34578 Navaho Lane

City:	Nampa	State:	NV	Zip Code:	89462

Insurance ID #:	44-3333 ABC
Insurance Name:	Winter Insurance Company
Insurance Group #:	36928
Employer Name:	ABC Corporation

Patient Information

Name:	Neil Norton
Address:	34578 Navaho Lane

City:	Nampa	State:	NV	Zip Code:	89462

Telephone #:	(702) 555-8946	Account #:	10050
Date of Birth:	12/02/CCYY-17	Gender:	Male
Marital Status:	Single	Relationship to Guarantor:	Child
Student Status:	☒ Full-time	☐ Part-time	
Insurance Type:	☒ Pvt ☐ M/care ☐ M/caid ☐ WC ☐ Other _____		
Hospitalization Date:	From: 11/10/CCYY	To: 11/12/CCYY	
Hospital Information:	Nampa Medical Center, P.O. Box 500, Nampa, NV 89462		

Authorization

☒ Authorization to Release Information
☒ Authorization for Assignment of Benefits
☐ Authorization for Consent for Treatment
☐ My insurance will be billed but there may be a balance due.

Signature: _Ned Norton_   Date: _11/10/CCYY_

Clinical Information

	DOS	POS	CPT® /HCPCS Description	ICD-9-CM (*Indicates diagnosis for all lines)	Amount
1	11/10/CCYY	Inpt Hosp	Biopsy of vestibule of mouth	Lesion in Vestibule of Mouth	$350.00
2					
3					
4					
5					
6					

Remarks:	Anesthesia Time: Start – 10:35am, Stop – 10:55am Surgeon: Butch M. N. Hackim, M.D. UPIN #: M42781

Previous Balance:		Payment:		Copay:		Adjustment:		
Total Fee:	$350.00	Cash ☐ Check ☐ Credit ☐		Cash ☐ Check ☐ Credit ☐		Remarks:	New Balance:	$350.00

Encounter Form

Provider Information

Name:	Nouri Nazari, M.D.
Address:	4100 Surgi-Center Drive
City:	Nampa · State: NV · Zip Code: 89462
Telephone #:	Fax #:
Medicare ID#:	UPIN #: I02284
Tax ID #:	88-8754493 · Accepts Medicare Assignment: ☒
Provider's Signature:	*Nouri Nazari, MD* Date: 12/30/CCYY

Appointment Information

Appointment Date:		Time:
Next Appt. Date:		Time:
Date of First Visit:		Date of Injury:
Referring Physician:	Butch M. N. Hackim, M.D.	

Guarantor Information

Name:	Ned Norton
Address:	34578 Navaho Lane
City: Nampa	State: NV · Zip Code: 89462
Insurance ID #:	44-3333 ABC
Insurance Name:	Winter Insurance Company
Insurance Group #:	36928
Employer Name:	ABC Corporation

Patient Information

Name:	Nancy Norton
Address:	34578 Navaho Lane
City:	Nampa · State: NV · Zip Code: 89462
Telephone #:	(702) 555-8946 · Account #: 10049
Date of Birth:	06/10/CCYY-49 · Gender: Female
Marital Status:	Married · Relationship to Guarantor: Spouse
Student Status:	☐ Full-time ☐ Part-time
Insurance Type:	☒ Pvt ☐ M/care ☐ M/caid ☐ WC ☐ Other
Hospitalization Date:	From: 12/30/CCYY To: 01/01/CCNY
Hospital Information:	Nampa Medical Center, P.O. Box 500, Nampa, NV 89462

Authorization

☒ Authorization to Release Information
☒ Authorization for Assignment of Benefits
☐ Authorization for Consent for Treatment
☐ My insurance will be billed but there may be a balance due.

Signature: *Nancy Norton* Date: 12/30/CCYY

Clinical Information

	DOS	POS	CPT® /HCPCS Description	ICD-9-CM (*Indicates diagnosis for all lines)	Amount
1	12/30/CCYY	Inpt Hosp	Cystoscopy/urethroscopy with biopsy	Cystitis	$350.00
2					
3					
4					
5					
6					

Remarks:	Anesthesia Time: Start – 6:35am, Stop – 7:10am		Surgeon: Butch M. N. Hackim, M.D. UPIN #: M42781	
Previous Balance:	$1950.00 · Payment: · Copay: · Adjustment:			
Total Fee:	$350.00 · Cash ☐ Check ☐ Credit ☐ · Cash ☐ Check ☐ Credit ☐ · Remarks:		New Balance:	$2300.00

Encounter Form

Provider Information

Name:	Nicole Nast, M.D.
Address:	6060 Nicollet Avenue
City:	Nathan · State: NV · Zip Code: 89122
Telephone #:	Fax #:
Medicare ID#:	UPIN #: J03350
Tax ID #:	88-8581793 · Accepts Medicare Assignment: ☐
Provider's Signature:	*Nicole Nast, MD* Date: 12/1/CCYY

Appointment Information

Appointment Date:		Time:
Next Appt. Date:		Time:
Date of First Visit:		Date of Injury:
Referring Physician:	Butch M. N. Hackim, M.D.	

Guarantor Information

Name:	Ned Norton
Address:	34578 Navaho Lane
City: Nampa	State: NV · Zip Code: 89462
Insurance ID #:	44-3333 ABC
Insurance Name:	Winter Insurance Company
Insurance Group #:	36928
Employer Name:	ABC Corporation

Patient Information

Name:	Nina Norton
Address:	34578 Navaho Lane
City:	Nampa · State: NV · Zip Code: 89462
Telephone #:	(702) 555-8946 · Account #: 10051
Date of Birth:	09/01/CCYY-18 · Gender: Female
Marital Status:	Single · Relationship to Guarantor: Child
Student Status:	☒ Full-time ☐ Part-time
Insurance Type:	☒ Pvt ☐ M/care ☐ M/caid ☐ WC ☐ Other
Hospitalization Date:	From: 12/01/CCYY To: 12/04/CCYY
Hospital Information:	Nampa Medical Center, P.O. Box 500, Nampa, NV 89462

Authorization

☒ Authorization to Release Information
☒ Authorization for Assignment of Benefits
☐ Authorization for Consent for Treatment
☐ My insurance will be billed but there may be a balance due.

Signature: *Ned Norton* Date: 12/1/CCYY

Clinical Information

	DOS	POS	CPT® /HCPCS Description	ICD-9-CM (*Indicates diagnosis for all lines)	Amount
1	12/01/CCYY	Inpt Hosp	Fissurectomy	Anal Fistula	$500.00
2					
3					
4					
5					
6					

Remarks:	Anesthesia Time: Start – 1:00pm, Stop – 2:05pm		Surgeon: Butch M. N. Hackim, M.D. UPIN #: M42781	
Previous Balance:	Payment: · Copay: · Adjustment:			
Total Fee:	$500.00 · Cash ☐ Check ☐ Credit ☐ · Cash ☐ Check ☐ Credit ☐ · Remarks:		New Balance:	$500.00

Anesthesia Claims Beginning Financials

WESTIN FAMILY

Insurance Plan	Ball Insurance Carriers—XYZ Corporation				
Patient:	**WILLIAM**	**WILMA**	**WENDY**	**WALLY**	
C/O DEDUCTIBLE				0.00	
DEDUCTIBLE	125.00	125.00	49.93	0.00	
COINSURANCE	7.19	13.28	13.60	0.00	
ACCIDENT BENEFIT					
LIFETIME MAXIMUM	989.95	5,053.14	6,825.89	961.20	
M/N OFFICE VISITS					
OFFICE VISITS	40.00	16.00	40.00	40.00	
HOSPITAL VISITS					
DXL	0.00	0.00	0.00	0.00	
SURGERY	0.00	0.00	0.00	0.00	
ASSISTANT SURGERY	0.00	0.00	175.00	0.00	
ANESTHESIA				0.00	
See Assistant Surgery Claims for other family members.					

Encounter Form

Provider Information

Name:	Winnie Whyme, M.D.
Address:	8457 White Avenue
City:	Walla Walla State: WA Zip Code: 98977
Telephone #:	Fax #:
Medicare ID#:	UPIN #: K50543
Tax ID #:	77-3445690 Accepts Medicare Assignment: ☒
Provider's Signature:	*Winnie Whyme, MD* Date: 1/25/CCYY

Appointment Information

Appointment Date:		Time:
Next Appt. Date:		Time:
Date of First Visit:		Date of Injury:
Referring Physician:	Butch M. N. Hackim, M.D.	

Guarantor Information

Name:	William Westin
Address:	Route 1 Box 83
City:	Walla Walla State: WA Zip Code: 98977
Insurance ID #:	77-7777 XYZ
Insurance Name:	Ball Insurance Carriers
Insurance Group #:	62958
Employer Name:	XYZ Corporation

Patient Information

Name:	Wendy Westin
Address:	Route 1 Box 83
City:	Walla Walla State: WA Zip Code: 98977
Telephone #:	(206) 555-9897 Account #: 10044
Date of Birth:	06/28/CCYY-10 Gender: Female
Marital Status:	Single Relationship to Guarantor: Child
Student Status:	☒ Full-time ☐ Part-time
Insurance Type:	☒ Pvt ☐ M/care ☐ M/caid ☐ WC ☐ Other _____
Hospitalization Date:	
Hospital Information:	White Memorial Center, P.O. Box 600, Walla Walla, WA 98977

Authorization

☒ Authorization to Release Information
☒ Authorization for Assignment of Benefits
☐ Authorization for Consent for Treatment
☐ My insurance will be billed but there may be a balance due.

Signature: *William Westin*   Date: 1/25/CCYY

Clinical Information

	DOS	POS	CPT® /HCPCS Description	ICD-9-CM (*Indicates diagnosis for all lines)	Amount
1	01/25/CCYY	Otpt Hosp	Excisional biopsy of mandible lesion w/ flap	Lesion of Face; Neck and; Trunk	$3150.00
2					
3					
4					
5					
6					

Remarks:	Anesthesia Time: Start – 9:10am, Stop – 11:45am Surgeon: Butch M. N. Hackim, M.D. UPIN #: M42781				
Previous Balance:	$800.00	Payment:	Copay:	Adjustment:	
Total Fee:	$3150.00	Cash ☐ Check ☐ Credit ☐	Cash ☐ Check ☐ Credit ☐	Remarks:	New Balance: $3950.00

Encounter Form

Provider Information

Name:	Wilford Wardell, M.D.
Address:	4444 Washington Avenue

City:	Walla Walla	State:	WA	Zip Code:	98977

Telephone #:		Fax #:	

Medicare ID#:		UPIN #:	L20202

Tax ID #:	11-7814784	Accepts Medicare Assignment:	☒

Provider's Signature:	*Wilford Wardell, MD*	Date: *10/12/CCYY*

Appointment Information

Appointment Date:		Time:	
Next Appt. Date:		Time:	
Date of First Visit:		Date of Injury:	
Referring Physician:	Butch M. N. Hackim, M.D.		

Guarantor Information

Name:	William Westin
Address:	Route 1 Box 83

City:	Walla Walla	State:	WA	Zip Code:	98977

Insurance ID #:	77-7777 XYZ
Insurance Name:	Ball Insurance Carriers
Insurance Group #:	62958
Employer Name:	XYZ Corporation

Patient Information

Name:	Wally Westin
Address:	Route 1 Box 83

City:	Walla Walla	State:	WA	Zip Code:	98977

Telephone #:	(206) 555-9897	Account #:	10053

Date of Birth:	10/16/CCYY-11	Gender:	Male

Marital Status:	Single	Relationship to Guarantor:	Child

Student Status:	☒ Full-time	☐ Part-time

Insurance Type:	☒ Pvt ☐ M/care ☐ M/caid ☐ WC ☐ Other

Hospitalization Date:	
Hospital Information:	White Memorial Center, P.O. Box 600, Walla Walla, WA 98977

Authorization

☒ Authorization to Release Information
☒ Authorization for Assignment of Benefits
☐ Authorization for Consent for Treatment
☐ My insurance will be billed but there may be a balance due.

Signature: *William Westin*   Date: *10/12/CCYY*

Clinical Information

	DOS	POS	CPT® /HCPCS Description	ICD-9-CM (*Indicates diagnosis for all lines)	Amount
1	10/12/CCYY	Otpt Hosp	Upper GI with brushing	Antral Ulcer; Gastritis	$1900.00
2					
3					
4					
5					
6					

Remarks:	Anesthesia Time: Start – 7:00am, Stop – 8:05am Surgeon: Butch M. N. Hackim, M.D. UPIN #: M42781

Previous Balance:		Payment:		Copay:		Adjustment:		
Total Fee:	$1900.00	Cash ☐ Check ☐ Credit ☐		Cash ☐ Check ☐ Credit ☐		Remarks:	New Balance:	$1900.00

Encounter Form

Provider Information

Name:	Wesley Whyme, M.D.
Address:	8457 White Avenue

City:	Walla Walla	State:	WA	Zip Code:	98977

Telephone #:		Fax #:	

Medicare ID#:		UPIN #:	M25580

Tax ID #:	77-3445555	Accepts Medicare Assignment:	☒

Provider's Signature:	*Wesley Whyme, MD*	Date: *12/9/CCYY*

Appointment Information

Appointment Date:		Time:	
Next Appt. Date:		Time:	
Date of First Visit:		Date of Injury:	
Referring Physician:	Butch M. N. Hackim, M.D.		

Guarantor Information

Name:	William Westin
Address:	Route 1 Box 83

City:	Walla Walla	State:	WA	Zip Code:	98977

Insurance ID #:	77-7777 XYZ
Insurance Name:	Ball Insurance Carriers
Insurance Group #:	62958
Employer Name:	XYZ Corporation

Patient Information

Name:	William Westin
Address:	Route 1 Box 83

City:	Walla Walla	State:	WA	Zip Code:	98977

Telephone #:	(206) 555-9897	Account #:	10042

Date of Birth:	04/03/CCYY-33	Gender:	Male

Marital Status:	Married	Relationship to Guarantor:	Self

Student Status:	☐ Full-time	☐ Part-time

Insurance Type:	☒ Pvt ☐ M/care ☐ M/caid ☐ WC ☐ Other

Hospitalization Date:	
Hospital Information:	White Memorial Center, P.O. Box 600, Walla Walla, WA 98977

Authorization

☒ Authorization to Release Information
☒ Authorization for Assignment of Benefits
☐ Authorization for Consent for Treatment
☐ My insurance will be billed but there may be a balance due.

Signature: *William Westin*   Date: *12/9/CCYY*

Clinical Information

	DOS	POS	CPT® /HCPCS Description	ICD-9-CM (*Indicates diagnosis for all lines)	Amount
1	12/09/CCYY	Otpt Hosp	Exc of left humerus bone cyst, exc olecranon bursa	Olecranon Bursitis	$1890.00
2					
3					
4					
5					
6					

Remarks:	Anesthesia Time: Start – 8:50am, Stop – 12:35pm Surgeon: Butch M. N. Hackim, M.D. UPIN #: M42781

Previous Balance:	$2650.00	Payment:		Copay:		Adjustment:		
Total Fee:	$1890.00	Cash ☐ Check ☐ Credit ☐		Cash ☐ Check ☐ Credit ☐		Remarks:	New Balance:	$4540.00

Encounter Form

Provider Information

Name:	Ward Winley, M.D.
Address:	3623 Wild Wind Drive
City:	Walla Walla State: WA Zip Code: 98977
Telephone #:	Fax #:
Medicare ID#:	UPIN #: A20558
Tax ID #:	11-7833334 Accepts Medicare Assignment: ☒
Provider's Signature:	*Ward Winley, MD* Date: 6/11/CCYY

Appointment Information

Appointment Date:		Time:	
Next Appt. Date:		Time:	
Date of First Visit:		Date of Injury:	
Referring Physician:	Butch M. N. Hackim, M.D.		

Guarantor Information

Name:	William Westin
Address:	Route 1 Box 83
City:	Walla Walla State: WA Zip Code: 98977
Insurance ID #:	77-7777 XYZ
Insurance Name:	Ball Insurance Carriers
Insurance Group #:	62958
Employer Name:	XYZ Corporation

Patient Information

Name:	Wendy Westin
Address:	Route 1 Box 83
City:	Walla Walla State: WA Zip Code: 98977
Telephone #:	(206) 555-9897 Account #: 10044
Date of Birth:	06/28/CCYY-10 Gender: Female
Marital Status:	Single Relationship to Guarantor: Child
Student Status:	☒ Full-time ☐ Part-time
Insurance Type:	☒ Pvt ☐ M/care ☐ M/caid ☐ WC ☐ Other ____
Hospitalization Date:	
Hospital Information:	White Memorial Center, P.O. Box 600, Walla Walla, WA 98977

Authorization

☒ Authorization to Release Information
☒ Authorization for Assignment of Benefits
☐ Authorization for Consent for Treatment
☐ My insurance will be billed but there may be a balance due.

Signature: *William Westin*   Date: 6/11/CCYY

Clinical Information

	DOS	POS	CPT® /HCPCS Description	ICD-9-CM (*Indicates diagnosis for all lines)	Amount
1	06/11/CCYY	Otpt Hosp	Rhinoplasty	*; *1; *2	$3125.00
2	06/11/CCYY	Otpt Hosp	Sinusotomy 3+	*Fracture of Nasal Bones; *1Hemorrhagic	$2000.00
3				Sinusitis; *2 Hypertrophy of nasal Turbinates	
4					
5					
6					
Remarks:	Anesthesia Time: Start – 13:10, Stop – 15:20			Surgeon: Butch M. N. Hackim, M.D. UPIN #: M42781	
Previous Balance:	$3950.00	Payment:		Copay:	Adjustment:	
Total Fee:	$5125.00	Cash ☐ Check ☐ Credit ☐	Cash ☐ Check ☐ Credit ☐	Remarks:	New Balance: $9075.00

Encounter Form

Provider Information

Name:	Wilbert Wagner, M.D.
Address:	6003 Waupok Way
City:	Western State: WA Zip Code: 98102
Telephone #:	Fax #:
Medicare ID#:	UPIN #: B45620
Tax ID #:	22-2222238 Accepts Medicare Assignment: ☒
Provider's Signature:	*Wilbert Wagner, MD* Date: 3/15/CCYY

Appointment Information

Appointment Date:		Time:	
Next Appt. Date:		Time:	
Date of First Visit:		Date of Injury:	
Referring Physician:	Butch M. N. Hackim, M.D.		

Guarantor Information

Name:	William Westin
Address:	Route 1 Box 83
City:	Walla Walla State: WA Zip Code: 98977
Insurance ID #:	77-7777 XYZ
Insurance Name:	Ball Insurance Carriers
Insurance Group #:	62958
Employer Name:	XYZ Corporation

Patient Information

Name:	Wilma Westin
Address:	Route 1 Box 83
City:	Walla Walla State: WA Zip Code: 989877
Telephone #:	(206) 555-9897 Account #: 10043
Date of Birth:	03/23/CCYY-31 Gender: Female
Marital Status:	Married Relationship to Guarantor: Spouse
Student Status:	☐ Full-time ☐ Part-time
Insurance Type:	☒ Pvt ☐ M/care ☐ M/caid ☐ WC ☐ Other ____
Hospitalization Date:	
Hospital Information:	White Memorial Center, P.O. Box 600, Walla Walla, WA 98977

Authorization

☒ Authorization to Release Information
☒ Authorization for Assignment of Benefits
☐ Authorization for Consent for Treatment
☐ My insurance will be billed but there may be a balance due.

Signature: *Wilma Westin*   Date: 3/15/CCYY

Clinical Information

	DOS	POS	CPT® /HCPCS Description	ICD-9-CM (*Indicates diagnosis for all lines)	Amount
1	03/15/CCYY	Otpt Hosp	Anesthesia, laparoscopy and salpingo-oophorectomy	Menorrhagia; Pelvis Pain; Ovarian Cyst	$1600.00
2					
3					
4					
5					
6					
Remarks:	Anesthesia Time: Start – 16:10, Stop – 17:25			Surgeon: Butch M. N. Hackim, M.D. UPIN #: M42781	
Previous Balance:	$1700.00	Payment:		Copay:	Adjustment:	
Total Fee:	$1600.00	Cash ☐ Check ☐ Credit ☐	Cash ☐ Check ☐ Credit ☐	Remarks:	New Balance: $3300.00

Health Claims Examining Exercises

(Instructor's Note: Medical Billing exercises in the entire text should be completed prior to students starting Health Claims Examining Exercise 7–A. New files should be set up for the Health Claims Examining exercises.)

Exercise 7-A

Directions: Complete an Insurance Coverage Form (located in the **Forms** chapter) and set up Family Files for all families in this chapter. Refer to the Family Data Tables **(Document 99)** located in the beginning of this chapter, and the Contracts located in the **Contracts, UCR Conversion Factor Report, and Relative Value Study** chapter.

Exercise 7-B

Directions: Complete a Payment Worksheet (located in the **Forms** chapter) for CMS-1500 claims **(Documents 101–105 and 107–111)** using the guidelines contained in the **Introduction** chapter and using the UCR Conversion Factor Report, Relative Value Study, and Contracts located in the **Contracts, UCR Conversion Factor Report, and Relative Value Study** chapter.

When processing claims, the Beginning Financials **(Documents 81, 87, and 93)** should be incorporated as payment history and claim calculations should be adjusted accordingly. Any carryover deductible listed should be included in the current year deductible for that individual. Therefore, in figuring current year deductible, students should be instructed to subtract the carryover deductible from the current year's amount.

Upon completion of each claim complete or update the Family Benefits Tracking Sheet (located in the **Forms** chapter) by compiling all of the claims payment data for the family.

8
Hospital Services

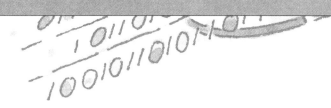

Medical Billing Exercises

Exercise 8-1

Directions: Complete Patient Information Sheets (leave **Assigned Provider** field blank), Ledger Cards, and Insurance Coverage Forms and set up patient charts for the following families using copies of the forms in the **Forms** chapter. Refer to the following Family Data Tables (**Documents 112–116**) for information.

   Individual folders with dividers may be used to store information for each family. One Patient Information Sheet and Insurance Coverage Form should be filled out for the entire family.

Document 112

FAMILY DATA TABLE

GONZALES FAMILY	INSURED'S INFORMATION	SPOUSE'S INFORMATION	CHILD #1	CHILD #2	CHILD #3
Name	Gary Gonzales	Ginnie Gonzales	Genara Gonzales	Gary Jr. Gonzales	Grace Gonzales
Address	56789 Garney Lane Garberville, GA 90012	56789 Garney Lane Garberville, GA 90012	56789 Garney Lane Garberville, GA 90012	56789 Garney Lane Garberville, GA 90012	56789 Garney Lane Garberville, GA 90012
Email Address	garyg@gonzales.com				
TELEPHONE #					
Home: Work: Cell:	(229) 555-2100 (229) 555-2101 (229) 555-2102	(229) 555-2100	(229) 555-2100	(229) 555-2100	(229) 555-2100
Date of Birth	07/27/CCYY-59	01/07/CCYY-57	10/17/CCYY-16	06/22/CCYY-18	08/20/CCYY-17
Social Security #	555-88-7777	555-88-7778	555-88-7779	555-88-7770	555-88-7771
Marital Status/Gender	Married/Male	Married/Female	Single/Female	Single/Male	Single/Female
Student Status			Full-time	Full-time	Full-time
Patient Account #	10056	10058	10057	10059	10060
Allergies/Medical Conditions	None	None	None	None	None
PRIMARY INSURANCE CARRIER					
Name Address	Winter Insurance Company 9763 Western Way Whittier, CO 82963	Winter Insurance Company 9763 Western Way Whittier, CO 82963	Winter Insurance Company 9763 Western Way Whittier, CO 82963	Winter Insurance Company 9763 Western Way Whittier, CO 82963	Winter Insurance Company 9763 Western Way Whittier, CO 82963
Effective Date	01/01/CCPY	01/01/CCPY	01/01/CCPY	01/01/CCPY	01/01/CCPY
Member's ID #	88-7777 ABC	88-7777 ABC	88-7777 ABC	88-7777 ABC	88-7777 ABC
Group Policy #	36928	36928	36928	36928	36928
Policy/Employer	ABC Corporation 1234 Whitaker Lane Colter, CO 81222				
OTHER INSURANCE CARRIER					
Name Address					
Effective Date					
Member's ID #					
Group Policy #					
Policy/Employer					
Responsible Party	Self	Self	Insured	Insured	Insured
EMERGENCY CONTACT					
Name Telephone # Address	Gill Galo (229) 555-2103 98765 Garney Lane Garberville, GA 90012	Gill Galo (229) 555-2103 98765 Garney Lane Garberville, GA 90012	Gill Galo (229) 555-2103 98765 Garney Lane Garberville, GA 90012	Gill Galo (229) 555-2103 98765 Garney Lane Garberville, GA 90012	Gill Galo (229) 555-2103 98765 Garney Lane Garberville, GA 90012

DOCUMENT 113

FAMILY DATA TABLE

LEVINE FAMILY	INSURED'S INFORMATION	SPOUSE'S INFORMATION	CHILD #1	CHILD #2	CHILD #3
Name	Larry Levine	Lannie Levine	Lloyd Levine	Lisa Levine	Lila Levine
Address	6780 Lodge Lane Lafayatte, LA 70513	6780 Lodge Lane Lafayatte, LA 70513	6780 Lodge Lane Lafayatte, LA 70513	6780 Lodge Lane Lafayatte, LA 70513	6780 Lodge Lane Lafayatte, LA 70513
Email Address	larryl@levine.com				
TELEPHONE #					
Home: **Work:** **Cell:**	(504) 555-7051 (504) 555-7052 (504) 555-7053	(504) 555-7051	(504) 555-7051	(504) 555-7051	(504) 555-7051
Date of Birth	10/10/CCYY-64	10/09/CCYY-54	09/19/CCYY-16	10/04/CCYY-17	09/21/CCYY-18
Social Security #	001-22-3333	001-22-3334	001-22-3335	001-22-3336	001-22-3337
Marital Status/Gender	Married/Male	Married/Female	Single/Male	Single/Female	Single/Female
Student Status			Full-time	Full-time	Full-time
Patient Account #	10061	10062	10063	10064	10065
Allergies/Medical Conditions	None	None	None	None	None
PRIMARY INSURANCE CARRIER					
Name **Address**	Rover Insurers, Inc. 5931 Rolling Road Ronson, CO 81369	Rover Insurers, Inc. 5931 Rolling Road Ronson, CO 81369	Rover Insurers, Inc. 5931 Rolling Road Ronson, CO 81369	Rover Insurers, Inc. 5931 Rolling Road Ronson, CO 81369	Rover Insurers, Inc. 5931 Rolling Road Ronson, CO 81369
Effective Date	01/01/CCPY	01/01/CCPY	01/01/CCPY	01/01/CCPY	01/01/CCPY
Member's ID #	22-3333 NIN	22-3333 NIN	22-3333 NIN	22-3333 NIN	22-3333 NIN
Group Policy #	21088	21088	21088	21088	21088
Policy/Employer	Ninja Enterprises 1234 Nockout Road Newton, NM 88012				
OTHER INSURANCE CARRIER					
Name **Address**					
Effective Date					
Member's ID #					
Group Policy #					
Policy/Employer					
Responsible Party	Self	Self	Insured	Insured	Insured
EMERGENCY CONTACT					
Name **Telephone #** **Address**	Layla Loronzo (504) 555-7054 876 Lodge Lane Lafayatte, LA 70513	Layla Loronzo (504) 555-7054 876 Lodge Lane Lafayatte, LA 70513	Layla Loronzo (504) 555-7054 876 Lodge Lane Lafayatte, LA 70513	Layla Loronzo (504) 555-7054 876 Lodge Lane Lafayatte, LA 70513	Layla Loronzo (504) 555-7054 876 Lodge Lane Lafayatte, LA 70513

FAMILY DATA TABLE

INGLES FAMILY	INSURED'S INFORMATION	SPOUSE'S INFORMATION	CHILD #1	CHILD #2	CHILD #3
Name	Inez Ingles	Irving Ingles	Irma Ingles	Ilene Ingles	
Address	987 Island Drive Inichi, IN 46623	987 Island Drive Inichi, IN 46623	987 Island Drive Inichi, IN 46623	987 Island Drive Inichi, IN 46623	
Email Address	inezi@ingles.com				
TELEPHONE #					
Home:	(219) 555-4662	(219) 555-4662	(219) 555-4662	(219) 555-4662	
Work:	(219) 555-4663				
Cell:	(219) 555-4664				
Date of Birth	08/17/CCYY-41	04/02/CCYY-46	10/17/CCYY-16	07/27/CCYY-18	
Social Security #	000-55-1111	000-55-1112	000-55-1113	000-55-1114	
Marital Status/Gender	Married/Female	Married/Male	Single/Female	Single/Female	
Student Status			Full-time	Full-time	
Patient Account #	10066	10067	10068	10069	
Allergies/Medical Conditions	None	None	None	None	
PRIMARY INSURANCE CARRIER					
Name Address	Ball Insurance Carriers 3895 Bubble Blvd. Ste. 283 Boxwood, CO 85926	Ball Insurance Carriers 3895 Bubble Blvd. Ste. 283 Boxwood, CO 85926	Ball Insurance Carriers 3895 Bubble Blvd. Ste. 283 Boxwood, CO 85926	Ball Insurance Carriers 3895 Bubble Blvd. Ste. 283 Boxwood, CO 85926	
Effective Date	01/01/CCPY	01/01/CCPY	01/01/CCPY	01/01/CCPY	
Member's ID #	55-1111 XYZ	55-1111 XYZ	55-1111 XYZ	55-1111 XYZ	
Group Policy #	62958	62958	62958	62958	
Policy/Employer	XYZ Corporation 9817 Bobcat Blvd. Bastion, CO 81319				
OTHR INSURANCE CARRIER					
Name Address					
Effective Date					
Member's ID #					
Group Policy #					
Policy/Employer					
Responsible Party	Self	Self	Insured	Insured	
EMERGENCY CONTACT					
Name	Isac Ilnoy	Isac Ilnoy	Isac Ilnoy	Isac Ilnoy	
Telephone #	(219) 555-4665	(219) 555-4665	(219) 555-4665	(219) 555-4665	
Address	789 Island Drive Inichi, IN 46623	789 Island Drive Inichi, IN 46623	789 Island Drive Inichi, IN 46623	789 Island Drive Inichi, IN 46623	

DOCUMENT 115

FAMILY DATA TABLE

JENNINGS FAMILY	INSURED'S INFORMATION	SPOUSE'S INFORMATION	CHILD #1	CHILD #2	CHILD #3
Name	Jack Jennings	Jennifer Jennings	Jaqueline Jennings	Julia Jennings	Janet Jennings
Address	4738 Jasmine Road Jersey, NJ 08077	4738 Jasmine Road Jersey, NJ 08077	4738 Jasmine Road Jersey, NJ 08077	4738 Jasmine Road Jersey, NJ 08077	4738 Jasmine Road Jersey, NJ 08077
Email Address	jackj@jennings.com				
TELEPHONE #					
Home:	(551) 555-0807	(551) 555-0807	(551) 555-0807	(551) 555-0807	(551) 555-0807
Work:	(551) 555-0808				
Cell:	(551) 555-0809				
Date of Birth	06/20/CCYY-43	10/04/CCYY-41	04/29/CCYY-17	10/07/CCYY-18	12/07/CCYY-15
Social Security #	111-77-9999	111-77-9901	111-77-9902	111-77-9903	111-77-9904
Marital Status/Gender	Married /Male	Married/Female	Single/Female	Single/Female	Single/Female
Student Status			Full-time	Full-time	Full-time
Patient Account #	10072	10073	10070	10071	10075
Allergies/Medical Conditions	None	None	None	None	None
PRIMARY INSURANCE CARRIER					
Name Address	Winter Insurance Company 9763 Western Way Whittier, CO 82963	Winter Insurance Company 9763 Western Way Whittier, CO 82963	Winter Insurance Company 9763 Western Way Whittier, CO 82963	Winter Insurance Company 9763 Western Way Whittier, CO 82963	Winter Insurance Company 9763 Western Way Whittier, CO 82963
Effective Date	01/01/CCPY	01/01/CCPY	01/01/CCPY	01/01/CCPY	01/01/CCPY
Member's ID #	77-9999 ABC	77-9999 ABC	77-9999 ABC	77-9999 ABC	77-9999 ABC
Group Policy #	36928	36928	36928	36928	36928
Policy/Employer	ABC Corporation 1234 Whitaker Lane Colter, CO 81222				
OTHER INSURANCE CARRIER					
Name Address					
Effective Date					
Member's ID #					
Group Policy #					
Policy/Employer					
Responsible Party	Self	Self	Insured	Insured	Insured
EMERGENCY CONTACT					
Name Telephone # Address	Jeffrey Johnson (551) 555-0810 8374 Jasmine Road Jersey, NJ 08077	Jeffrey Johnson (551) 555-0810 8374 Jasmine Road Jersey, NJ 08077	Jeffrey Johnson (551) 555-0810 8374 Jasmine Road Jersey, NJ 08077	Jeffrey Johnson (551) 555-0810 8374 Jasmine Road Jersey, NJ 08077	Jeffrey Johnson (551) 555-0810 8374 Jasmine Road Jersey, NJ 08077

FAMILY DATA TABLE

DOCUMENT 116

FURY FAMILY	INSURED'S INFORMATION	SPOUSE'S INFORMATION	CHILD #1	CHILD #2	CHILD #3
Name	Fred Fury	Fay Fury	Fern Fury	Forrest Fury	
Address	5555 Fairlane Blvd. Folley, FL 32208	5555 Fairlane Blvd. Folley, FL 32208	5555 Fairlane Blvd. Folley, FL 32208	5555 Fairlane Blvd. Folley, FL 32208	
Email Address	fredf@fury.com				
TELEPHONE #					
Home:	(407) 555-3220	(407) 555-3220	(407) 555-3220	(407) 555-3220	
Work:	(407) 555-3221				
Cell:	(407) 555-3222				
Date of Birth	11/07/CCYY-56	09/30/CCYY-60	11/05/CCYY-17	09/08/CCYY-18	
Social Security #	222-44-6666	222-44-6667	222-44-6668	222-44-6669	
Marital Status/Gender	Married/Male	Married/Female	Single/Female	Single/Male	
Student Status			Full-time	Full-time	
Patient Account #	10077	10076	10078	10079	
Allergies/Medical Conditions	None	None	None	None	
PRIMARY INSURANCE CARRIER					
Name Address	Rover Insurers, Inc. 5931 Rolling Road Ronson, CO 81369	Rover Insurers, Inc. 5931 Rolling Road Ronson, CO 81369	Rover Insurers, Inc. 5931 Rolling Road Ronson, CO 81369	Rover Insurers, Inc. 5931 Rolling Road Ronson, CO 81369	
Effective Date	01/01/CCPY	01/01/CCPY	01/01/CCPY	01/01/CCPY	
Member's ID #	44-6666 NIN	44-6666 NIN	44-6666 NIN	44-6666 NIN	
Group Policy #	21088	21088	21088	21088	
Policy/Employer	Ninja Enterprises 1234 Nockout Road Newton, NM 88012				
OTHER INSURANCE CARRIER					
Name Address					
Effective Date					
Member's ID #					
Group Policy #					
Policy/Employer					
Responsible Party	Self	Self	Insured	Insured	
EMERGENCY CONTACT					
Name	Felicia Fisher	Felicia Fisher	Felicia Fisher	Felicia Fisher	
Telephone #	(407) 555-3223	(407) 555-3223	(407) 555-3223	(407) 555-3223	
Address	4444 Fairlane Blvd. Folley, FL 32208	4444 Fairlane Blvd. Folley, FL 32208	4444 Fairlane Blvd. Folley, FL 32208	4444 Fairlane Blvd. Folley, FL 32208	

Exercise **8-2**

Directions: Complete a UB-92 for each of the Hospital Admission Forms (**Documents 118–122, 124–128, 130–134, 136–141, and 143–147**) in this chapter. UB-92 forms may be provided by your instructor or purchased from a stationery store.

After completion of each UB-92 form, complete a Patient Receipt (if a payment was made), and post the transaction(s) to the patient Ledger Card/Statement of Account previously created.

Enter either **Inpt Hospital Svcs** or **Otpt Hospital Svcs** in the **Description of Service** column on the Ledger Card/Statement of Account for hospital claims.

Exercise **8-3**

Directions: Upon completion of all of the activities in Exercise 8–2, complete a Bank Deposit Slip/Ticket (located in the **Forms** chapter) for all payments made on the patient's account in this chapter.

Exercise **8-4**

Directions: Using an Insurance Claims Register (located in the **Forms** chapter) list all claims that have been fully prepared and are ready for submission to the insurance carrier for payment. Enter the date that you created the CMS-1500 in the **Date Claim Filed** column.

Exercise **8-5**

Directions: Complete an Insurance Tracer Form (located in the **Forms** chapter) for the following claim. For additional information refer to the Family Data Table (**Document 23**), completed claim form, or the Encounter Form.

Patient	Date Billed	Date of Service	Date of Illness	Diagnosis	Claim #
Felecia Francisco	10/31/CCYY	10/02/CCYY	10/02/CCYY	250.00	Document 33

Hospital Claims Beginning Financials
GONZALES FAMILY

Insurance Plan	Winter Insurance Company—ABC Corporation				

Patient:	GARY	GINNIE	GENARA	GARY JR.	GRACE
C/O DEDUCTIBLE	0.00	0.00	0.00	0.00	0.00
DEDUCTIBLE	21.00	0.00	35.00	0.00	0.00
COINSURANCE	0.00	0.00	0.00	0.00	0.00
ACCIDENT BENEFIT	0.00	0.00	0.00	0.00	0.00
LIFETIME MAXIMUM	298,012.23	995.33	34.00	2,234.65	456.00
M/N OFFICE VISITS					
OFFICE VISITS					
HOSPITAL VISITS					
DXL					
SURGERY					
ASSISTANT SURGERY					
ANESTHESIA					

Hospital Admission Form

Provider Information

Name:	Garnier General Hospital
Address:	3829 Gage Lane
City:	Garnier	State: GA	Zip Code: 30186
Telephone#:	Fax#:
Medicare ID#:	110001	UPIN#:
Tax ID #:	99-8395710	Accepts Medicare Assignment: ☐
Provider Rep:	Betty Biller	Date: 10/9/CCYY

Patient Information

Name:	Gary Gonzales
Address:	56789 Garney Lane
City:	Garberville	State: GA	Zip Code: 30012
Telephone#:	(229) 555-2100	Patient Control #: 10056
Date of Birth:	07/27/CCYY-59	Gender: Male
Marital Status:	Married	Relationship to Guarantor: Self
Student Status:	☐ Full-time	☐ Part-time
Insurance Type:	☒ Pvt ☐ M/care ☐ M/caid ☐ WC ☐ Other _____

Admission Information

Admission Date:	10/09/CCYY	Time: 7:00 AM
Discharge Date:	10/09/CCYY	Time: 10:00 PM
Attending Phy's ID#:	C08544	Date of Injury:
Attending Physician:	Gilbert Granville, M.D.

Guarantor Information

Name:	Gary Gonzales
Address:	56789 Garney Lane
City:	Garberville	State: GA	Zip Code: 30012
Insurance ID #:	88-7777 ABC	SSN: 555-88-7777
Insurance Name:	Winter Insurance Company
Insurance Group #:	36928
Employer Name:	ABC Corporation

Authorization

☒ Authorization to Release Information
☒ Authorization for Assignment of Benefits
☐ Authorization for Consent for Treatment
☐ My insurance will be billed but there may be a balance due.
Signature: Gary Gonzales   Date: 10/9/CCYY

Clinical Information

Principal Diagnosis:	Ganglion of tendon sheath
Other Diagnosis:	
Surgical Procedure:	Excision of lesion, tendon; sheath hand 10/09/CCYY
Other Procedures:	
Remarks:	
Previous Balance:	Payment:	Copay:	Adjustment:	
Total Fee:	$3361.25	Cash ☐ Check ☐ Credit ☐	Cash ☐ Check ☐ Credit ☐	Remarks:	New Balance: $3361.25

Garnier General Hospital
3829 Gage Lane
Garnier, GA 30186

Patient Name	Patient No.	Sex	Date of Birth	Admission Date	Discharge Date	Page No.
GARY GONZALES	10056	M	07/27/CCYY-59	10/09/CCYY	10/09/CCYY	1

Guarantor Name and Address
GARY GONZALES
56789 GARNEY LANE
GARBERVILLE, GA 30012

Insurance Company: WINTER INSURANCE CO.
Claim Number: DOCUMENT 118
Attending Physician: GILBERT GRANVILLE, M.D.

Date of Service	Description of Hospital Services	Service Code	Qty.	Charges	Total Charges
	DETAIL OF CURRENT CHARGES				
10/09/CCYY	MIN SURG TIME 1.00 HR	40200529	1	630.00	
10/09/CCYY	SUR-MONITR EKG CHG	40200784	1	58.00	
10/09/CCYY	SURG-BOVIE	40200826	1	32.00	
10/09/CCYY	RECOV EMERG	40202384	1	236.00	
10/09/CCYY	MINOR TRAY	40205049	1	436.00	
10/09/CCYY	PULSE OXIMETER	40205189	1	46.00	
10/09/CCYY	SUTURE MINOR 1-5	40205403	1	63.00	
10/09/CCYY	SUR-MONITR 8/P CHG	40205460	1	58.00	
10/09/CCYY	PACU VS MONITORING	40205635	1	95.00	
	TOTAL SURGERY AND RECOVERY				**1,654.00**
10/09/CCYY	OBSERVATION ROOM	40300014	1	150.00	
	TOTAL DAY CARE SERVICES				**150.00**
10/09/CCYY	NITROUS 60 MIN	40404824	1	160.00	
10/09/CCYY	FORANE 60 MIN	40405110	1	156.00	
10/09/CCYY	OXYGEN 60 MIN	40405318	1	65.00	
10/09/CCYY	ANESTH UNIT	40405912	1	260.00	
10/09/CCYY	ANES 02/SENSOR	40405920	1	150.00	
	TOTAL ANESTHESIOLOGY				**791.00**
10/09/CCYY	AIR WAY	40503062	1	8.50	
10/09/CCYY	BNDG ELASTOMULL 3 IN	40515983	1	7.50	
10/09/CCYY	KIT OUTPATIENT SURG	40518276	1	32.75	
10/09/CCYY	DRSNG GZE 4X4(10)	40525289	1	5.75	
10/09/CCYY	DRESS-TELFA 3X4	40525909	1	1.25	
10/09/CCYY	ELECTRODE DISPERS (BOVIE PAD)	40528085	1	28.50	
10/09/CCYY	GLOVES SURG	40532053	2	4.50	
10/09/CCYY	KLEENEX	40542086	1	1.25	
10/09/CCYY	O$_2$ MASK	40549412	1	20.50	
10/09/CCYY	O$_2$ HUMIDIFIER	40549420	1	30.25	
10/09/CCYY	PAC-BASIC SET UP	40550055	1	87.50	
10/09/CCYY	PILLOW DISP	40555252	1	12.25	
10/09/CCYY	SOL-IRRIGT NS 1L	40564189	1	11.00	

Garnier General Hospital
3829 Gage Lane
Garnier, GA 30186

Patient Name	Patient No.	Sex	Date of Birth	Admission Date	Discharge Date	Page No.
GARY GONZALES	10056	M	07/27/CCYY-59	07/27/CCYY	10/09/CCYY	2

Guarantor Name and Address
GARY GONZALES
56789 GARNEY LANE
GARBERVILLE, GA 30012

Insurance Company: WINTER INSURANCE CO.
Claim Number: DOCUMENT 118
Attending Physician: GILBERT GRANVILLE, M.D.

Date of Service	Description of Hospital Services	Service Code	Qty.	Charges	Total Charges
10/09/CCYY	STCKNEIT, STER 4-6	40567125	1	19.75	
10/09/CCYY	SUCTN FRAZIER	40569388	1	12.25	
10/09/CCYY	SUCTN LINER 2000	40569279	1	26.75	
10/09/CCYY	SUCTION YANKAUR HANDL	40569303	1	38.50	
10/09/CCYY	TRAY SKIN PREP W/PVP I	40577579	1	26.75	
10/09/CCYY	TBE CONNENCTGN 120	40578189	1	14.00	
10/09/CCYY	PACK TOWEL (6)	40579039	1	14.00	
10/09/CCYY	THERMOMETER GLASS	40579096	1	4.50	
10/09/CCYY	URINE CUP	40580037	1	2.25	
	TOTAL CENTRAL SUPPLY				**410.25**
10/09/CCYY	PATH DIAG, SM PART-A	40705105	1	70.00	
10/09/CCYY	PATH HANDLING PART-A	40705196	1	35.50	
	TOTAL PATH LAB				**105.50**
10/09/CCYY	ANECTINE GTTS	41742800	1	24.00	
10/09/CCYY	PENTOTHAL SDM 1GM	41756305	1	77.50	
	TOTAL PHARMACY				**101.50**
10/09/CCYY	IV CATHETER	47136049	1	24.00	
10/09/CCYY	IV START KIT	47137195	1	36.00	
10/09/CCYY	IV TUBING EXTENSION SET	47137278	1	14.00	
10/09/CCYY	IV TUBING PRIMARY SET	47137534	1	31.00	
10/09/CCYY	SOL-D-5 LR 500ML	47138169	1	44.00	
	TOTAL IV THERAPY				**149.00**

Garnier General Hospital
3829 Gage Lane
Garnier, GA 30186

Patient Name	Patient No.	Sex	Date of Birth	Admission Date	Discharge Date	Page No.
GARY GONZALES	10056	M	07/27/CCYY-59	07/27/CCYY	10/09/CCYY	3

Guarantor Name and Address
GARY GONZALES
56789 GARNEY LANE
GARBERVILLE, GA 30012

Insurance Company: WINTER INSURANCE CO
Claim Number: DOCUMENT 118
Attending Physician: GILBERT GRANVILLE, M.D.

Date of Service	Description of Hospital Services	Service Code	Qty.	Charges	Total Charges
	SUMMARY OF CHARGES				
	PHARMACY			101.50	
	IV THERAPY			149.00	
	MED-SURG SUPPLIES			1,198.25	
	PATHOLOGY LAB OR (PATH LAB)			105.50	
	OR SERVICES			630.00	
	ANESTHESIA			791.00	
	AMBUL SURG			150.00	
	RECOVERY ROOM			236.00	
	SUBTOTAL OF CHARGES				3,361.25
	PAYMENTS AND ADJUSTMENTS			NONE	
	SUBTOTAL PAYMENTS/ADJ				NONE
	BALANCE				3,361.25
	BALANCE DUE				3,361.25

Hospital Admission Form

Provider Information

Name:	Garberville Surgi-Center
Address:	P.O. Box 9923
City:	Garberville	State: GA	Zip Code: 30015
Telephone#:		Fax#:
Medicare ID#:	110002	UPIN#:
Tax ID #:	99-7493742	Accepts Medicare Assignment: ☐
Provider Rep:	*Betty Biller*	Date: *10/18/CCYY*

Admission Information

Admission Date:	10/18/CCYY	Time:	9:00 AM
Discharge Date:	10/18/CCYY	Time:	11:00 PM
Attending Phy's ID#:	D55660	Date of Injury:	
Attending Physician:	Gus Gannon, M.D.		

Guarantor Information

Name:	Gary Gonzales		
Address:	56789 Garney Lane		
City:	Garberville	State: GA	Zip Code: 30012
Insurance ID #:	88-7777 ABC	SSN:	555-88-7777
Insurance Name:	Winter Insurance Company		
Insurance Group #:	36928		
Employer Name:	ABC Corporation		

Patient Information

Name:	Genara Gonzales		
Address:	56789 Garney Lane		
City:	Garberville	State: GA	Zip Code: 30012
Telephone#:	(229) 555-2100	Patient Control #:	10057
Date of Birth:	10/17/CCYY-16	Gender:	Female
Marital Status:	Single	Relationship to Guarantor:	Child
Student Status:	☒ Full-time	☐ Part-time	
Insurance Type:	☒ Pvt ☐ M/care ☐ M/caid ☐ WC ☐ Other _____		

Authorization

☒ Authorization to Release Information
☒ Authorization for Assignment of Benefits
☐ Authorization for Consent for Treatment
☐ My insurance will be billed but there may be a balance due.

Signature: *Gary Gonzales*   Date: *10/18/CCYY*

Clinical Information

Principal Diagnosis:	Pterygium
Other Diagnosis:	
Surgical Procedure:	Excision of Pterygium with Corneal Graft 10/18/CCYY
Other Procedures:	
Remarks:	

Previous Balance:		Payment:		Copay:		Adjustment:		
Total Fee:	$2507.50	Cash ☐ Check ☐ Credit ☐		Cash ☐ Check ☐ Credit ☐		Remarks:	New Balance:	$2507.50

Garberville Surgi-Center
P.O. Box 9923
Garberville, GA 30015

Patient Name	Patient No.	Sex	Admission Date	Discharge Date	Page No.
GENARA GONZALES	10057	F	10/18/CCYY	10/18/CCYY	1

Guarantor Name and Address
GARY GONZALES
56789 GARNEY LANE
GARBERVILLE, GA 30012

Insurance Company: WINTER INSURANCE CO.
Claim Number: DOCUMENT 119
Attending Physician: GUS GANNON, M.D.

Date of Service	Description of Hospital Services	Service Code	Qty.	Charges	Total Charges
	DETAIL OF CURRENT CHARGES				
10/18/CCYY	MIN SURG TIME .75 HR	40200503	1	473.00	
10/18/CCYY	SUR-MONITR EKG CHG	40200784	1	58.00	
10/18/CCYY	MICROSCOPE	40200792	1	158.00	
10/18/CCYY	SURG-BOVIE	40200826	1	32.00	
10/18/CCYY	RECOV EMERG	40202384	1	236.00	
10/18/CCYY	MINOR TRAY	40205049	1	436.00	
10/18/CCYY	PULSE OXIMETER	40205189	1	46.00	
10/18/CCYY	SUTURE MINOR 1-5	40205403	1	63.00	
10/18/CCYY	SUR-MONITR B/P CHG	40205460	1	58.00	
10/18/CCYY	PACU VS MONITORING	40205635	1	95.00	
	TOTAL SURGERY AND RECOVERY				**1,655.00**
10/18/CCYY	OBSERVATION ROOM	40300014	1	150.00	
	TOTAL DAY CARE SERVICES				**150.00**
10/18/CCYY	OXYGEN 45 MIN	40405300	1	55.00	
	TOTAL ANESTHESIOLOGY				**55.00**
10/18/CCYY	BED PAN	40511081	1	8.50	
10/18/CCYY	BED PAN	40511081	1	8.50	
10/18/CCYY	CATH W/DELEE TRAP	40515231	1	11.00	
10/18/CCYY	KIT OUTPATIENT SURG	40518276	1	32.75	
10/18/CCYY	DRS-GAUZE XEY 4X4	40525446	1	9.75	
10/18/CCYY	GLOVES SURG	40532053	1	2.25	
10/18/CCYY	KLEENEX	40542086	1	1.25	
10/18/CCYY	O$_2$ MASK	40542086	1	20.50	
10/18/CCYY	PCK DRAPE SHE MED	40550139	2	55.50	
10/18/CCYY	PACK X LARGE GOWN	40550147	2	51.00	
10/18/CCYY	PAD-EYE	40552150	1	1.25	
10/18/CCYY	PAD-EYE	40552150	2	2.50	
10/18/CCYY	PILLOW DISP	40555252	1	12.25	
10/18/CCYY	SYRINGE 1CC TO 10 CC W/NEEDLE	40572166	1	4.75	
10/18/CCYY	TRAY SKIN PREP W/PVP	40577579	1	26.75	

Garberville Surgi-Center
P.O. Box 9923
Garberville, GA 30015

Patient Name	Patient No.	Sex	Admission Date	Discharge Date	Page No.
GENARA GONZALES	10057	F	10/18/CCYY	10/18/CCYY	2

Guarantor Name and Address
GARY GONZALES
56789 GARNEY LANE
GARBERVILLE, GA 30012

Insurance Company: WINTER INSURANCE CO.
Claim Number: DOCUMENT 119
Attending Physician: GUS GANNON, M.D.

Date of Service	Description of Hospital Services	Service Code	Qty.	Charges	Total Charges
10/18/CCYY	PACK TOWEL (6)	40579039	2	28.00	
10/18/CCYY	THERMOMETER GLASS	40579096	1	4.50	
10/18/CCYY	URINE CUP	40580037	1	2.25	
10/18/CCYY	URINE CUP	40580037	1	2.25	
10/18/CCYY	EYE SPEAR WECK	40582009	1	2.75	
10/18/CCYY	EYE SPEAR WECK	40582009	1	2.75	
	TOTAL CENTRAL SUPPLY				**291.00**
10/18/CCYY	PATH DIAG, SM PART-A	40705105	1	70.00	
10/18/CCYY	PATH HANDLING PART-A	40705196	1	35.50	
	TOTAL LAB PATH				**105.50**
10/18/CCYY	INNOVAR 2 ML	41750456	1	37.00	
10/18/CCYY	XYLOCAINE 1% EPI	47162931	1	13.50	
10/18/CCYY	MAXITRL OPTH DR5C	41771007	1	32.00	
10/18/CCYY	TETRACAINE OPTH	41776402	1	17.50	
	TOTAL PHARMACY				**100.00**
10/18/CCYY	IV CATHETER	47136049	1	24.00	
10/18/CCYY	IV START KIT	47137195	1	36.00	
10/18/CCYY	IV TUBING EXTENSION SET	47137278	1	14.00	
10/18/CCYY	IV TUBING PRIMARY SET	47137534	1	31.00	
10/18/CCYY	SOL-D-5 LR 1000 ML	47138177	1	46.00	
	TOTAL IV THERAPY				**151.00**

Garberville Surgi-Center
P.O. Box 9923
Garberville, GA 30015

Patient Name	Patient No.	Sex	Admission Date	Discharge Date	Page No.
GENARA GONZALES	10057	F	10/18/CCYY	10/18/CCYY	3

Guarantor Name and Address
GARY GONZALES
56789 GARNEY LANE
GARBERVILLE, GA 30012

Insurance Company: WINTER INSURANCE CO.
Claim Number: DOCUMENT 119
Attending Physician: GUS GANNON, M.D.

Date of Service	Description of Hospital Services	Service Code	Qty.	Charges	Total Charges
	SUMMARY OF CHARGES				
	PHARMACY			100.00	
	IV THERAPY			151.00	
	MED-SURG SUPPLIES			1,237.00	
	PATHOLOGY LAB OR (PATH LAB)			105.50	
	OR SERVICES			473.00	
	ANESTHESIA			55.00	
	AMBUL SURG			150.00	
	RECOVERY ROOM			236.00	
	SUBTOTAL OF CHARGES				2,507.50
	PAYMENTS AND ADJUSTMENTS			NONE	
	SUBTOTAL PAYMENTS/ADJ				NONE
	BALANCE				2,507.50
	BALANCE DUE				2,507.50

Hospital Admission Form

DOCUMENT 120

Provider Information

Name:	Garberville Main Hospital
Address:	567 Grapevine Road

City:	Garberville	State:	GA	Zip Code:	30025

Telephone#:	Fax#:	
Medicare ID#:	110003	UPIN#:

Tax ID #:	99-5730375	Accepts Medicare Assignment: ☐
Provider Rep:	*Betty Biller*	Date: *10/19/CCYY*

Patient Information

Name:	Ginnie Gonzales
Address:	56789 Garney Lane

City:	Garberville	State:	GA	Zip Code:	30012
Telephone#:	(229) 555-2100	Patient Control #:	10058		
Date of Birth:	01/07/CCYY-57	Gender:	Female		
Marital Status:	Married	Relationship to Guarantor:		Spouse	
Student Status:	☐ Full-time	☐ Part-time			
Insurance Type:	☒ Pvt ☐ M/care ☐ M/caid ☐ WC ☐ Other _____				

Admission Information

Admission Date:	10/19/CCYY	Time:	10:00 AM
Discharge Date:	10/19/CCYY	Time:	3:00 PM
Attending Phy's ID#:	E84560	Date of Injury:	
Attending Physician:	Grace Gleason, M.D.		

Guarantor Information

Name:	Gary Gonzales
Address:	56789 Garney Lane

City:	Garberville	State:	GA	Zip Code:	30012

Insurance ID #:	88-7777 ABC	SSN:	555-88-7777
Insurance Name:	Winter Insurance Company		
Insurance Group #:	36928		
Employer Name:	ABC Corporation		

Authorization

☒ Authorization to Release Information
☒ Authorization for Assignment of Benefits
☐ Authorization for Consent for Treatment
☐ My insurance will be billed but there may be a balance due.

Signature: *Ginnie Gonzales*   Date: *10/19/CCYY*

Clinical Information

Principal Diagnosis:	Other Specified Gastritis without Hemmorrhage	
Other Diagnosis:	Diaphragmatic Hernia	
Surgical Procedure:	EGD with closed biopsy	10/19/CCYY
Other Procedures:	Colonoscopy	10/19/CCYY
Remarks:		

Previous Balance:		Payment:		Copay:		Adjustment:			
Total Fee:	$2671.75	Cash ☐ Check ☐ Credit ☐		Cash ☐ Check ☐ Credit ☐		Remarks:		New Balance:	$2671.75

Garberville Main Hospital
567 Grapevine Road
Garberville, GA 30025

Patient Name	Patient No.	Sex	Date of Birth	Admission Date	Discharge Date	Page No.
GINNIE GONZALES	10058	F	01/07/CCYY-57	01/07/CCYY	10/19/CCYY	1

Guarantor Name and Address
GARY GONZALES
56789 GARNEY LANE
GARBERVILLE, GA 30012

Insurance Company: WINTER INSURANCE CO.
Claim Number: DOCUMENT 120
Attending Physician: GRACE GLEASON, M.D.

Date of Service	Description of Hospital Services	Service Code	Qty.	Charges	Total Charges
	DETAIL OF CURRENT CHARGES				
10/19/CCYY	MIN SURG TIME 1.00HR	40200529	1	630.00	
10/19/CCYY	SUR-MONITR EKG CHG	40200784	1	58.00	
10/19/CCYY	RECOV EMERG	40202384	1	236.00	
10/19/CCYY	MINOR TRAY	40205049	1	436.00	
10/19/CCYY	PULSLE OXIMETER	40205189	1	46.00	
10/19/CCYY	GASTROINTESTINALSCOPE	40205270	1	86.00	
10/19/CCYY	COLONOSCOPE	40205304	1	86.00	
10/19/CCYY	SUR-MONITR B/P CHG	40205460	1	58.00	
10/19/CCYY	PACU VS MONITORING	40205635	1	95.00	
	TOTAL SURGERY AND RECOVERY				**1,731.00**
10/19/CCYY	OBSERVATION ROOM	40300014	1	150.00	
	TOTAL DAY CARE SERVICES				**150.00**
10/19/CCYY	OXYGEN 60 MIN	40405318	1	65.00	
	TOTAL ANESTHESIOLOGY				**65.00**
10/19/CCYY	KIT OUTPATIENT SURG	40518276	1	32.75	
10/19/CCYY	DRS-CAUZE XRY 4X4	40525446	1	9.75	
10/19/CCYY	GLOVES EUDERM	40532079	2	30.00	
10/19/CCYY	KLEENEX	40542086	1	1.25	
10/19/CCYY	O_2 MASK	40549412	1	20.50	
10/19/CCYY	O_2 HUMIDIFIER	40549420	1	30.25	
10/19/CCYY	PCK DRAPE SHE MED	40550139	1	27.75	
10/19/CCYY	PILLOW DISP	40555252	1	12.25	
10/19/CCYY	SUCTN LINER 2000	40569279	1	26.75	
10/19/CCYY	SUCTION YANKAUR HNDL	40569303	1	38.50	
10/19/CCYY	SYRINGE 1 CC TO 10 CC W/NEEDLE	40572166	1	4.75	
10/19/CCYY	TBE CONNECTGN	40578189	1	14.00	
10/19/CCYY	PACK TOWEL (6)	40579039	1	14.00	
10/19/CCYY	THERMOMETER GLASS	40579096	1	4.50	
10/19/CCYY	URINE CUP	40580037	1	2.25	
	TOTAL CENTRAL SUPPLY				**269.25**

Garberville Main Hospital
567 Grapevine Road
Garberville, GA 30025

Patient Name	Patient No.	Sex	Date of Birth	Admission Date	Discharge Date	Page No.
GINNIE GONZALES	10058	F	01/07/CCYY-57	01/07/CCYY	10/19/CCYY	2

Guarantor Name and Address
GARY GONZALES
56789 GARNEY LANE
GARBERVILLE, GA 30012

Insurance Company: WINTER INSURANCE CO.
Claim Number: DOCUMENT 120
Attending Physician: GRACE GLEASON, M.D.

Date of Service	Description of Hospital Services	Service Code	Qty.	Charges	Total Charges
10/19/CCYY	GROSS & MICRO PART-A	40705097	1	65.50	
10/19/CCYY	PATH HANDLING PART-A	40705196	1	35.50	
	TOTAL PATH LAB				**101.00**
10/19/CCYY	GO-LIGHTLY	41715103	1	73.00	
10/19/CCYY	DEMEROL INJ	41746900	1	17.00	
10/19/CCYY	MISCELLANEOUS INJ	41753609	1	10.00	
	DIPRIVAN		1		
10/19/CCYY	STADOL 2 MG IM	41759457	1	11.50	
	TOTAL PHARMACY				**111.50**
10/19/CCYY	OXYGEN SET-UP	41801952	1	62.00	
10/19/CCYY	OXYGEN PER HOUR	41802208	1	11.00	
	TOTAL INHALATION THERAPY				**73.00**
10/19/CCYY	IV CATHETER	47136049	1	24.00	
10/19/CCYY	IV START KIT	47137195	1	36.00	
10/19/CCYY	IV START KIT	47137195	1	36.00	
10/19/CCYY	IV TUBING PRIMARY SET	47137534	1	31.00	
10/19/CCYY	SOL-D-5-W 500 ML	47138060	1	44.00	
	TOTAL IV THERAPY				**171.00**

Garberville Main Hospital
567 Grapevine Road
Garberville, GA 30025

Patient Name	Patient No.	Sex	Date of Birth	Admission Date	Discharge Date	Page No.
GINNIE GONZALES	10058	F	01/07/CCYY-57	01/07/CCYY	10/19/CCYY	3

Guarantor Name and Address
GARY GONZALES
56789 GARNEY LANE
GARBERVILLE, GA 30012

Insurance Company: WINTER INSURANCE CO.
Claim Number: DOCUMENT 120
Attending Physician: GRACE GLEASON, M.D.

Date of Service	Description of Hospital Services	Service Code	Qty.	Charges	Total Charges
	SUMMARY OF CHARGES				
	PHARMACY			111.50	
	IV THERAPY			171.00	
	MED-SURG SUPPLIES			1,134.25	
	PATHOLOGY LAB OR (PATH LAB)			101.00	
	OR SERVICES			630.00	
	ANESTHESIA			65.00	
	RESPIRATORY SVC			73.00	
	AMBUL SURG			150.00	
	RECOVERY ROOM			236.00	
	SUBTOTAL OF CHARGES				2,671.75
	PAYMENTS AND ADJUSTMENTS			NONE	
	SUBTOTAL PAYMENTS/ADJ				NONE
	BALANCE				2,671.75
	BALANCE DUE				2,671.75

Hospital Admission Form

Provider Information

Name:	Garberville General Hospital
Address:	1234 Gary Lane

City:	Garberville	State:	GA	Zip Code:	30014

Telephone#:		Fax#:	
Medicare ID#:	110004	UPIN#:	
Tax ID #:	99-3847205	Accepts Medicare Assignment:	☐
Provider Rep:	*Betty Biller*	Date:	*9/18/CCYY*

Admission Information

Admission Date:	09/18/CCYY	Time:	8:00 AM
Discharge Date:	09/18/CCYY	Time:	9:00 PM
Attending Phy's ID#:	F70980	Date of Injury:	9/17/CCYY
Attending Physician:	Gene Gaston, M.D.		

Guarantor Information

Name:	Gary Gonzales
Address:	56789 Garney Lane

City:	Garberville	State:	GA	Zip Code:	30012

Patient Information

Name:	Gary Gonzales, Jr.
Address:	56789 Garney Lane

City:	Garberville	State:	GA	Zip Code:	30012
Telephone#:	(229) 555-2100	Patient Control #:	10059		
Date of Birth:	06/22/CCYY-18	Gender:	Male		
Marital Status:	Single	Relationship to Guarantor:		Child	
Student Status:	☒ Full-time	☐ Part-time			
Insurance Type:	☒ Pvt ☐ M/care ☐ M/caid ☐ WC ☐ Other _____				

Insurance ID #:	88-7777 ABC	SSN:	555-88-7777
Insurance Name:	Winter Insurance Company		
Insurance Group #:	36928		
Employer Name:	ABC Corporation		

Authorization

☒ Authorization to Release Information
☒ Authorization for Assignment of Benefits
☐ Authorization for Consent for Treatment
☐ My insurance will be billed but there may be a balance due.

Signature: *Gary Gonzales*   Date: *9/18/CCYY*

Clinical Information

Principal Diagnosis:	Open wound knee/leg with tendon tear	
Other Diagnosis:		
Surgical Procedure:	Excision knee semilunar cartilage	9/18/CCYY
Other Procedures:	Knee arthroscopy	9/18/CCYY
Remarks:	Fell at home on concrete driveway on 9/17/CCYY.	

Previous Balance:		Payment:		Copay:		Adjustment:			
Total Fee:	$8910.00	Cash ☐ Check ☐ Credit ☐		Cash ☐ Check ☐ Credit ☐		Remarks:		New Balance:	$8910.00

Garberville General Hospital
1234 Gary Lane
Garberville, GA 30014

Patient Name	Patient No.	Sex		Admission Date	Discharge Date	Page No.
GARY GONZALES JR.	10059	M		09/18/CCYY	09/18/CCYY	1

Guarantor Name and Address
GARY GONZALES
56789 GARNEY LANE
GARBERVILLE, GA 30012

Insurance Company: WINTER INSURANCE CO.
Claim Number: DOCUMENT 121
Attending Physician: GENE GASTON, M.D.

Date of Service	Description of Hospital Services	Service Code	Qty.	Unit Price	Total Charges
09/18/CCYY	ANCEF 1 GM VIAL	4170161	3	32.00	96.00
09/18/CCYY	ANCEF 1 GM VIAL	4170161	3	32.00	96.00
09/18/CCYY	HEXADROL 10 MG INJ	4170597	1	55.00	55.00
09/18/CCYY	ETHRANE MIN CHRG	4170672	1	25.00	25.00
09/18/CCYY	PENTOTHAL PER 100 MG	4170710	3	24.00	72.00
09/18/CCYY	HYPOQUE 60% INJ	4170712	1	55.00	55.00
09/18/CCYY	PAVULON PER CC	4170728	4	15.00	60.00
09/18/CCYY	BETADINE OINT 1 OZ	4170803	1	12.00	12.00
09/18/CCYY	XYLOCAINE 2% JELLY	4170855	1	17.00	17.00
09/18/CCYY	DEMEROL TUBEX INJ	4171076	2	16.00	32.00
09/18/CCYY	DEMEROL TUBEX INJ	4171076	2	16.00	32.00
09/18/CCYY	ETHRANE PER 5 MIN	4172403	39	8.00	312.00
09/18/CCYY	INAPSINE 2 CC INJ	4172498	1	12.00	12.00
	PHARMACY **SUBTOTAL**	** 250			**876.00**
09/18/CCYY	D5.45 NS 500 ML	4171333	2	28.00	56.00
09/18/CCYY	D5.45 NS 500 ML	4171333	1	28.00	28.00
09/18/CCYY	.9 N/S IRRIG 1000/2000 ML	4171344	3	28.00	84.00
09/18/CCYY	D5LR 500 ML	4172402	2	28.00	56.00
09/18/CCYY	D5W 50 ML	4174046	2	28.00	56.00
09/18/CCYY	D5W 50 ML	4174046	3	28.00	84.00
	IV SOLUTIONS **SUBTOTAL**	** 258			**364.00**
09/18/CCYY	I.V. SERVICE FEE	4172419	2	23.00	46.00
09/18/CCYY	I.V. SERVICE FEE	4172419	3	23.00	69.00
	I.V. THERAPY **SUBTOTAL**	** 260			**115.00**
09/18/CCYY	GOWN STERILE	4050009	1	12.00	12.00
09/18/CCYY	ANESTH BREATHIN CIRC	4050014	1	25.00	25.00
09/18/CCYY	ANESTH MASK DISP	4050047	1	20.00	20.00
09/18/CCYY	KNEE IMMOBILIZER-ALL SIZES	4050797	1	63.00	63.00
09/18/CCYY	CASSETTE COVERS DISP	4050807	1	13.00	13.00
09/18/CCYY	FRAZIER SUCTION TIP	4050833	1	13.00	13.00
09/18/CCYY	YANKAUER SUCTION TIP	4050835	1	11.00	11.00
09/18/CCYY	TELFA ALL SIZES	4050893	1	6.00	6.00
09/18/CCYY	ANGIOCATH	4051000	2	12.00	24.00

Garberville General Hospital
1234 Gary Lane
Garberville, GA 30014

Patient Name	Patient No.	Sex	Admission Date	Discharge Date	Page No.
GARY GONZALES JR.	10059	M	09/18/CCYY	09/18/CCYY	2

Guarantor Name and Address
GARY GONZALES
56789 GARNEY LANE
GARBERVILLE, GA 30012

Insurance Company: WINTER INSURANCE CO.
Claim Number: DOCUMENT 121
Attending Physician: GENE GASTON, M.D.

Date of Service	Description of Hospital Services	Service Code	Qty.	Unit Price	Total Charges
09/18/CCYY	MIDSTREAM KIT	4051052	1	9.00	9.00
09/18/CCYY	CRUTCHES ADULT	4051059	1	58.00	58.00
09/18/CCYY	AIRWAYS ALL SIZES	4051071	1	8.00	8.00
09/18/CCYY	SUCTION SET 10 FT	4051129	3	26.00	78.00
09/18/CCYY	ENDOTRACH TUBE	4051160	1	28.00	28.00
09/18/CCYY	IV START PAK	4051190	1	12.00	12.00
09/18/CCYY	RAZOR DISP	4051231	1	2.00	2.00
09/18/CCYY	RAYTEC 4X4 SPONGE 10	4051232	2	11.00	22.00
09/18/CCYY	URINAL	4051369	1	6.00	6.00
09/18/CCYY	O$_2$ MASK	4051410	1	13.00	13.00
09/18/CCYY	ESOPHAGEAL SETH DISP	4051460	1	25.00	25.00
09/18/CCYY	SPECIMEN CONTAINER	4051535	1	4.00	4.00
09/18/CCYY	SUCTION LINER DISP	4053009	3	17.00	51.00
09/18/CCYY	KERLEX ROLL K6730	4053010	1	7.00	7.00
09/18/CCYY	O$_2$ HUMIDIFIER	4053048	1	19.00	19.00
09/18/CCYY	DRAPE SHEET MEDIUM	4053063	1	10.00	10.00
09/18/CCYY	SUTURE ETHILON	4053136	3	13.00	39.00
09/18/CCYY	SUTURE VICRYL	4053137	2	14.00	28.00
09/18/CCYY	MAYO COVER	4053222	3	22.00	66.00
09/18/CCYY	UNDERPAD PER SIX	4053319	1	10.00	10.00
09/18/CCYY	ADDITIVE SET, V1444	4053320	1	16.00	16.00
09/18/CCYY	SECONDARY IV V1903 T	4053325	1	21.00	21.00
09/18/CCYY	DIAL A FLO	4053329	1	28.00	28.00
09/18/CCYY	SPECIMEN STOCKING	4054005	2	9.00	18.00
	MED/SURG SUPPLIES **SUBTOTAL**	** 270			**765.00**
09/18/CCYY	ARTHROSOCOPY BLADE	4054060	1	150.00	150.00
	SUPPLY/OTHER **SUBTOTAL**	** 279			**150.00**
09/18/CCYY	COMPLETE BLOOD COUNT 85023	4060117	1	53.00	53.00
09/18/CCYY	A.P.T.T. PATIENT 85730	4060245	1	50.00	50.00
09/18/CCYY	PROTIME 85610	4060318	1	50.00	50.00
09/18/CCYY	ROUTINE URINALYSIS 81000	4060487	1	46.00	46.00
09/18/CCYY	ELECTROLYTES PANEL 80004	4062177	1	171.00	171.00
	LABORATORY **SUBTOTAL**	** 300			**370.00**

Garberville General Hospital
1234 Gary Lane
Garberville, GA 30014

Patient Name	Patient No.	Sex		Admission Date	Discharge Date	Page No.
GARY GONZALES JR.	10059	M		09/18/CCYY	09/18/CCYY	3

Guarantor Name and Address
GARY GONZALES
56789 GARNEY LANE
GARBERVILLE, GA 30012

Insurance Company: WINTER INSURANCE CO.
Claim Number: DOCUMENT 121
Attending Physician: GENE GASTON, M.D.

Date of Service	Description of Hospital Services	Service Code	Qty.	Unit Price	Total Charges
09/18/CCYY	CHEST 2 VIEWS EA 71020	4140063	1	105.00	105.00
09/18/CCYY	KNEE COMPLETE EACH 73564	4140116	3	85.00	255.00
09/18/CCYY	PORTABLE X-RAY	4140208	3	40.00	120.00
	DX X-RAY **SUBTOTAL**	** 320			**480.00**
09/18/CCYY	RECOVERY ROOM 1ST HOUR	4020059	1	233.00	233.00
09/18/CCYY	CLASS III 1ST HOUR	4020505	1	1,109.00	1,109.00
09/18/CCYY	CLASS III ADD 15 MIN	4020506	12	277.00	3,324.00
	OR SERVICES **SUBTOTAL**	** 360			**4,666.00**
09/18/CCYY	ANESTHESIA ADD'L 15 MINUTES	4041001	12	55.00	660.00
09/18/CCYY	ANESTHESIA FIRST HOUR	4041004	1	253.00	253.00
	ANESTHESIA **SUBTOTAL**	** 370			**913.00**
09/18/CCYY	GAIT TRAINING 97116	4200024	1	36.00	36.00
	PHYSICAL THERP **SUBTOTAL**	** 420			**36.00**
09/18/CCYY	OUT-PT SURG DAY CARE	3370001	1	150.00	150.00
	PHYSICAL THERAPY **SUBTOTAL**	** 490			**150.00**
09/18/CCYY	OUT PATIENT KIT	4054052	1	25.00	25.00
	PT CONVENIENCE **SUBTOTAL**	** 990			**25.00**

Hospital Admission Form

Provider Information

Name:	Garberville Women's Clinic
Address:	P.O. Box 7777

City:	Garberville	State:	GA	Zip Code:	30013

Telephone#:		Fax#:	

Medicare ID#:	110005	UPIN#:	

Tax ID #:	99-4739479	Accepts Medicare Assignment:	☐

Provider Rep:	*Betty Biller*	Date: 8/24/CCYY

Patient Information

Name:	Grace Gonzales
Address:	56789 Garney Lane

City:	Garberville	State:	GA	Zip Code:	30012

Telephone#:	(229) 555-2100	Patient Control #:	10060

Date of Birth:	08/20/CCYY-17	Gender:	Female

Marital Status:	Single	Relationship to Guarantor:	Child

Student Status:	☒ Full-time	☐ Part-time

Insurance Type:	☒ Pvt ☐ M/care ☐ M/caid ☐ WC ☐ Other _____

Admission Information

Admission Date:	08/24/CCYY	Time:	7:00 AM
Discharge Date:	08/24/CCYY	Time:	7:00 PM

Attending Phy's ID#:	G80405	Date of Injury:	
Attending Physician:	Graciela Greene, M.D.		

Guarantor Information

Name:	Gary Gonzales
Address:	56789 Garney Lane

City:	Garberville	State:	GA	Zip Code:	30012

Insurance ID #:	88-7777 ABC	SSN:	555-88-7777
Insurance Name:	Winter Insurance Company		
Insurance Group #:	36928		
Employer Name:	ABC Corporation		

Authorization

☒ Authorization to Release Information
☒ Authorization for Assignment of Benefits
☐ Authorization for Consent for Treatment
☐ My insurance will be billed but there may be a balance due.

Signature: *Gary Gonzales*   Date: 8/24/CCYY

Clinical Information

Principal Diagnosis:	Female stress incontinence	
Other Diagnosis:	Prolapse of vagina	
Surgical Procedure:	Cystocele/Rectocele Repair	8/24/CCYY
Other Procedures:	Cervical Lesion Destruction	8/24/CCYY

Remarks:	

Previous Balance:		Payment:		Copay:		Adjustment:			
Total Fee:	$6137.75	Cash ☐ Check ☐ Credit ☐		Cash ☐ Check ☐ Credit ☐		Remarks:		New Balance:	$6137.75

Garberville Women's Clinic
P.O. Box 7777
Garberville, GA 30013

Patient Name	Patient No.	Sex		Admission Date	Discharge Date	Page No.
GRACE GONZALES	10060	F		08/24/CCYY	08/24/CCYY	1

Guarantor Name and Address
GARY GONZALES
56789 GARNEY LANE
GARBERVILLE, GA 30012

Insurance Company: WINTER INSURANCE CO.
Claim Number: DOCUMENT 122
Attending Physician: GRACIELA GREENE, M.D.

Date of Service	Description of Hospital Services	Service Code	Qty.	Charges	Total Charges
	DETAIL OF CURRENT CHARGES				
08/24/CCYY	ROOM & BOARD	99020505	0	0.00	
	TOTAL ROOM & BOARD				**0.00**
08/24/CCYY	MAJ SURGTIME 1.50 HR	40200149	1	935.00	
08/24/CCYY	SUR-MONITR EKG CHG	40200784	1	58.00	
08/24/CCYY	SURG-BOVIE	40200826	1	32.00	
08/24/CCYY	RECOV EMERG	40202384	1	236.00	
08/24/CCYY	MAJOR TRAY	40205015	1	809.00	
08/24/CCYY	PULSE OXIMETER	40205189	1	46.00	
08/24/CCYY	SUTURE MAJOR 6-15	40205445	1	86.00	
08/24/CCYY	SUR-MONITR B/P CHG	40205460	1	58.00	
08/24/CCYY	HERZOG ARGON LASER	40205536	1	578.00	
08/24/CCYY	GYNCATH 600 EA	40205569	1	368.00	
08/24/CCYY	PACU VS MONITORING	40205635	1	95.00	
	TOTAL SURGERY AND RECOVERY				**3,301.00**
08/24/CCYY	NITROUS 90 MIN	40404840	1	237.00	
08/24/CCYY	FORANE 90 MIN	40405136	1	234.00	
08/24/CCYY	OXYGEN 90 MIN	40405334	1	86.00	
08/24/CCYY	ANESTH UNIT	40405932	1	260.00	
08/24/CCYY	ANES O2/SENSOR	40405920	1	150.00	
	TOTAL ANESTHESIOLOGY				**967.00**
08/24/CCYY	ADMIT KITS	40503021	1	42.00	
08/24/CCYY	AIR WAY	40503062	1	8.50	
08/24/CCYY	BAG VAGINAL IRRIG	40504359	1	18.00	
08/24/CCYY	CONNECTOR TRANS-JET	40519383	1	4.50	
08/24/CCYY	DRS-GAUZE XRY	40525446	1	9.75	
08/24/CCYY	ELECTRODE DISPERS (BOVIE PAD)	40528085	1	28.50	
08/24/CCYY	GLOVES SURG	40532053	4	9.00	
08/24/CCYY	KLEENEX	40542086	1	1.25	
	TOTAL GENERAL SUPPLY				**121.50**

Garberville Women's Clinic
P.O. Box 7777
Garberville, GA 30013

Patient Name	Patient No.	Sex	Admission Date	Discharge Date	Page No.
GRACE GONZALES	10060	F	08/24/CCYY	08/24/CCYY	2

Guarantor Name and Address
GARY GONZALES
56789 GARNEY LANE
GARBERVILLE, GA 30012

Insurance Company: WINTER INSURANCE CO.
Claim Number: DOCUMENT 122
Attending Physician: GRACIELA GREENE, M.D.

Date of Service	Description of Hospital Services	Service Code	Qty.	Charges	Total Charges
08/24/CCYY	CEFTIZOXIME PBK-2 GM* PINPSK	41750065	7	206.50	
08/24/CCYY	MED PIGGY BACKS	41710047	1	28.50	
08/24/CCYY	MEFOXIN 2 GM	41753062	1	92.00	
08/24/CCYY	MEFOXIN 2 GM	41753062	4	368.00	
08/24/CCYY	PENTOTHAL SDM 1 GM	41756305	1	77.50	
08/24/CCYY	PITRESSIN 20 UNIT	41756503	1	26.50	
08/24/CCYY	SUBLIMAZE 2 CC	41759804	1	21.50	
08/24/CCYY	TRACIUM 50 MG AMP	41761669	1	70.00	
08/24/CCYY	PROFILE SERV CHRG	41763756		14.00	
08/24/CCYY	SULTRIN VAG CREAM	41775206	1	32.00	
	TOTAL PHARMACY				**936.50**
08/24/CCYY	OXYGEN SET-UP	41808952	1	62.00	
08/24/CCYY	OXYGEN PER IIOUR	41802208	1	11.00	
	TOTAL INHALATION THERAPY				**73.00**
08/24/CCYY	IV CATHETER	47136049	1	24.00	
08/24/CCYY	IV START KIT	47137195	1	36.00	
08/24/CCYY	IV TUBING EXTENSION SET	47137278	1	14.00	
08/24/CCYY	IV TUBING PRIMARY SET	47137534	1	31.00	
08/24/CCYY	SOL-D-5 LR 1000 ML	47138177	1	46.00	
08/24/CCYY	SOL-D-5 LR 1000 ML	47138177	1	46.00	
08/24/CCYY	SP;-O.9NS 500 ML	47138292	1	39.00	
	TOTAL IV THERAPY				**236.00**
08/24/CCYY	URINE ROUTINE	40170110	1	36.00	
08/24/CCYY	UROTHROMBIN TIME	40150674	1	51.25	
08/24/CCYY	BTT	40150934	1	59.50	
08/24/CCYY	CDC	40150393	1	64.75	
08/24/CCYY	CREATININE	40151331	1	50.50	
08/24/CCYY	BUN	40154863	1	49.50	
08/24/CCYY	TYPE & RH	45110009	1	37.50	
08/24/CCYY	ANTIBODY SCREEN	40110132	1	61.00	
08/24/CCYY	X-MATCH	40110181	1	92.75	
	TOTAL LABORATORY-PRIMARY				**502.75**

Garberville Women's Clinic
P.O. Box 7777
Garberville, GA 30013

Patient Name	Patient No.	Sex	Admission Date	Discharge Date	Page No.
GRACE GONZALES	10060	F	08/24/CCYY	08/24/CCYY	3

Guarantor Name and Address
GARY GONZALES
56789 GARNEY LANE
GARBERVILLE, GA 30012

Insurance Company: WINTER INSURANCE CO.
Claim Number: DOCUMENT 122
Attending Physician: GRACIELA GREENE, M.D.

Date of Service	Description of Hospital Services	Service Code	Qty.	Charges	Total Charges
	SUMMARY OF CHARGES				
	PHARMACY			936.50	
	IV THERAPY			236.00	
	MED-SUR SUPPLIES			2,251.50	
	PATHOLOGY LAB OR (PATH LAB)			502.75	
	OR SERVICES			935.00	
	ANESTHESIA			967.00	
	RESPIRATORY SVC			73.00	
	RECOVERY ROOM			236.00	
	SUBTOTAL OF CHARGES				6,137.75
	PAYMENTS AND ADJUSTMENTS			NONE	
	SUBTOTAL PAYMENTS/ADJ				NONE
	BALANCE				6,137.75
	BALANCE DUE				6,137.75

Hospital Claims Beginning Financials

LEVINE FAMILY

Insurance Plan	Rover Insurers, Inc.—Ninja Enterprises				

Patient:	LARRY	LANNIE	LLOYD	LISA	LILA
C/O DEDUCTIBLE	0.00	0.00	0.00	0.00	0.00
DEDUCTIBLE	50.00	75.00	20.00	0.00	5.46
COINSURANCE	0.00	0.00	0.00	0.00	0.00
ACCIDENT BENEFIT	0.00	157.50	0.00	0.00	0.00
LIFETIME MAXIMUM	3,005.00	154,602.92	4,027.60	2,767.60	11,226.00
M/N OFFICE VISITS					
OFFICE VISITS					
HOSPITAL VISITS					
DXL					
SURGERY					
ASSISTANT SURGERY					
ANESTHESIA					

Hospital Admission Form

Provider Information

Name:	Lafayette General Hospital
Address:	5566 Lopez Street
City:	Lafayette — State: LA — Zip Code: 70517
Telephone#:	Fax#:
Medicare ID#:	190006 — UPIN#:
Tax ID #:	88-2233456 — Accepts Medicare Assignment: ☐
Provider Rep:	*Betty Biller* — Date: *9/19/CCYY*

Patient Information

Name:	Larry Levine
Address:	6780 Lodge Lane
City:	Lafayette — State: LA — Zip Code: 70513
Telephone#:	(504) 555-7051 — Patient Control #: 10061
Date of Birth:	10/10/CCYY-64 — Gender: Male
Marital Status:	Married — Relationship to Guarantor: Self
Student Status:	☐ Full-time ☐ Part-time
Insurance Type:	☒ Pvt ☐ M/care ☐ M/caid ☐ WC ☐ Other _____

Admission Information

Admission Date:	09/19/CCYY — Time: 8:00 AM
Discharge Date:	09/19/CCYY — Time: 11:00 AM
Attending Phy's ID#:	H25547 — Date of Injury:
Attending Physician:	Linda La Russo, M.D.

Guarantor Information

Name:	Larry Levine
Address:	6780 Lodge Lane
City:	Lafayette — State: LA — Zip Code: 70513
Insurance ID #:	22-3333 NIN — SSN: 001-22-3333
Insurance Name:	Rover Insurers, Inc.
Insurance Group #:	21088
Employer Name:	Ninja Enterprises

Authorization

☒ Authorization to Release Information
☒ Authorization for Assignment of Benefits
☐ Authorization for Consent for Treatment
☐ My insurance will be billed but there may be a balance due.
Signature: *Larry Levine* — Date: *9/19/CCYY*

Clinical Information

Principal Diagnosis:	Calculus of Kidney
Other Diagnosis:	
Surgical Procedure:	Insertion of urethral stent — 9/19/CCYY
Other Procedures:	
Remarks:	

Previous Balance:	Payment:	Copay:	Adjustment:	
Total Fee: $862.60	Cash ☐ Check ☐ Credit ☐	Cash ☐ Check ☐ Credit ☐	Remarks:	New Balance: $862.60

Lafayette General Hospital
5566 Lopez Street
Lafayette, LA 70517

Patient Name	Patient No.	Sex	Date of Birth	Admission Date	Discharge Date	Page No.
LARRY LEVINE	10061	M	10/10/CCYY-64	09/19/CCYY	09/19/CCYY	1

Guarantor Name and Address
LARRY LEVINE
6780 LODGE LANE
LAFAYETTE, LA 70513

Insurance Company: ROVER INSURERS, INC.
Claim Number: DOCUMENT 124
Attending Physician: LINDA LA RUSSO, M.D.

Date of Service	Description of Hospital Services	Service Code	Qty.	Charges	Total Charges
09/19/CCYY	XYLO EPI 1.5% 30M90749-95	50100866	1	37.45	
09/19/CCYY	XYLOCAINE 1.5% 2090749-95	50100593	1	40.35	
09/19/CCYY	VERSED 5 YR 2 ML 90749-95	50110873	1	55.55	
09/19/CCYY	SUBLIMAZE 2 ML 90749-95	50100270	1	31.05	
	TOTAL PHARMACY-INJECTABLES			–	164.40
09/19/CCYY	IV LACT RINGERS 100099	50271105	2	126.10	
09/19/CCYY	SET IVAC PRIMARY 00920	50290295	1	47.85	
09/19/CCYY	SET, IV EXTENSION 00920	50290576	1	36.40	
	TOTAL IV & IRRIGATION SOLUTION			–	210.35
09/19/CCYY	TRAY, IRRIGATION 00099	62022298	1	36.40	
09/19/CCYY	TRAY, EPIDURAL C000099	62023304	1	75.90	
09/19/CCYY	TRAY, CATH FOLEY 00099	62022066	1	94.65	
09/19/CCYY	CANNULA, NASAL 00099	62011028	1	13.10	
09/19/CCYY	CATH URETHRAL AM00099	62054168	1	142.00	
09/19/CCYY	CATH, IV PLACEMEN00099	62054093	1	72.80	
09/19/CCYY	DRESSING, TEGADER00099	62014030	2	53.00	
	TOTAL CENTRAL STORES/EQUIP			–	487.85
	SUB-TOTAL OF CHARGES				862.60
	PAY THIS AMOUNT				862.60

*** DEPARTMENT SUMMARY ***

PHARMACY-INJECTABLES			–	164.40
IV & IRRIGATION SOLUTION			–	210.35
CENTRAL STORES/EQUIP			–	487.85
PAY THIS AMOUNT				862.60

Hospital Admission Form

DOCUMENT *125*

Provider Information

Name:	La Moore Women's Clinic
Address:	123 LaForge Street

City:	Lafayette	State:	LA	Zip Code:	70513
Telephone#:		Fax#:			

Medicare ID#:	190007	UPIN#:	
Tax ID #:	88-8227310	Accepts Medicare Assignment:	☐
Provider Rep:	*Betty Biller*	Date:	*9/18/CCYY*

Patient Information

Name:	Lannie Levine
Address:	6780 Lodge Lane

City:	Lafayette	State:	LA	Zip Code:	70513
Telephone#:	(504) 555-7051	Patient Control #:	10062		
Date of Birth:	10/09/CCYY-54	Gender:	Female		
Marital Status:	Married	Relationship to Guarantor:			Spouse
Student Status:	☐ Full-time		☐ Part-time		
Insurance Type:	☒ Pvt ☐ M/care ☐ M/caid ☐ WC ☐ Other _____				

Admission Information

Admission Date:	09/18/CCYY	Time:	10:00 AM
Discharge Date:	09/18/CCYY	Time:	5:00 PM
Attending Phy's ID#:	I64545	Date of Injury:	
Attending Physician:	Luke Longwood, M.D.		

Guarantor Information

Name:	Larry Levine
Address:	6780 Lodge Lane

City:	Lafayette	State:	LA	Zip Code:	70513
Insurance ID #:	22-3333 NIN	SSN:	001-22-3333		
Insurance Name:	Rover Insurers, Inc.				
Insurance Group #:	21088				
Employer Name:	Ninja Enterprises				

Authorization

☒ Authorization to Release Information
☒ Authorization for Assignment of Benefits
☐ Authorization for Consent for Treatment
☐ My insurance will be billed but there may be a balance due.

Signature: *Lannie Levine*   Date: *9/18/CCYY*

Clinical Information

Principal Diagnosis:	Hyperemesis Gravidarum			
Other Diagnosis:	Inflammatory disease of uterus			
Surgical Procedure:	D & C	9/18/CCYY		
Other Procedures:	Ultrasound, O.B.	9/18/CCYY	Electrocardiogram	9/18/CCYY
Remarks:				
Previous Balance:		Payment:	Copay:	Adjustment:
Total Fee:	$1897.80	Cash ☐ Check ☐ Credit ☐	Cash ☐ Check ☐ Credit ☐	Remarks:	New Balance: $1897.80

La Moore Women's Clinic
123 LaForge Street
Lafayette, LA 70513

Patient Name	Patient No.	Sex	Date of Birth	Admission Date	Discharge Date	Page No.
LANNIE LEVINE	10062	F	10/09/CCYY-54	09/18/CCYY	09/18/CCYY	1

Guarantor Name and Address
LARRY LEVINE
6780 LODGE LANE
LAFAYETTE, LA 70513

Insurance Company: ROVER INSURERS, INC.
Claim Number: DOCUMENT 125
Attending Physician: LUKE LONGWOOD, M.D.

Date of Service	Description of Hospital Services	Service Code	Qty.	Unit Price	Total Charges
09/18/CCYY	POT CHLORIDE INJ	4170703	2	10.00	20.00
09/18/CCYY	MONISTAT 7 CREAM	4170914	1	25.00	25.00
	PHARMACY **SUBTOTAL**	** 250			45.00
09/18/CCYY	D5.45 WS 5000 ML	4171333	2	28.00	56.00
	IV SOLUTIONS **SUBTOTAL**	** 258			56.00
09/18/CCYY	I.V. SERVICE FEE	4172419	2	23.00	46.00
	I.V. THERAPY **SUBTOTAL**	** 260			46.00
09/18/CCYY	ANGIOCATH	4051000	1	12.00	12.00
09/18/CCYY	MIDSTREAM KIT	4051052	1	9.00	9.00
09/18/CCYY	IV START PAK	4051190	1	12.00	12.00
09/18/CCYY	RAZOR DISP.	4051231	1	2.00	2.00
09/18/CCYY	AEROBIC CULTURETTE	4051541	2	4.00	8.00
09/18/CCYY	GLOVES STERILE	4051550	1	4.00	4.00
09/18/CCYY	ADDITIVE SET, V1444	4053320	1	16.00	16.00
09/18/CCYY	SECONDARY IV V1903 T	4053325	1	21.00	21.00
09/18/CCYY	DIAL A FLO	4053329	1	28.00	28.00
09/18/CCYY	PAP SMEAR KIT	4054007	1	15.00	15.00
	MED/SURG SUPPLIES **SUBTOTAL**	** 270			127.00
09/18/CCYY	SMA-24 80019	4060070	1	270.00	270.00
09/18/CCYY	COMPLETE BLOOD COUNT 85023	4060117	1	53.00	53.00
09/18/CCYY	CREATININE SERUM 82565	4060120	1	46.00	46.00
09/18/CCYY	GLUCOSE 82947	4060148	1	46.00	46.00
09/18/CCYY	GRAM STAIN [SMEAR] 87205	4060431	1	42.00	42.00
09/18/CCYY	WET MOUNT 87210	4060484	1	35.00	35.00
09/18/CCYY	ROUTINE URINALYSIS 81000	4060487	1	46.00	46.00
09/18/CCYY	BUN [UREA NITROGEN] 84520	4060497	1	46.00	46.00
09/18/CCYY	R P R [VDRL] QUAL. 86592	4060507	1	42.00	42.00
09/18/CCYY	G C CULTURE 87070	4062144	1	90.00	90.00

La Moore Women's Clinic
123 LaForge Street
Lafayette, LA 70513

Patient Name	Patient No.	Sex	Date of Birth	Admission Date	Discharge Date	Page No.
LANNIE LEVINE	10062	F	10/09/CCYY-54	09/18/CCYY	09/18/CCYY	2

Guarantor Name and Address
LARRY LEVINE
6780 LODGE LANE
LAFAYETTE, LA 70513

Insurance Company: ROVER INSURERS, INC.
Claim Number: DOCUMENT 125
Attending Physician: LUKE LONGWOOD, M.D.

Date of Service	Description of Hospital Services	Service Code	Qty.	Unit Price	Total Charges
09/18/CCYY	CULTURE URINE 87086	4062168	1	79.00	79.00
09/18/CCYY	PREGNANCY TEST SERUM 84703	4062173	1	65.00	65.00
09/18/CCYY	ELECTROLYTES PANEL 80004	4062177	1	171.00	171.00
	LABORATORY **SUBTOTAL**	** 300			1,031.00
09/18/CCYY	CHLAMYDIA DNA	4090164	1	82.80	82.80
	OTHER LAB **SUBTOTAL**	** 309			82.80
09/18/CCYY	O.B. ULTRASOUND 76805	4150339	1	400.00	400.00
	ULTRASOUND **SUBTOTAL**	** 402			400.00
09/18/CCYY	EKG STANDARD 93005	4110061	1	85.00	85.00
	EKG/ECG **SUBTOTAL**	** 730			85.00
09/18/CCYY	OUT PATIENT KIT	4054052	1	25.00	25.00
	PT CONVENIENCE **SUBTOTAL**	** 990			25.00
	TOTAL				1,897.80
	PLEASE PAY THIS AMOUNT				1,897.80

Hospital Admission Form

Provider Information

Name:	Lafayette Surgical Center				
Address:	222 Lipton Lane				
City:	Lafayette	State:	LA	Zip Code:	70513
Telephone#:		Fax#:			
Medicare ID#:	190008	UPIN#:			
Tax ID #:	88-7799090	Accepts Medicare Assignment:	☐		
Provider Rep:	*Betty Biller*	Date:	*9/5/CCYY*		

Admission Information

Admission Date:	09/05/CCYY	Time:	5:00 PM
Discharge Date:	09/05/CCYY	Time:	12 midnight
Attending Phy's ID#:	J20006	Date of Injury:	09/05/CCYY
Attending Physician:	Lincoln Lansing, M.D.		

Patient Information

Name:	Lloyd Levine				
Address:	6780 Lodge Lane				
City:	Lafayette	State:	LA	Zip Code:	70513
Telephone#:	(504) 555-7051	Patient Control #:	10063		
Date of Birth:	09/19/CCYY-16	Gender:	Male		
Marital Status:	Single	Relationship to Guarantor:			Child
Student Status:	☒ Full-time	☐ Part-time			
Insurance Type:	☒ Pvt ☐ M/care ☐ M/caid ☐ WC ☐ Other ___				

Guarantor Information

Name:	Larry Levine				
Address:	6780 Lodge Lane				
City:	Lafayette	State:	LA	Zip Code:	70513
Insurance ID #:	22-3333 NIN	SSN:	001-22-3333		
Insurance Name:	Rover Insurers, Inc.				
Insurance Group #:	21088				
Employer Name:	Ninja Enterprises				

Authorization

☒ Authorization to Release Information
☒ Authorization for Assignment of Benefits
☐ Authorization for Consent for Treatment
☐ My insurance will be billed but there may be a balance due.

Signature: *Larry Levine*   Date: *9/5/CCYY*

Clinical Information

Principal Diagnosis:	Open wound tongue/mouth floor
Other Diagnosis:	
Surgical Procedure:	Suture of tongue laceration 9/05/CCYY
Other Procedures:	
Remarks:	Fell off sofa at home on 09/05/CCYY and bit tongue.

Previous Balance:		Payment:		Copay:		Adjustment:			
Total Fee:	$3069.05	Cash ☐ Check ☐ Credit ☐		Cash ☐ Check ☐ Credit ☐		Remarks:		New Balance:	$3069.05

Lafayette Surgical Center
222 Lipton Lane
Lafayette, LA 70513

Patient Name	Patient No.	Sex	Date of Birth	Admission Date	Discharge Date	Page No.
LLOYD LEVINE	10063	M	09/19/CCYY-19	09/05/CCYY	09/05/CCYY	1

Guarantor Name and Address
LARRY LEVINE
6780 LODGE LANE
LAFAYETTE, LA 70513

Insurance Company: ROVER INSURERS, INC.
Claim Number: DOCUMENT 126
Attending Physician: LINCOLN LANSING, M.D.

Date of Service	Description of Hospital Services	CPT®	Service Code	Qty.	Unit Price	Total Charges
09/05/CCYY	OUTPATIENT SURGERY ROOM	77	20401	1	213.05	213.05
09/05/CCYY	SURGERY – MINOR 30 MIN	55	20035	1	250.70	250.70
09/05/CCYY	SURGERY – MINOR EA ADD 15 MIN		20041	1	125.30	125.30
09/05/CCYY	SURGERY – MINOR EA ADD 15 MIN		20041	1	125.30	125.30
09/05/CCYY	SURGERY MAJOR SET-UP		20020	1	268.00	268.00
09/05/CCYY	SURGERY – CALL BACK		20027	1	382.45	382.45
09/05/CCYY	ANESTHESIA EQUIP. 1 HR MINIMUM		26014	1	299.75	299.75
09/05/CCYY	RECOVERY ROOM – 1 HOUR	66	20303	1	255.85	255.85
09/05/CCYY	SUTURE SPECIALTY		50348	4	52.95	211.80
09/05/CCYY	SUCTION CANNISTERS EVACUPAC		52299	1	18.10	18.10
09/05/CCYY	CAUTERY SET-UP		51545	1	69.80	69.80
09/05/CCYY	MONITOR CADRIAC		54051	1	43.95	43.95
09/05/CCYY	ELECTRODE CARDIAC		51712	1	16.80	16.80
09/05/CCYY	TUBE ENDOTRACH ALL		52372	1	24.55	24.55
09/05/CCYY	IV IRRIG SOL NACL 1000 R5200		58387	1	50.40	50.40
09/05/CCYY	SUCTION YANKAUR		52666	1	7.75	7.75
09/05/CCYY	STYLET 6FR		50205	1	12.55	12.55
09/05/CCYY	ANESTHESIA BREATHING CIRCUIT		51144	1	45.45	45.45
09/05/CCYY	PAD GROUNDING DESERT ADULT		51918	1	18.10	18.10
09/05/CCYY	DRESSING RAYTEC		51680	1	3.15	3.15
09/05/CCYY	PACK EENT		52794	1	74.15	74.15
09/05/CCYY	TUBE CONNECTING		52371	1	9.50	9.50
09/05/CCYY	TUBE SUCTION COAGULATION ELE		52399	1	33.15	33.15
09/05/CCYY	TUBE CONNECTING		52371	1	9.50	9.50
09/05/CCYY	SUCTION YANKAUR		52666	2	7.75	15.50
09/05/CCYY	GLOVE SURGICAL STERILE ALL S		58411	3	4.90	14.70
09/06/CCYY	ANECTINE 11-20 ML INJ		39086	1	17.25	17.25
09/06/CCYY	DOPRAM 10 MG\1 ML		40038	1	205.65	205.65
09/06/CCYY	PENTO 500 MG INJ ANES		41454	1	58.30	58.30
09/05/CCYY	DEMEROL 25 MG INJ		39335	1	11.25	11.25
09/05/CCYY	ATRIOUBE 0.4 IM		40023	1	11.25	11.25
09/05/CCYY	ACETOMINOPHEN LIQ 160 MG/5 ML		42079	2	3.40	6.80
09/05/CCYY	BLOOD COUNT CBC	85022	37547	1	39.35	39.35
09/05/CCYY	PRO TIME	85610	37731	1	47.80	47.80
09/05/CCYY	P.T.T.	85730	37733	1	59.75	59.75
09/05/CCYY	RT – OXYGEN		59092	1	12.35	12.35

Lafayette Surgical Center
222 Lipton Lane
Lafayette, LA 70513

Patient Name	Patient No.	Sex	Date of Birth	Admission Date	Discharge Date	Page No.
LLOYD LEVINE	10063	M	09/19/CCYY-19	09/05/CCYY	09/05/CCYY	2

Guarantor Name and Address
LARRY LEVINE
6780 LODGE LANE
LAFAYETTE, LA 70513

Insurance Company: ROVER INSURERS, INC.
Claim Number: DOCUMENT 126
Attending Physician: LINCOLN LANSING, M.D.

Date of Service	Description of Hospital Services	CPT®	Service Code	Qty.	Unit Price	Total Charges
	TOTAL SURGERY					1,407.60
	TOTAL PATIENT ROOM					213.05
	TOTAL LABORATORY-CLINICAL					146.90
	TOTAL RESPIRATORY SERVICES					12.35
	TOTAL ANESTHESISA EQUIPMENT					299.75
	TOTAL PHARMACY					360.90
	TOTAL MED/SURG SUPPLIES & DEVICES					628.50
	AMOUNT DUE					3,069.05

Hospital Admission Form

Provider Information

Name:	Lasker Memorial Hospital
Address:	7878 Lotus Avenue

City:	Lafayette	State:	LA	Zip Code:	70511

Telephone#:		Fax#:	
Medicare ID#:	190009	UPIN#:	

Tax ID #:	88-3384756	Accepts Medicare Assignment:	☐

Provider Rep:	Betty Biller	Date: 10/27/CCYY

Patient Information

Name:	Lisa Levine
Address:	6780 Lodge Lane

City:	Lafayette	State:	LA	Zip Code:	70513

Telephone#:	(504) 555-7051	Patient Control #:	10064
Date of Birth:	10/04/CCYY-17	Gender:	Female

Marital Status:	Single	Relationship to Guarantor:	Child
Student Status:	☒ Full-time	☐ Part-time	
Insurance Type:	☒ Pvt ☐ M/care ☐ M/caid ☐ WC ☐ Other _____		

Admission Information

Admission Date:	10/27/CCYY	Time:	4:00 AM
Discharge Date:	10/27/CCYY	Time:	9:00 AM
Attending Phy's ID#:	K88800	Date of Injury:	
Attending Physician:	Leroy Larson, M.D.		

Guarantor Information

Name:	Larry Levine
Address:	6780 Lodge Lane

City:	Lafayette	State:	LA	Zip Code:	70513

Insurance ID #:	22-3333 NIN	SSN:	001-22-3333
Insurance Name:	Rover Insurers, Inc.		
Insurance Group #:	21088		
Employer Name:	Ninja Enterprises		

Authorization

☒ Authorization to Release Information
☒ Authorization for Assignment of Benefits
☐ Authorization for Consent for Treatment
☐ My insurance will be billed but there may be a balance due.

Signature: Larry Levine	Date: 10/27/CCYY

Clinical Information

Principal Diagnosis:	Sinusitis
Other Diagnosis:	
Surgical Procedure:	
Other Procedures:	
Remarks:	

Previous Balance:		Payment:		Copay:		Adjustment:	
Total Fee:	$851.00	Cash ☐ Check ☐ Credit ☐		Cash ☐ Check ☐ Credit ☐		Remarks:	New Balance: $851.00

Lasker Memorial Hospital
7878 Lotus Avenue
Lafayette, LA 70511

Patient Name	Patient No.	Sex	Admission Date	Discharge Date	Page No.
LISA LEVINE	10064	F	10/27/CCYY	10/27/CCYY	1

Guarantor Name and Address
LARRY LEVINE
6780 LODGE LANE
LAFAYETTE, LA 70513

Insurance Company: ROVER INSURERS, INC.
Claim Number: DOCUMENT 127
Attending Physician: LEROY LARSON, M.D.

Date of Service	Description of Hospital Services	Service Code	Qty.	Unit Price	Total Charges
	SUMMARY OF CHARGES				
	PHARMACY	250	1		3.00
	LABORATORY OR (LAB)	300	6		308.00
	DX X-RAY	320	3		354.00
	EMERG ROOM	450	2		186.00
	TOTAL CHARGES	001			851.00

Hospital Admission Form

Provider Information

Name:	Lafayette Medical Center
Address:	3434 Lockwood Drive

City:	Lafayette	State:	LA	Zip Code:	70513

Telephone#:		Fax#:	
Medicare ID#:	190010	UPIN#:	

Tax ID #:	88-8998887	Accepts Medicare Assignment: ☐
Provider Rep:	_Betty Biller_	Date: _9/30/CCYY_

Patient Information

Name:	Lila Levine
Address:	6780 Lodge Lane

City:	Lafayette	State:	LA	Zip Code:	70513

Telephone#:	(504) 555-7051	Patient Control #:	10065
Date of Birth:	09/21/CCYY-18	Gender:	Female

Marital Status:	Single	Relationship to Guarantor:	Child
Student Status:	☒ Full-time	☐ Part-time	
Insurance Type:	☒ Pvt ☐ M/care ☐ M/caid ☐ WC ☐ Other _____		

Admission Information

Admission Date:	09/30/CCYY	Time:	10:00 AM
Discharge Date:	09/30/CCYY	Time:	7:00 PM
Attending Phy's ID#:	L54560	Date of Injury:	
Attending Physician:	Lewis Latour, M.D.		

Guarantor Information

Name:	Larry Levine
Address:	6780 Lodge Lane

City:	Lafayette	State:	LA	Zip Code:	70513

Insurance ID #:	22-3333 NIN	SSN:	001-22-3333
Insurance Name:	Rover Insurers, Inc.		
Insurance Group #:	21088		
Employer Name:	Ninja Enterprises		

Authorization

☒ Authorization to Release Information
☒ Authorization for Assignment of Benefits
☐ Authorization for Consent for Treatment
☐ My insurance will be billed but there may be a balance due.

Signature: _Larry Levine_ Date: _9/30/CCYY_

Clinical Information

Principal Diagnosis:	Abdominal Pain
Other Diagnosis:	Cholelithiasis
Surgical Procedure:	Abdominal Ultrasound 9/30/CCYY
Other Procedures:	
Remarks:	

Previous Balance:		Payment:		Copay:		Adjustment:			
Total Fee:	$1268.00	Cash ☐ Check ☐ Credit ☐		Cash ☐ Check ☐ Credit ☐		Remarks:		New Balance:	$1268.00

Lafayette Medical Center
3434 Lockwood Drive
Lafayette, LA 70513

Patient Name	Patient No.	Sex		Admission Date	Discharge Date	Page No.
LILA LEVINE	10065	F		09/30/CCYY	09/30/CCYY	1

Guarantor Name and Address
LARRY LEVINE
6780 LODGE LANE
LAFAYETTE, LA 70513

Insurance Company: ROVER INSURERS, INC.
Claim Number: DOCUMENT 128
Attending Physician: LEWIS LATOUR, M.D.

Date of Service	Description of Hospital Services	Service Code	Qty.	Unit Price	Total Charges
09/30/CCYY	AMYLASE SERUM 82150	4060006	1	58.00	58.00
09/30/CCYY	CREATININE SERUM 82565	4060120	1	46.00	46.00
09/30/CCYY	GLUCOSE 82947	4060148	1	46.00	46.00
09/30/CCYY	LIVER FUNCTION TEST 80058	4060214	1	226.00	226.00
09/30/CCYY	ROUTINE URINALYSIS 81000	4060487	1	46.00	46.00
09/30/CCYY	BUN [UREA NITROGEN] 84520	4060497	1	46.00	46.00
09/30/CCYY	STAT TEST CHARGE	4060580	1	30.00	30.00
09/30/CCYY	ELECTROLYTES PANEL 80004	4062177	1	171.00	171.00
	LABORATORY **SUBTOTAL**	** 300			669.00
09/30/CCYY	CHEST 2 VIEWS EA 71020	4140063	1	105.00	105.00
09/30/CCYY	TECH CALL AFTER HOURS 99052	4140206	1	44.00	44.00
	DX X-RAY **SUBTOTAL**	** 320			149.00
09/30/CCYY	STAT FEE – ULTRASOUND	4150230	1	50.00	50.00
09/30/CCYY	ABD. SURVEY 76700	4150248	1	400.00	400.00
	ULTRASOUND **SUBTOTAL**	** 402			450.00

TOTAL   **1,268.00**

PLEASE PAY THIS AMOUNT   1,268.00

Hospital Claims Beginning Financials

INGLES FAMILY

Insurance Plan	Ball Insurance Carriers—XYZ Corporation

Patient:	INEZ	IRVING	IRMA	ILENE	
C/O DEDUCTIBLE	0.00	0.00	0.00	0.00	
DEDUCTIBLE	120.00	50.00	27.00	2.00	
COINSURANCE	0.00	0.00	0.00	0.00	
ACCIDENT BENEFIT	0.00	0.00	0.00	0.00	
LIFETIME MAXIMUM	2,627.00	27,224.00	3,940.00	5,929.92	
M/N OFFICE VISITS					
OFFICE VISITS					
HOSPITAL VISITS					
DXL					
SURGERY					
ASSISTANT SURGERY					
ANESTHESIA					

Hospital Admission Form

Provider Information

Name:	Inichi General Hospital
Address:	234 Imperial Highway
City:	Inichi	State:	IN	Zip Code:	46623
Telephone#:		Fax#:	
Medicare ID#:	150011	UPIN#:	
Tax ID #.	77-8502857	Accepts Medicare Assignment: ☐
Provider Rep:	*Betty Biller*	Date: 9/5/CCYY

Admission Information

Admission Date:	09/05/CCYY	Time:	10:00 AM
Discharge Date:	09/05/CCYY	Time:	4:00 PM
Attending Phy's ID#:	M58705	Date of Injury:	
Attending Physician:	Isabel Ingram, M.D.		

Patient Information

Name:	Inez Ingles
Address:	987 Island Drive
City:	Inichi	State:	IN	Zip Code:	46623
Telephone#:	(219) 555-4662	Patient Control #:	10066
Date of Birth:	08/17/CCYY-41	Gender:	Female
Marital Status:	Married	Relationship to Guarantor:	Self
Student Status:	☐ Full-time	☐ Part-time
Insurance Type:	☒ Pvt ☐ M/care ☐ M/caid ☐ WC ☐ Other _____

Guarantor Information

Name:	Inez Ingles
Address:	987 Island Drive
City:	Inichi	State:	IN	Zip Code:	46623
Insurance ID #:	55-1111 XYZ	SSN:	000-55-1111
Insurance Name:	Ball Insurance Carriers
Insurance Group #:	62958
Employer Name:	XYZ Corporation

Authorization

☒ Authorization to Release Information
☒ Authorization for Assignment of Benefits
☐ Authorization for Consent for Treatment
☐ My insurance will be billed but there may be a balance due.
Signature: *Inez Ingles*   Date: 9/5/CCYY

Clinical Information

Principal Diagnosis:	Hallux Valgus, Bunion Acquired		
Other Diagnosis:			
Surgical Procedure:	Bunionectomy, Osteotomy Metatarsal	9/05/CCYY	
Other Procedures:	Internal Fixation of Bone	9/05/CCYY	Electrocardiogram 9/05/CCYY
Remarks:			

Previous Balance:		Payment:		Copay:		Adjustment:		
Total Fee:	$7863.60	Cash ☐ Check ☐ Credit ☐		Cash ☐ Check ☐ Credit ☐		Remarks:	New Balance:	$7863.60

Inichi General Hospital
234 Imperial Highway
Inichi, IN 46623

Patient Name	Patient No.	Sex		Admission Date	Discharge Date	Page No.
INEZ INGLES	10066	F		09/05/CCYY	09/05/CCYY	1

Guarantor Name and Address
INEZ INGLES
987 ISLAND DRIVE
INICHI, IN 46623

Insurance Company: BALL INSURANCE CARRIERS
Claim Number: DOCUMENT 130
Attending Physician: ISABEL INGRAM, M.D.

Date of Service	Description of Hospital Services	Service Code	Qty.	Charges	Total Charges
09/05/CCYY	MINOR SET-UP	40200701	1	352.00	
09/05/CCYY	SURG-LOCAL WITH CMAC	40200800	1	56.00	
09/05/CCYY	MAJOR SURG. 2 ¼	40201352	1	2,009.00	
09/05/CCYY	RECOVERY RM 1 HR	40202509	1	380.00	
09/05/CCYY	EKG MONITOR OR	40202657	1	77.00	
09/05/CCYY	O2 MONITOR OR	40202681	1	56.00	
09/05/CCYY	BP MONITOR OR	40202707	1	67.00	
09/05/CCYY	TRAY-PODIATRY	40202731	1	626.00	
09/05/CCYY	OR SET	40202871	1	86.00	
09/05/CCYY	MICRO-AIRE POWER EQUIPMENT	40203226	1	69.00	
09/05/CCYY	RECOVERY RM BP MONITOR	40203267	1	67.00	
09/05/CCYY	RECOVERY RM EKG MONITOR	40203275	1	77.00	
09/05/CCYY	RECOVERY RM TEMP MONITOR	40203283	1	18.00	
09/05/CCYY	RECOVERY RM PULSE MONITOR	40203291	1	33.00	
09/05/CCYY	OR-O2 SET UP	40203333	1	48.00	
	TOTAL SURGERY & RECOVERY				**4,021.00**
09/05/CCYY	LOCAL ANESTH SET	40405979	1	35.00	
09/05/CCYY	OR-O2 1ST HOUR	40406282	1	38.00	
	TOTAL ANESTHESIOLOGY				**73.00**
09/05/CCYY	BANDAGE 4X5 YDS/CU	40501702	1	18.85	
09/05/CCYY	POST OP SURG BOOT	40515959	1	39.40	
09/05/CCYY	SURG-ACE BANDAGE	40519258	1	20.30	
09/05/CCYY	SURG-ESMARK/BNDG	40521379	1	100.55	
09/05/CCYY	SURG-NITROGEN TAN	40522500	1	69.10	
09/05/CCYY	SURG-SAW BLADES-DISP	40523011	1	78.70	
09/05/CCYY	SURG-SKIN SKRIBE	40523500	1	8.10	
09/05/CCYY	SURG-WEBRIL SOFT	40524159	1	10.10	
09/05/CCYY	SURG-XEROFORM GAU	40524209	1	12.20	
09/05/CCYY	BED PAN-REG	40528945	1	10.50	
09/05/CCYY	SURG-PREP TRAY	40528952	1	25.40	
09/05/CCYY	SURG-SINGLE BASIN PACK	40529752	1	112.00	
09/05/CCYY	SURG-SUTURE SET MINOR	40529794	1	86.65	
09/05/CCYY	SURG-BEAVER BLADE #6700	40530511	1	15.25	

Inichi General Hospital
234 Imperial Highway
Inichi, IN 46623

Patient Name	Patient No.	Sex		Admission Date	Discharge Date	Page No.
INEZ INGLES	10066	F		09/05/CCYY	09/05/CCYY	2

Guarantor Name and Address
INEZ INGLES
987 ISLAND DRIVE
INICHI, IN 46623

Insurance Company: BALL INSURANCE CARRIERS
Claim Number: DOCUMENT 130
Attending Physician: ISABEL INGRAM, M.D.

Date of Service	Description of Hospital Services	Service Code	Qty.	Unit Price	Total Charges
09/05/CCYY	SURG-DISP T DRAPE	40530693	1	27.20	
09/05/CCYY	SURG-PACK PODIATRY	40531071	1	265.80	
09/05/CCYY	SURG-TOURNIQUET	40532418	1	407.70	
09/05/CCYY	SURG-TENS ELECTRODE	40532434	1	67.50	
09/05/CCYY	PACK, SHORT STAY OR	40532640	1	28.75	
09/05/CCYY	SURG-ACUFLEX ROD	40533598	1	412.00	
	TOTAL CENTRAL SUPPLY				**1,816.05**
09/04/CCYY	CHEM-SMA 6	40609851	1	157.30	
09/04/CCYY	HEMA-CBC	40611956	1	50.60	
09/04/CCYY	HEMA-PTT	40613358	1	51.70	
09/04/CCYY	URIN-URINALYSIS COMPLETE	40620502	1	34.10	
	TOTAL LAB COUNCIL				**293.70**
09/05/CCYY	PATH-HANDLING CHG	40702003	1	36.30	
09/05/CCYY	PATH-PROCESS BLOCK A C LABORATORY	40702011	1	5.50	
09/05/CCYY	PATH-PROCESS IDLE A C LABORATORY	40702029	1	1.20	
09/05/CCYY	PATH-PROCESS DECAL A C LABORATORY	40702045	1	2.40	
09/05/CCYY	PATH-REPRT TRANSCR	40702086	1	16.50	
	TOTAL PATH LAB				**61.90**
09/04/CCYY	EKG ROUTINE	41100454	1	100.00	
	TOTAL CARDIOLOGY				**100.00**
09/04/CCYY	CHEST 2 V AP/LA	41402009	1	113.00	
09/05/CCYY	FOOT LID LTD	41404450	2	106.00	
09/05/CCYY	X-RAY PORTBLE CHARGE	41410507	1	44.00	
	TOTAL RADIOLOGY				**263.00**

Inichi General Hospital
234 Imperial Highway
Inichi, IN 46623

Patient Name	Patient No.	Sex	Admission Date	Discharge Date	Page No.
INEZ INGLES	10066	F	09/05/CCYY	09/05/CCYY	3

Guarantor Name and Address
INEZ INGLES
987 ISLAND DRIVE
INICHI, IN 46623

Insurance Company: BALL INSURANCE CARRIERS
Claim Number: DOCUMENT 130
Attending Physician: ISABEL INGRAM, M.D.

Date of Service	Description of Hospital Services	Service Code	Qty.	Unit Price	Total Charges
09/05/CCYY	IV ADD	41700071	1	20.65	
09/05/CCYY	ANCEF 1 GM IV/IM	41703109	1	84.90	
09/05/CCYY	BACITRACIN 50,000 H	47105500	1	46.00	
09/05/CCYY	IRRICATING 2000 ML	41732215	1	38.85	
09/05/CCYY	IRRIGATING 500-1000 ML	41732249	1	32.75	
09/05/CCYY	IV DUAL INJ SET	41733171	1	29.10	
09/05/CCYY	IV EXTENSION SET	41733379	1	20.65	
09/05/CCYY	MARCAINE INJ.	41739303	1	35.80	
09/05/CCYY	POLYMXN IV 500,000 UNITS	41754359	1	33.65	
09/05/CCYY	VITAMIN TAB	41775909	1	2.40	
09/05/CCYY	XYLOCAINE INJ.	41777202	1	19.40	
09/05/CCYY	IV D5/LR 100 ML	41778952	1	47.95	
09/05/CCYY	IV D5W 50-250 ML PF	41778986	1	47.95	
09/05/CCYY	VERSED 10 MG H	41780156	1	23.70	
09/05/CCYY	ORUDIS 75 MG 0	41781469	1	2.40	
09/05/CCYY	DIPRIVAN 20 ML	41783341	1	40.45	
	TOTAL PHARMACY				**526.60**
09/05/CCYY	EVAL-COMPLETE	42000505	1	96.85	
09/05/CCYY	GAIT (STANDARD)	42000653	1	71.00	
09/05/CCYY	1 PROCEDURE	42001156	1	71.00	
	TOTAL PHYSICAL THERAPY				**238.85**
09/05/CCYY	DAY CARE	42300111	1	256.00	
	TOTAL EMERGENCY ROOM				**256.00**
	SUB-TOTAL OF CHARGES				7,650.10
	ADDITIONAL CHARGES				
09/05/CCYY	SURG-MONITOR CHARGE	40202251	1	51.00	
	TOTAL SURGERY & RECOVERY				**51.00**
09/05/CCYY	OR-O2 ADD 15 MIN	40406305	1	60.00	
	TOTAL ANESTHESIOLOGY				**60.00**

Inichi General Hospital
234 Imperial Highway
Inichi, IN 46623

Patient Name	Patient No.	Sex		Admission Date	Discharge Date	Page No.
INEZ INGLES	10066	F		09/05/CCYY	09/05/CCYY	4

Guarantor Name and Address
INEZ INGLES
987 ISLAND DRIVE
INICHI, IN 46623

Insurance Company: BALL INSURANCE CARRIERS
Claim Number: DOCUMENT 130
Attending Physician: ISABEL INGRAM, M.D.

Date of Service	Description of Hospital Services	Service Code	Qty.	Unit Price	Total Charges
09/05/CCYY	SURG-CAUT W/PAD/PEN	40519753	1	94.40	
09/05/CCYY	SPEC CONTAINR 4 OZ	40529273	1	8.10	
	TOTAL CENTRAL SUPPLY				**102.50**
	SUB-TOTAL ADDITIONAL CHARGES			213.50	
	TOTAL CHARGES				**7863.60**
	BALANCE DUE				7863.60

Inichi General Hospital
234 Imperial Highway
Inichi, IN 46623

Patient Name	Patient No.	Sex	Admission Date	Discharge Date	Page No.
INEZ INGLES	10066	F	09/05/CCYY	09/05/CCYY	5

Guarantor Name and Address
INEZ INGLES
987 ISLAND DRIVE
INICHI, IN 46623

Insurance Company: BALL INSURANCE CARRIERS
Claim Number: DOCUMENT 130
Attending Physician: ISABEL INGRAM, M.D.

Date of Service	Description of Hospital Services	Service Code	Qty.	Unit Price	Total Charges
	SUMMARY OF CHARGES				
	OR SERVICES			4,072.00	
	ANESTHESIA			133.00	
	MED-SUR SUPPLIES			1,920.95	
	LABORATORY OR (LAB)			293.70	
	PATHOLOGY LAB (PATH LAB)			61.90	
	EKG/ECG			100.00	
	DX X-RAY			263.00	
	PHARMACY			524.20	
	PHYSICAL THERP			238.85	
	AMBUL SURG			256.00	
	SUB-TOTAL OF CHARGES				7,863.60
	PAYMENTS/ADJUSTMENTS				NONE
	SUBTOTAL PAYMENTS/ADJUSTMENTS				NONE
	BALANCE				7,863.60
	BALANCE DUE				7,863.60

Hospital Admission Form

DOCUMENT 131

Provider Information

Name:	Inichi Main Hospital
Address:	5863 Itasca Drive

City:	Inichi	State:	IN	Zip Code:	46623
Telephone#:		Fax#:			

Medicare ID#:	150012
UPIN#:	

Tax ID #:	77-0020304	Accepts Medicare Assignment:	☐
Provider Rep:	*Betty Biller*	Date: 9/5/CCYY	

Patient Information

Name:	Irving Ingles
Address:	987 Island Drive

City:	Inichi	State:	IN	Zip Code:	46623
Telephone#:	(219) 555-4662	Patient Control #:	10067		

Date of Birth:	04/02/CCYY-46	Gender:	Male
Marital Status:	Married	Relationship to Guarantor:	Spouse
Student Status:	☐ Full-time	☐ Part-time	
Insurance Type:	☒ Pvt ☐ M/care ☐ M/caid ☐ WC ☐ Other _____		

Admission Information

Admission Date:	09/05/CCYY	Time:	10:00 AM
Discharge Date:	09/05/CCYY	Time:	11:00 PM
Attending Phy's ID#:	A87754	Date of Injury:	9/05/CCYY
Attending Physician:	Iola Ithica, M.D.		

Guarantor Information

Name:	Inez Ingles
Address:	987 Island Drive

City:	Inichi	State:	IN	Zip Code:	46623
Insurance ID #:	55-1111 XYZ	SSN:	000-55-1111		
Insurance Name:	Ball Insurance Carriers				
Insurance Group #:	62958				
Employer Name:	XYZ Corporation				

Authorization

☒ Authorization to Release Information
☒ Authorization for Assignment of Benefits
☐ Authorization for Consent for Treatment
☐ My insurance will be billed but there may be a balance due.

Signature: *Irving Ingles* Date: 9/5/CCYY

Clinical Information

Principal Diagnosis:	Open wound knee/leg with tendon	
Other Diagnosis:		
Surgical Procedure:	Excision knee semilunar cartilage	9/05/CCYY
Other Procedures:	Knee arthroscopy	9/05/CCYY
Remarks:	Fell while skiing.	

Previous Balance:		Payment:		Copay:		Adjustment:			
Total Fee:	$8910.00	Cash ☐ Check ☐ Credit ☐		Cash ☐ Check ☐ Credit ☐		Remarks:		New Balance:	$8910.00

Inichi Main Hospital
5863 Itasca Drive
Inichi, IN 46623

Patient Name	Patient No.	Sex	Admission Date	Discharge Date	Page No.
IRVING INGLES	10067	M	09/05/CCYY	09/05/CCYY	1

Guarantor Name and Address
INEZ INGLES
987 ISLAND DRIVE
INICHI, IN 46623

Insurance Company: BALL INSURANCE CARRIERS
Claim Number: DOCUMENT 131
Attending Physician: IOLA ITHICA, M.D.

Date of Service	Description of Hospital Services	Service Code	Qty.	Charges	Total Charges
	SUMMARY OF CHARGES				
	PHARMACY	250	62		876.00
	IV SOLUTIONS	258	13		364.00
	I.V. THERAPY	260	5		115.00
	MED/SURG SUPPLIES	270	45		765.00
	SUPPLY/OTHER	279	1		150.00
	LABORATORY	300	5		370.00
	DX X-RAY	320	7		480.00
	OR SERVICES	360	14		4,666.00
	ANESTHESIA	370	13		913.00
	PHYSICAL THERAPY	420	1		36.00
	AMBUL SURG	490	1		150.00
	PT CONVENIENCE	990	1		25.00
	TOTAL CHARGES				8,910.00

Hospital Admission Form

Provider Information

Name:	Inichi Surgical Center
Address:	4692 Ibarra Blvd.

City:	Inichi	State:	IN	Zip Code:	46623

Telephone#:		Fax#:	
Medicare ID#:	150013	UPIN#:	
Tax ID #:	77-3499812	Accepts Medicare Assignment:	☐
Provider Rep:	*Betty Biller*	Date: *10/19/CCYY*	

Patient Information

Name:	Irma Ingles
Address:	987 Island Drive

City:	Inichi	State:	IN	Zip Code:	46623
Telephone#:	(219) 555-4662	Patient Control #:	10068		
Date of Birth:	10/17/CCYY-16	Gender:	Female		
Marital Status:	Single	Relationship to Guarantor:		Child	
Student Status:	☒ Full-time	☐ Part-time			
Insurance Type:	☒ Pvt ☐ M/care ☐ M/caid ☐ WC ☐ Other _____				

Admission Information

Admission Date:	10/19/CCYY	Time:	10:00 AM
Discharge Date:	10/19/CCYY	Time:	3:00 PM
Attending Phy's ID#:	B12331	Date of Injury:	
Attending Physician:	Iris Inwood, M.D.		

Guarantor Information

Name:	Inez Ingles
Address:	987 Island Drive

City:	Inichi	State:	IN	Zip Code:	46623
Insurance ID #:	55-1111 XYZ	SSN:	000-55-1111		
Insurance Name:	Ball Insurance Carriers				
Insurance Group #:	62958				
Employer Name:	XYZ Corporation				

Authorization

☒ Authorization to Release Information
☒ Authorization for Assignment of Benefits
☐ Authorization for Consent for Treatment
☐ My insurance will be billed but there may be a balance due.

Signature: _*Inez Ingles*_   Date: *10/19/CCYY*

Clinical Information

Principal Diagnosis:	Pterygium
Other Diagnosis:	
Surgical Procedure:	Pterygium Excision Conjunctiva Free Graft 10/19/CCYY
Other Procedures:	
Remarks:	

Previous Balance:		Payment:		Copay:		Adjustment:			
Total Fee:	$2507.50	Cash ☐ Check ☐ Credit ☐		Cash ☐ Check ☐ Credit ☐		Remarks:		New Balance:	$2507.50

Inichi Surgical Center
4692 Ibarra Blvd.
Inichi, IN 46623

Patient Name	Patient No.	Sex	Admission Date	Discharge Date	Page No.
IRMA INGLES	10068	F	10/19/CCYY	10/19/CCYY	1

Guarantor Name and Address
INEZ INGLES
987 ISLAND DRIVE
INICHI, IN 46623

Insurance Company: BALL INSURANCE CARRIERS
Claim Number: DOCUMENT 132
Attending Physician: IRIS INWOOD, M.D.

Date of Service	Description of Hospital Services	Service Code	Qty.	Charges	Total Charges
	SUMMARY OF CHARGES				
	PHARMACY	250	4		100.00
	IV THERAPY	260	5		151.00
	MED-SURG SUPPLIES	270	33		1,237.00
	PATHOLOGY LAB (PATH L)	310	2		105.50
	OR SERVICES	360	1		473.00
	ANESTHESIA	370	1		55.00
	AMBUL SURG	490	1		150.00
	RECOVERY ROOM	710	1		236.00
	TOTAL CHARGES	001			2,507.50

Hospital Admission Form
DOCUMENT 133

Provider Information

Name:	Inichi Valley Hospital
Address:	1000 Igloo Blvd.

City:	Inichi	State:	IN	Zip Code:	46625

Telephone#:		Fax#:	

Medicare ID#:	150014	UPIN#:	

Tax ID #:	77-2233456	Accepts Medicare Assignment:	☐

Provider Rep:	*Betty Biller*	Date: *12/18/CCYY*

Patient Information

Name:	Inez Ingles
Address:	987 Island Drive

City:	Inichi	State:	IN	Zip Code:	46623

Telephone#:	(219) 555-4662	Patient Control #:	10066

Date of Birth:	08/17/CCYY-41	Gender:	Female

Marital Status:	Married	Relationship to Guarantor:	Self

Student Status:	☐ Full-time	☐ Part-time

Insurance Type:	☒ Pvt ☐ M/care ☐ M/caid ☐ WC ☐ Other _____

Admission Information

Admission Date:	12/18/CCYY	Time:	10:00 AM
Discharge Date:	12/18/CCYY	Time:	4:00 PM
Attending Phy's ID#:	C56468	Date of Injury:	
Attending Physician:	Ivy Imperial, M.D.		

Guarantor Information

Name:	Inez Ingles
Address:	987 Island Drive

City:	Inichi	State:	IN	Zip Code:	46623

Insurance ID #:	55-1111 XYZ	SSN:	000-55-1111
Insurance Name:	Ball Insurance Carriers		
Insurance Group #:	62958		
Employer Name:	XYZ Corporation		

Authorization

☒ Authorization to Release Information
☒ Authorization for Assignment of Benefits
☐ Authorization for Consent for Treatment
☐ My insurance will be billed but there may be a balance due.

Signature:	*Inez Ingles*	Date: *12/18/CCYY*

Clinical Information

Principal Diagnosis:	Bronchitis	
Other Diagnosis:		
Surgical Procedure:	Diagnostic ultrasound of thorax	12/18/CCYY
Other Procedures:		
Remarks:		

Previous Balance:	$7863.60	Payment:		Copay:		Adjustment:			
Total Fee:	$1834.00	Cash ☐ Check ☐ Credit ☐		Cash ☐ Check ☐ Credit ☐		Remarks:		New Balance:	$9697.60

Inichi Valley Hospital
1000 Igloo Blvd.
Inichi, IN 46625

Patient Name	Patient No.	Sex	Admission Date	Discharge Date	Page No.
INEZ INGLES	10066	F	12/18/CCYY	12/18/CCYY	1

Guarantor Name and Address
INEZ INGLES
987 ISLAND DRIVE
INICHI, IN 46623

Insurance Company: BALL INSURANCE CARRIERS
Claim Number: DOCUMENT 133
Attending Physician: IVY IMPERIAL, M.D.

Date of Service	Description of Hospital Services	Service Code	Qty.	Charges	Total Charges
	SUMMARY OF CHARGES				
	PHARMACY	250	5		240.00
	IV SOLUTIONS	258	5		105.00
	IV THERAPY	260	5		98.00
	MED/SURG SUPPLIES	270	4		66.00
	LABORATORY	300	8		612.00
	DX X-RAY	320	2		143.00
	ULTRASOUND	402	1		375.00
	TREATMENT ROOM	760	1		170.00
	PAT CONVENIENCE	990	1		25.00
	TOTAL CHARGES				1,834.00

Hospital Admission Form

DOCUMENT *134*

Provider Information

Name:	Inichi Medical Center
Address:	1234 Irish Drive

City:	Inichi	State:	IN	Zip Code:	46623
Telephone#:		Fax#:			
Medicare ID#:	150015	UPIN#:			
Tax ID #:	77-3398276	Accepts Medicare Assignment:	☐		
Provider Rep:	*Betty Biller*	Date: *1/6/CCYY*			

Patient Information

Name:	Ilene Ingles
Address:	987 Island Drive

City:	Inichi	State:	IN	Zip Code:	46623
Telephone#:	(219) 555-4662	Patient Control #:	10069		
Date of Birth:	07/27/CCYY-18	Gender:	Female		
Marital Status:	Single	Relationship to Guarantor:	Child		
Student Status:	☒ Full-time	☐ Part-time			
Insurance Type:	☒ Pvt ☐ M/care ☐ M/caid ☐ WC ☐ Other ___				

Admission Information

Admission Date:	01/06/CCYY	Time:	8:00 AM
Discharge Date:	01/06/CCYY	Time:	12:00 Noon
Attending Phy's ID#:	D31850	Date of Injury:	
Attending Physician:	Ivan Ironwood, M.D.		

Guarantor Information

Name:	Inez Ingles
Address:	987 Island Drive

City:	Inichi	State:	IN	Zip Code:	46623
Insurance ID #:	55-1111 XYZ	SSN:	000-55-1111		
Insurance Name:	Ball Insurance Carriers				
Insurance Group #:	62958				
Employer Name:	XYZ Corporation				

Authorization

☒ Authorization to Release Information
☒ Authorization for Assignment of Benefits
☐ Authorization for Consent for Treatment
☐ My insurance will be billed but there may be a balance due.

Signature: *Inez Ingles* Date: *1/6/CCYY*

Clinical Information

Principal Diagnosis:	Ganglion of Tendon Sheath
Other Diagnosis:	
Surgical Procedure:	Excision of lesion tendon sheath/hand 01/06/CCYY
Other Procedures:	
Remarks:	

Previous Balance:		Payment:		Copay:		Adjustment:			
Total Fee:	$3361.25	Cash ☐ Check ☐ Credit ☐		Cash ☐ Check ☐ Credit ☐		Remarks:		New Balance:	$3361.25

Inichi Medical Center
1234 Irish Drive
Inichi, IN 46623

Patient Name	Patient No.	Sex	Date of Birth	Admission Date	Discharge Date	Page No.
ILENE INGLES	10069	F	07/27/83	01/06/CCYY	01/06/CCYY	1

Guarantor Name and Address
INEZ INGLES
987 ISLAND DRIVE
INICHI, IN 46623

Insurance Company: BALL INSURANCE CARRIERS
Claim Number: DOCUMENT 134
Attending Physician: IVAN IRONWOOD, M.D.

Date of Service	Description of Hospital Services	Service Code	Qty.	Charges	Total Charges
	SUMMARY OF CHARGES				
	PHARMACY	250	2		101.50
	IV THERAPY	260	5		149.00
	MED-SUR SUPPLIES	270	30		1,198.25
	PATHOLOGY LAB OR (PATH L)	310	2		105.50
	OR SERVICES	360	1		630.00
	ANESTHESIA	370	5		791.00
	AMBUL SURG	490	1		150.00
	RECOVERY ROOM	710	1		236.00
	TOTAL CHARGES	001			3,361.25

Hospital Claims Beginning Financials
JENNINGS FAMILY

Insurance Plan	Winter Insurance Company—ABC Corporation				

Patient:	JACK	JENNIFER	JACQUELINE	JULIA	JANET
C/O DEDUCTIBLE	0.00	0.00	0.00	0.00	0.00
DEDUCTIBLE	27.00	0.00	27.00	62.00	2.70
COINSURANCE	0.00	0.00	0.00	0.00	0.00
ACCIDENT BENEFIT	0.00	0.00	0.00	0.00	0.00
LIFETIME MAXIMUM	424.24	2,027.20	9,724.14	980.00	375.26
M/N OFFICE VISITS					
OFFICE VISITS					
HOSPITAL VISITS					
DXL					
SURGERY					
ASSISTANT SURGERY					
ANESTHESIA					

Hospital Admission Form

Provider Information

Name:	Jersey Medical Center
Address:	555 Jaramillo Drive
City:	Jersey	State: NJ	Zip Code: 08074
Telephone#:	Fax#:
Medicare ID#:	310016	UPIN#:
Tax ID #:	94-3865496	Accepts Medicare Assignment: ☐
Provider Rep:	Betty Biller	Date: 6/25/CCYY

Admission Information

Admission Date:	06/22/CCYY	Time:	3:00 PM
Discharge Date:	06/25/CCYY	Time:	3:00 PM
Attending Phy's ID#:	E34101	Date of Injury:	
Attending Physician:	Joyce Johnson, M.D.		

Guarantor Information

Name:	Jack Jennings
Address:	4738 Jasmine Road
City: Jersey	State: NJ	Zip Code: 08077
Insurance ID #:	77-9999 ABC	SSN: 111-77-9999
Insurance Name:	Winter Insurance Company
Insurance Group #:	36928
Employer Name:	ABC Company

Patient Information

Name:	Jacqueline Jennings
Address:	4738 Jasmine Road
City:	Jersey	State: NJ	Zip Code: 08077
Telephone#:	(551) 555-0807	Patient Control #: 10070
Date of Birth:	04/29/CCYY-17	Gender: Female
Marital Status:	Single	Relationship to Guarantor: Child
Student Status:	☒ Full-time ☐ Part-time
Insurance Type:	☒ Pvt ☐ M/care ☐ M/caid ☐ WC ☐ Other _____

Authorization

☒ Authorization to Release Information
☒ Authorization for Assignment of Benefits
☐ Authorization for Consent for Treatment
☐ My insurance will be billed but there may be a balance due.
Signature: Jack Jennings   Date: 6/22/CCYY

Clinical Information

Principal Diagnosis:	Sprain Hip & Thigh
Other Diagnosis:	
Surgical Procedure:	Other C.A.T. Scan 6/22/CCYY
Other Procedures:	
Remarks:	

Previous Balance:		Payment:		Copay:		Adjustment:		
Total Fee:	$8035.45	Cash ☐ Check ☐ Credit ☐		Cash ☐ Check ☐ Credit ☐		Remarks:	New Balance:	$8035.45

Jersey Medical Center
5555 Jaramillo Drive
Jersey, NJ 08074

Patient Name	Patient No.	Sex	Admission Date	Discharge Date	Page No.
JACQUELINE JENNINGS	10070	F	06/22/CCYY	06/25/CCYY	1

Guarantor Name and Address
JACK JENNINGS
4738 JASMINE ROAD
JERSEY, NJ 08077

Insurance Company: WINTER INSURANCE CO.
Claim Number: DOCUMENT 136
Attending Physician: JOYCE JOHNSON, M.D.

Date of Service	Description of Hospital Services	Service Code	Qty.	Charges	Total Charges
	SUMMARY OF CHARGES				
	ROOM-BOARD/3 & 4 BED	130	3		1,185.00
	PHARMACY	250	43		747.95
	IV THERAPY	260	7		204.00
	MED-SUR SUPPLIES	270	15		331.75
	LABORATORY OR (LAB)	300	9		577.00
	DX X-RAY	320	2		204.00
	NUCLEAR MEDICINE OR (NUC)	340	6		1,505.75
	CT SCAN	350	4		2,980.00
	EKG/ECG	730	1		75.00
	TELEMETRY	732	1		225.00
	TOTAL CHARGES	001			8,035.45

Hospital Admission Form

DOCUMENT *137*

Provider Information					
Name:	Jackson Medical Center				
Address:	4444 Jumping Jack Lane				
City:	Jersey	State:	NJ	Zip Code:	08073
Telephone#:		Fax#:			
Medicare ID#:	310017	UPIN#:			
Tax ID #:	94-6678998	Accepts Medicare Assignment:	☐		
Provider Rep:	*Betty Biller*		Date: *4/13/CCYY*		

Admission Information			
Admission Date:	04/12/CCYY	Time:	1:00 AM
Discharge Date:	04/13/CCYY	Time:	4:00 PM
Attending Phy's ID#:	F14546	Date of Injury:	
Attending Physician:	James Justice, M.D.		

Guarantor Information					
Name:	Jack Jennings				
Address:	4738 Jasmine Road				
City:	Jersey	State:	NJ	Zip Code:	08077
Insurance ID #:	77-9999 ABC	SSN:	111-77-9999		
Insurance Name:	Winter Insurance Company				
Insurance Group #:	36928				
Employer Name:	ABC Company				

Patient Information					
Name:	Julia Jennings				
Address:	4738 Jasmine Road				
City:	Jersey	State:	NJ	Zip Code:	08077
Telephone#:	(551) 555-0807	Patient Control #:	10071		
Date of Birth:	10/07/CCYY-18	Gender:		Female	
Marital Status:	Single	Relationship to Guarantor:		Child	
Student Status:	☒ Full-time	☐ Part-time			
Insurance Type:	☒ Pvt ☐ M/care ☐ M/caid ☐ WC ☐ Other _____				

Authorization
☒ Authorization to Release Information
☒ Authorization for Assignment of Benefits
☐ Authorization for Consent for Treatment
☐ My insurance will be billed but there may be a balance due.
Signature: *Jack Jennings*   Date: *4/12/CCYY*

Clinical Information								
Principal Diagnosis:	Acute Bronchitis							
Other Diagnosis:	Obstructive Chronic Bronchitis							
Surgical Procedure:								
Other Procedures:								
Remarks:								
Previous Balance:		Payment:		Copay:		Adjustment:		
Total Fee:	$2471.85	Cash ☐ Check ☐ Credit ☐		Cash ☐ Check ☐ Credit ☐		Remarks:	New Balance:	$2471.85

Jackson Medical Center
4444 Jumping Jack Lane
Jersey, NJ 08073

Patient Name	Patient No.	Sex	Admission Date	Discharge Date	Page No.
JULIA JENNINGS	10071	F	04/12/CCYY	04/13/CCYY	1

Guarantor Name and Address
JACK JENNINGS
4738 JASMINE ROAD
JERSEY, NJ 08077

Insurance Company: WINTER INSURANCE CO.
Claim Number: DOCUMENT 137
Attending Physician: JAMES JUSTICE, M.D.

Date of Service	Description of Hospital Services	Service Code	Qty.	Charges	Total Charges
	DETAIL OF CURRENT CHARGES				
04/13/CCYY	ROOM & BOARD	99011009	1	-395.00	
04/13/CCYY	ROOM & BOARD	99011504	1	395.00	
04/12/CCYY	ROOM & BOARD	99011009	1	395.00	
	TOTAL ROOM & BOARD				**395.00**
04/12/CCYY	ADMIT KITS	40503021	1	40.00	
04/12/CCYY	MIDSTREAM URINE COLLECTOR	40546178	1	7.75	
04/12/CCYY	PILLOW DISP	40555252	1	11.75	
04/12/CCYY	SYRINGE 1 CC TO 10 CC W/NEEDLE	40572166	1	4.50	
04/12/CCYY	SLIPPERS/PILLOW PAWS	40573149	1	3.75	
04/12/CCYY	SPECIPAN	40573156	1	13.25	
04/12/CCYY	URINE CUP	40588037	1	2.25	
04/13/CCYY	IMED PUMP RENTAL DAILY 01	40586393	2	110.50	
04/12/CCYY	IMED PRIMARY SET CS20	40584401	1	24.25	
04/12/CCYY	IMED PRIMARY SET CS20	40584407	1	24.25	
	TOTAL CENTRAL SUPPLY				**242.25**
04/12/CCYY	CHEM-AMYLASE	40600959	1	49.50	
04/12/CCYY	CH-CREATININE BLD	40603151	1	40.00	
04/12/CCYY	C-HCG SERUM PREG	40605503	1	95.50	
04/12/CCYY	SMA 12	40609505	1	158.00	
04/12/CCYY	CHEM-SMA 6	40609752	1	135.50	
04/13/CCYY	CH-THEOPHYLLINE	40610206	1	82.00	
04/12/CCYY	HEMA-CBC	40611600	1	43.00	
04/12/CCYY	H-PROTHROMBINTIME	40612756	1	38.50	
04/12/CCYY	HEMA-PTT	40612855	1	48.50	
04/13/CCYY	MCR URINE CULTURE	40518241	1	63.50	
04/13/CCYY	URIN-ROUTINE UA	59619355	1	29.50	
04/12/CCYY	VENI-PUNCTURE	40619611	1	17.00	
04/13/CCYY	VENI-PUNCTURE	40619611	1	17.00	
	TOTAL LAB CLINICAL				**817.50**

Jackson Medical Center
4444 Jumping Jack Lane
Jersey, NJ 08073

Patient Name	Patient No.	Sex	Admission Date	Discharge Date	Page No.
10071	10071	F	04/12/CCYY	04/13/CCYY	2

Guarantor Name and Address
JACK JENNINGS
4738 JASMINE ROAD
JERSEY, NJ 08077

Insurance Company: WINTER INSURANCE CO.
Claim Number: DOCUMENT 137
Attending Physician: JAMES JUSTICE, M.D.

Date of Service	Description of Hospital Services	Service Code	Qty.	Charges	Total Charges
04/12/CCYY	ABG KIT	40900052	1	36.00	
04/12/CCYY	ABG PUNCTURE	40900102	1	56.00	
04/12/CCYY	ABG STUDY	40900201	1	200.00	
	TOTAL LABORATORY BLOOD GASES				**292.00**
04/13/CCYY	IV ADDITIVE FEE	41705369	6	105.60	
04/13/CCYY	MED. PIGGY BACKS	41710047	2	54.50	
04/13/CCYY	AMINOPHYLLIN INJ	41742255	4	52.00	
04/13/CCYY	PROFILE SERV CHRG	41763756	1	13.50	
04/12/CCYY	3 CC NS/ALUPNT.3 CC	41774209	2	17.00	
04/13/CCYY	3CC NS/ALUPNT.3 CC	41774209	2	17.00	
04/13/CCYY	ZINACEF 750 MG	41777624	2	64.00	
	TOTAL PHARMACY				**323.60**
04/12/CCYY	H H N CURCUIT	41800806	1	26.50	
04/13/CCYY	H H N CIRCUIT	41800806	1	26.50	
04/12/CCYY	H H N TREATMENT	41800855	2	66.00	
04/13/CCYY	H H N TREATMENT	41800855	2	66.00	
	TOTAL INHALATION THERAPY				**185.00**
04/12/CCYY	IV CATHETER	47136049	1	23.00	
04/12/CCYY	IV CATHETER	47136049	1	23.00	
04/12/CCYY	IV TUBING EXTENSION SET	47137278	1	13.00	
04/12/CCYY	IV TUBING SECONDARY SET	47137567	1	33.00	
04/12/CCYY	SOL-D-5-W 500 ML	47138060	1	41.50	
04/12/CCYY	SOL-D-5-W 500 ML	47138060	1	41.50	
04/12/CCYY	SOL D-5-0.45NS 1000 ML	47138136	1	41.50	
	TOTAL IV THERAPY				**216.50**
	BALANCE DUE				2,471.85

Jackson Medical Center
4444 Jumping Jack Lane
Jersey, NJ 08073

Patient Name	Patient No.	Sex	Admission Date	Discharge Date	Page No.
JULIA JENNINGS	10071	F	04/12/CCYY	04/13/CCYY	3

Guarantor Name and Address
JACK JENNINGS
4738 JASMINE ROAD
JERSEY, NJ 08077

Insurance Company: WINTER INSURANCE CO.
Claim Number: DOCUMENT 137
Attending Physician: JAMES JUSTICE, M.D.

Date of Service	Description of Hospital Services	Service Code	Qty.	Charges	Total Charges
	SUMMARY OF CHARGES				
	ROOM & BOARD			395.00	
	PHARMACY			323.60	
	IV THERAPY			216.50	
	MED-SUR SUPPLIES			242.25	
	LABORATORY OR (LAB)			1,109.50	
	RESPIRATORY SVC			185.00	
	SUBTOTAL OF CHARGES				2,471.85
	PAYMENTS AND ADJUSTMENTS			NONE	
	SUBTOTAL PAYMENTS/ADJ				NONE
	BALANCE DUE				2,471.85

Hospital Admission Form

DOCUMENT 138

Provider Information

Name:	Jersey Medical Center					
Address:	2222 Johnson Road					
City:	Jersey	State:	NJ	Zip Code:	08079	
Telephone#:		Fax#:				
Medicare ID#:	310018	UPIN#:				
Tax ID #:	94-1623477	Accepts Medicare Assignment:	☐			
Provider Rep:	Betty Biller		Date: 11/16/CCYY			

Admission Information

Admission Date:	11/13/CCYY	Time:	6:00 PM
Discharge Date:	11/16/CCYY	Time:	4:00 PM
Attending Phy's ID#:	G12513	Date of Injury:	
Attending Physician:	Joe Jenkins, M.D.		

Guarantor Information

Name:	Jack Jennings				
Address:	4738 Jasmine Road				
City:	Jersey	State:	NJ	Zip Code:	08077
Insurance ID #:	77-9999 ABC	SSN:	111-77-9999		
Insurance Name:	Winter Insurance Company				
Insurance Group #:	36928				
Employer Name:	ABC Company				

Patient Information

Name:	Jack Jennings				
Address:	4738 Jasmine Road				
City:	Jersey	State:	NJ	Zip Code:	08077
Telephone#:	(551) 555-0807	Patient Control #:	10072		
Date of Birth:	06/20/CCYY-43	Gender:	Male		
Marital Status:	Married	Relationship to Guarantor:		Self	
Student Status:	☐ Full-time	☐ Part-time			
Insurance Type:	☒ Pvt ☐ M/care ☐ M/caid ☐ WC ☐ Other				

Authorization

☒ Authorization to Release Information
☒ Authorization for Assignment of Benefits
☐ Authorization for Consent for Treatment
☐ My insurance will be billed but there may be a balance due.

Signature: Jack Jennings   Date: 11/13/CCYY

Clinical Information

Principal Diagnosis:	Acute Duodenal Ulcer	
Other Diagnosis:	Single Liveborn	
Surgical Procedure:	EGD with closed biopsy	11/13/CCYY
Other Procedures:		
Remarks:		

Previous Balance:		Payment:		Copay:		Adjustment:			
Total Fee:	$3768.75	Cash ☐ Check ☐ Credit ☐		Cash ☐ Check ☐ Credit ☐		Remarks:		New Balance:	$3768.75

Jersey Medical Center
2222 Johnson Road
Jersey, NJ 08079

Patient Name	Patient No.	Sex	Admission Date	Discharge Date	Page No.
JACK JENNINGS	10072	M	11/13/CCYY	11/16/CCYY	1

Guarantor Name and Address
JACK JENNINGS
4738 JASMINE ROAD
JERSEY, NJ 08077

Insurance Company: WINTER INSURANCE CO.
Claim Number: DOCUMENT 138
Attending Physician: JOE JENKINS, M.D.

Date of Service	Description of Hospital Services	Service Code	Qty.	Charges	Total Charges
	SUMMARY OF CHARGES				
	ROOM-BOARD/SEMI	120	3	465.00	1,395.00
	PHARMACY	250	34		447.55
	MED/SURG SUPPLIES	270	3		32.80
	CLINICAL LABORATORY	300	7		425.30
	PATHOLOGY LAB	310	1		34.70
	DX X-RAY	320	5		1,051.30
	GASTR-INTS SERVICE	750	4		382.10
	TOTAL CHARGES	001			3,768.75

Hospital Admission Form   DOCUMENT 139

Provider Information					
Name:	Jaffe Memorial Hospital				
Address:	1111 Jerome Street				
City:	Jersey	State:	NJ	Zip Code:	08078
Telephone#:		Fax#:			
Medicare ID#:	310019	UPIN#:			
Tax ID #:	94-2922301	Accepts Medicare Assignment:	☐		
Provider Rep:	*Betty Biller*	Date: *10/21/CCYY*			

Admission Information			
Admission Date:	10/20/CCYY	Time:	1:00 AM
Discharge Date:	10/21/CCYY	Time:	7:00 PM
Attending Phy's ID#:	H15564	Date of Injury:	
Attending Physician:	Jacob Jefferson, M.D.		

Guarantor Information				
Name:	Jack Jennings			
Address:	4738 Jasmine Road			
City:	Jersey	State:	NJ	Zip Code: 08077

Patient Information

Name:	Jennifer Jennings				
Address:	4738 Jasmine Road				
City:	Jersey	State:	NJ	Zip Code:	08077
Telephone#:	(551) 555-0807	Patient Control #:	10073		
Date of Birth:	10/04/CCYY-41	Gender:	Female		
Marital Status:	Married	Relationship to Guarantor:		Spouse	
Student Status:	☐ Full-time	☐ Part-time			
Insurance Type:	☒ Pvt ☐ M/care ☐ M/caid ☐ WC ☐ Other _____				

Insurance ID #:	77-9999 ABC	SSN:	111-77-9999
Insurance Name:	Winter Insurance Company		
Insurance Group #:	36928		
Employer Name:	ABC Company		

Authorization

☒ Authorization to Release Information
☒ Authorization for Assignment of Benefits
☐ Authorization for Consent for Treatment
☐ My insurance will be billed but there may be a balance due.

Signature: *Jennifer Jennings*   Date: *10/20/CCYY*

Clinical Information

Principal Diagnosis:	Normal Delivery
Other Diagnosis:	Pregnant State; Single Liveborn
Surgical Procedure:	Manual Assist Delivery 10/20/CCYY
Other Procedures:	
Remarks:	

Previous Balance:		Payment:		Copay:		Adjustment:		
Total Fee:	$1409.02	Cash ☐ Check ☐ Credit ☐		Cash ☐ Check ☐ Credit ☐		Remarks:	New Balance:	$1409.02

Jaffe Memorial Hospital
1111 Jerome Street
Jersey, NJ 08078

Patient Name	Patient No.	Sex	Admission Date	Discharge Date	Page No.
JENNIFER JENNINGS	10073	F	10/20/CCYY	10/21/CCYY	1

Guarantor Name and Address
JACK JENNINGS
4738 JASMINE ROAD
JERSEY, NJ 08077

Insurance Company: WINTER INSURANCE CO.
Claim Number: DOCUMENT 139
Attending Physician: JACOB JEFFERSON, M.D.

Date of Service	Description of Hospital Services	Service Code	Qty.	Unit Price	Total Charges
10/20/CCYY	14-01 OB/GYN ROOM		1	411.30	411.30
	TOTAL ROOM AND BOARD CHARGES				411.30
10/20/CCYY	ANTIBODY SCREEN	37210	1	55.60	55.60
10/20/CCYY	BLOOD COUNT CBC	37547	1	39.35	39.35
10/20/CCYY	PRO TIME	37731	1	47.80	47.80
10/20/CCYY	P.T.T.	37733	1	59.75	59.75
10/20/CCYY	TYPE & RH	37742	1	58.15	58.15
10/20/CCYY	VDRL RPR	37814	1	36.20	36.20
	TOTAL LABORATORY-CLINICAL				296.85
10/20/CCYY	AMERICAINE SPRAY	39048	1	20.25	20.25
10/20/CCYY	AQUAMEP .1 MG/.5 ML INJ	39106	1	11.25	11.25
10/20/CCYY	MASSE BREAST CRM 60 G	41206	1	30.00	30.00
10/20/CCYY	METHERGINE 0.2 MG TAB	41230	4	2.50	10.00
10/20/CCYY	METHERGINE 0.2 MG TAB	41230	4	2.50	10.00
10/20/CCYY	METHERGINE 0.2 MG TAB	41230	2	2.50	5.00
10/20/CCYY	PITOCIN 10 U INJ	41504	2	11.24	22.48
10/20/CCYY	TUCKS PADS #40 TOP	41877	1	20.15	20.15
10/20/CCYY	TYLENOL/COD 30 MG TAB	41886	1	2.25	2.25
10/20/CCYY	TYLENOL/COD 30 MG TAB	41886	2	2.25	4.50
10/20/CCYY	ERYTHROMYCIN OPTH OINT 3.5 GM	42099	1	11.24	11.24
10/20/CCYY	BOTTLE PERI	54092	1	2.85	2.85
10/20/CCYY	IV SOL DEXT 5% LACT RINGER 10	58300	1	38.20	38.20
10/20/CCYY	IV IRRIG SOL WATER 2000 R5005	58376	1	43.85	43.85
	TOTAL PHARMACY				232.02
10/20/CCYY	KIT PERSONAL COMFORT MH	50290	1	5.85	5.85
10/20/CCYY	BELT SANITARY	51223	1	10.35	10.35
10/20/CCYY	BELT SANITARY	51223	1	10.35	10.35
10/20/CCYY	TUBING IV PRIMARY IVAC	51810	1	16.40	16.40
10/20/CCYY	PACK DELIVERED VAGINAL CUSTOM	51929	1	140.35	140.35
10/20/CCYY	PACK COLD ABCO	51935	1	4.50	4.50
10/20/CCYY	PAD STERILE PK 12	51961	1	9.20	9.20
10/20/CCYY	PAD STERILE PK 12	51961	1	9.20	9.20

Jaffe Memorial Hospital
1111 Jerome Street
Jersey, NJ 08078

Patient Name	Patient No.	Sex	Admission Date	Discharge Date	Page No.
JENNIFER JENNINGS	10073	F	10/20/CCYY	10/21/CCYY	2

Guarantor Name and Address
JACK JENNINGS
4738 JASMINE ROAD
JERSEY, NJ 08077

Insurance Company: WINTER INSURANCE CO.
Claim Number: DOCUMENT 139
Attending Physician: JACOB JEFFERSON, M.D.

Date of Service	Description of Hospital Services	Service Code	Qty.	Unit Price	Total Charges
10/21/CCYY	PAD PERI STERILE PK 12	51961	1	9.20	9.20
10/20/CCYY	RAZOR DISP TOMAC	52153	1	3.90	3.90
10/20/CCYY	SUCTION CATHETER CUTTER 10FR	52173	1	3.40	3.40
10/20/CCYY	UNDERPADS ADULT PK6	52480	1	6.20	6.20
10/20/CCYY	UNDERPADS ADULT PK6	52480	1	6.20	6.20
10/20/CCYY	UNDERPADS ADULT PK6	52480	1	6.20	6.20
10/21/CCYY	UNDERPADS ADULT PK6	52480	1	6.20	6.20
10/20/CCYY	IV CATH QUIK (ALL SIZES)	52731	1	13.45	13.45
10/20/CCYY	IV START PACK 18 11/4	52765	1	14.65	14.65
10/20/CCYY	IV START PACK 18 11/4	52765	1	14.65	14.65
10/20/CCYY	TRAY PREP SURGICAL EZ	53167	1	29.90	29.90
10/20/CCYY	TRAY PREP SOAP/WATER	52308	1	25.85	25.85
10/20/CCYY	TRAY PARACERVICAL PUDENDAL PH	52354	1	74.20	74.20
10/20/CCYY	MONITOR IVAC DAILY	54051	1	28.10	28.10
10/20/CCYY	AMNIHOOK MEMBRANE PERFORATOR	56137	1	5.85	5.85
10/20/CCYY	GLOVE SURGICAL STERILE ALL SI	58411	1	4.90	4.90
10/20/CCYY	GLOVE SURGICAL STERILE ALL SI	58411	1	4.90	4.90
10/20/CCYY	GLOVE SURGICAL STERILE ALL SI	58411	1	4.90	4.90
	TOTAL MED-SUR SUPPLIES & DEVICES				468.85
	TOTAL ROOM & BOARD CHARGES		1		411.30
	TOTAL LABORATORY-CLINICAL				296.85
	TOTAL PHARMACY				232.02
	TOTAL MED-SUR SUPPLIES & DEVICES				468.85
	AMOUNT DUE				1,409.02

Hospital Admission Form

DOCUMENT 140

Provider Information						Admission Information			
Name:	Jaffe Memorial Hospital					Admission Date:	10/20/CCYY	Time:	4:00 AM
Address:	1111 Jerome Street					Discharge Date:	10/21/CCYY	Time:	7:00 PM
City:	Jersey	State:	NJ	Zip Code:	08078	Attending Phy's ID#:	H15564	Date of Injury:	
Telephone#:		Fax#:				Attending Physician:	Jacob Jefferson, M.D.		
Medicare ID#:	310019	UPIN#:				**Guarantor Information**			
Tax ID #:	94-2922301	Accepts Medicare Assignment:		☐		Name:	Jack Jennings		
Provider Rep:	*Betty Biller*		Date: *10/21/CCYY*			Address:	4738 Jasmine Road		

Patient Information								
						City:	Jersey	State: NJ Zip Code: 08077
Name:	Baby Boy Jennings					Insurance ID #:	77-9999 ABC	SSN: 111-77-9999
Address:	4738 Jasmine Road					Insurance Name:	Winter Insurance Company	
City:	Jersey	State:	NJ	Zip Code:	08077	Insurance Group #:	36928	
Telephone#:	(551) 555-0807	Patient Control #:	10074			Employer Name:	ABC Company	

Date of Birth: 10/20/CCYY-0   Gender: Male

Authorization

Marital Status: Single   Relationship to Guarantor: Child

☒ Authorization to Release Information
☒ Authorization for Assignment of Benefits
☐ Authorization for Consent for Treatment
☐ My insurance will be billed but there may be a balance due.

Student Status: ☐ Full-time   ☐ Part-time

Insurance Type: ☒ Pvt ☐ M/care ☐ M/caid ☐ WC ☐ Other _____

Signature: *Jack Jennings*   Date: *10/20/CCYY*

Clinical Information	
Principal Diagnosis:	Single Liveborn
Other Diagnosis:	
Surgical Procedure:	
Other Procedures:	
Remarks:	

Previous Balance:		Payment:		Copay:		Adjustment:			
Total Fee:	$479.85	Cash ☐ Check ☐ Credit ☐		Cash ☐ Check ☐ Credit ☐		Remarks:		New Balance:	$479.85

Jaffe Memorial Hospital
1111 Jerome Street
Jersey, NJ 08078

Patient Name	Patient No.	Sex	Age	Admission Date	Discharge Date	Page No.
BABY BOY JENKINS	10074	M	00	10/20/CCYY	10/21/CCYY	1

Guarantor Name and Address
JACK JENNINGS
4738 JASMINE ROAD
JERSEY, NJ 08077

Insurance Company: WINTER INSURANCE CO.
Claim Number: DOCUMENT 140
Attending Physician: JACOB JEFFERSON, M.D.

Date of Service	Description of Hospital Services	Service Code	Qty.	Unit Price	Total Charges
10/20/CCYY	1400-01 NURSERY		1	240.60	240.60
	TOTAL ROOM & BOARD CHARGES				240.60
10/21/CCYY	DEL RM NEWBORN SCREENING	21002	1	41.00	41.00
	TOTAL LABOR ROOM/DELIVERY				41.00
10/21/CCYY	RADIOLOGY-PORTABLE STUDIES 76499	30289	1	51.70	51.70
10/21/CCYY	RADIOLOGY-SKULL, 2 VIEWS 70250	30500	1	95.50	95.50
	TOTAL RADIOLOGY-DIAGNOSTIC				147.20
10/20/CCYY	TRIPLE DYE	40183	1	11.25	11.25
10/20/CCYY	VASELINE OINT 60 OZ	40184	1	12.90	12.90
10/20/CCYY	WASHCLOTH BABY MOIST	55247	1	10.80	10.80
	TOTAL PHARMACY				34.95
10/20/CCYY	PAMPERS NEWBORN	52481	1	16.10	16.10
	TOTAL MED-SUR SUPPLIES & DEVICES				16.10

Jaffe Memorial Hospital
1111 Jerome Street
Jersey, NJ 08078

Patient Name	Patient No.	Sex	Age	Admission Date	Discharge Date	Page No.
BABY BOY JENNINGS	10074	M	00	10/20/CCYY	10/21/CCYY	2

Guarantor Name and Address
JACK JENNINGS
4738 JASMINE ROAD
JERSEY, NJ 08077

Insurance Company: WINTER INSURANCE CO.
Claim Number: DOCUMENT 140
Attending Physician: JACOB JEFFERSON, M.D.

Date of Service	Description of Hospital Services	Service Code	Qty.	Unit Price	Total Charges
	TOTAL ROOM AND BOARD CHARGES		1		240.60
	TOTAL LABOR ROOM/DELIVERY				41.00
	TOTAL RADIOLOGY-DIAGNOSTIC				147.20
	TOTAL PHARMACY				34.95
	TOTAL MED-SUR SUPPLIES & DEVICES				16.10
	AMOUNT DUE				479.85

Hospital Admission Form

Provider Information

Name:	Jersey Main Hospital				
Address:	3333 Jager Blvd.				
City:	Jersey	State:	NJ	Zip Code:	08071
Telephone#:		Fax#:			
Medicare ID#:	310021	UPIN#:			
Tax ID #:	94-3388827	Accepts Medicare Assignment:	☐		
Provider Rep:	*Betty Biller*		Date: *10/17/CCYY*		

Patient Information

Name:	Janet Jennings				
Address:	4738 Jasmine Road				
City:	Jersey	State:	NJ	Zip Code:	08077
Telephone#:	(551) 555-0807	Patient Control #:	10075		
Date of Birth:	12/07/CCYY-15	Gender:	Female		
Marital Status:	Single	Relationship to Guarantor:		Child	
Student Status:	☒ Full-time	☐ Part-time			
Insurance Type:	☒ Pvt ☐ M/care ☐ M/caid ☐ WC ☐ Other _____				

Admission Information

Admission Date:	10/15/CCYY	Time:	6:00 PM
Discharge Date:	10/17/CCYY	Time:	12:00 Noon
Attending Phy's ID#:	J21302	Date of Injury:	
Attending Physician:	Jenna Jackson, M.D.		

Guarantor Information

Name:	Jack Jennings				
Address:	4738 Jasmine Road				
City:	Jersey	State:	NJ	Zip Code:	08077
Insurance ID #:	77-9999 ABC	SSN:	111-77-9999		
Insurance Name:	Winter Insurance Company				
Insurance Group #:	36928				
Employer Name:	ABC Company				

Authorization

☒ Authorization to Release Information
☒ Authorization for Assignment of Benefits
☐ Authorization for Consent for Treatment
☐ My insurance will be billed but there may be a balance due.
Signature: *Jack Jennings* Date: *10/15/CCYY*

Clinical Information

Principal Diagnosis:	Acute gastritis	
Other Diagnosis:	Hypovelomia; Abdominal Pain	
Surgical Procedure:	Diagnostic ultrasound of digestive system	10/15/CCYY
Other Procedures:	Upper GI Series	10/16/CCYY
Remarks:		

Previous Balance:		Payment:		Copay:		Adjustment:			
Total Fee:	$4783.00	Cash ☐ Check ☐ Credit ☐		Cash ☐ Check ☐ Credit ☐		Remarks:		New Balance:	$4783.00

Jersey Main Hospital
3333 Jager Blvd.
Jersey, NJ 08071

Patient Name	Patient No.	Sex	Admission Date	Discharge Date	Page No.
JANET JENNINGS	10075	F	10/15/CCYY	10/17/CCYY	1

Guarantor Name and Address
JACK JENNINGS
4738 JASMINE ROAD
JERSEY, NJ 08077

Insurance Company: WINTER INSURANCE CO.
Claim Number: DOCUMENT 141
Attending Physician: JENNA JACKSON, M.D.

Date of Service	Description of Hospital Services	Service Code	Qty.	Charges	Total Charges
10/15/CCYY	ROOM & BOARD	99020802	1	395.00	
10/16/CCYY	ROOM & BOARD	99020802	1	395.00	
	TOTAL ROOM & BOARD				**790.00**
10/15/CCYY	PED ADMIT KIT CS 12	40525602	1	38.75	
10/15/CCYY	IV ARM SUPPORT	40539090	1	5.00	
10/15/CCYY	MISC CENTRAL SUPPLY	40545303	1	4.00	
	ENSURE IT DRESS				
10/15/CCYY	MIDSTREAM URINE COLLELCTOR	40546178	1	8.25	
10/15/CCYY	PILLOW DISP	40555252	1	12.25	
10/16/CCYY	SYRINGE 1 CC TO 10 CC W/NEEDLE	40572166	1	4.75	
10/15/CCYY	SLIPPERS/PILLOW PAWS	40573149	1	4.00	
10/16/CCYY	EZ BARIUM CUP 12 OZ	40583809	1	16.00	
10/16/CCYY	EZ BARIUM CUP 12 OZ	40583809	1	16.00	
10/15/CCYY	IMED BURETROL SET 10	40584377	1	35.00	
10/16/CCYY	IMED PUMP RENTAIL DAILY 01	40584393	1	116.00	
10/17/CCYY	IMED PUMP RENTAL DAILY 01	40584393	3	174.00	
	TOTAL CENTRAIL SUPPLY				**434.00**
10/15/CCYY	CH-CREATININE BLD	40603151	1	42.00	
10/15/CCYY	SMA 12	40609505	1	166.00	
10/15/CCYY	CHEM-SMA 6	40609752	1	142.50	
10/15/CCYY	HEMA-CBC	40611600	1	45.00	
10/16/CCYY	HEMA-CBC	40611600	1	45.00	
10/15/CCYY	HEMA-DIFFERENTIAL	40611907	1	23.00	
10/15/CCYY	H-PROTHROMBINTIME	40612756	1	40.50	
10/15/CCYY	HEMA-PTT	40612855	1	51.00	
10/15/CCYY	MC-ROUTINE CULTURE	40618001	1	81.50	
10/15/CCYY	MCR URINE CULTURE	40618241	1	66.50	
10/15/CCYY	URIN-ROUTINE UA	40619355	1	31.00	
10/15/CCYY	VENI-PUNCTURE	40619611	1	18.00	

Jersey Main Hospital
3333 Jager Blvd.
Jersey, NJ 08071

Patient Name	Patient No.	Sex	Admission Date	Discharge Date	Page No.
JANET JENNINGS	10075	F	10/15/CCYY	10/17/CCYY	2

Guarantor Name and Address
JACK JENNINGS
4738 JASMINE ROAD
JERSEY, NJ 08077

Insurance Company: WINTER INSURANCE CO.
Claim Number: DOCUMENT 141
Attending Physician: JENNA JACKSON, M.D.

Date of Service	Description of Hospital Services	Service Code	Qty.	Charges	Total Charges
	DETAIL OF CURRENT CHARGES				
10/16/CCYY	VENI-PUNCTURE	40619611	1	18.00	
	TOTAL LAB CLINICAL				**770.00**
10/16/CCYY	ABDMN FLAT KUB IV	41400557	1	85.00	
10/15/CCYY	ABDOMEN SERIES 2V	41400607	1	143.00	
10/15/CCYY	CHEST 2V AP & LAT	41401902	1	113.00	
10/16/CCYY	SML BOWEL SERIES	41408204	1	173.00	
10/16/CCYY	UPPER GI	41410002	1	275.00	
10/15/CCYY	X-RAY EMERGNCY CAL	41410408	1	39.00	
	TOTAL RADIOLOGY				**828.00**
10/15/CCYY	IV ADDITIVE FEE	41705369	2	37.00	
10/16/CCYY	IV ADDITIVE FEE	41705369	2	37.00	
10/15/CCYY	MVI-12	41754151	2	32.00	
10/16/CCYY	MVI-12	41754151	2	32.00	
	TOTAL PHARMACY				**138.00**
10/15/CCYY	ABDOMEN-GENERAL	42500017	1	475.00	
10/15/CCYY	ULTRASND-PELVIS	42501403	1	475.00	
10/15/CCYY	ULTRASOUND KIDNEY	42501650	1	475.00	
10/15/CCYY	ULTRASOUND-CALL B	42501759	1	160.00	
	TOTAL ULTRA SOUND				**1,585.00**
10/15/CCYY	IV CATHETER	47136049	1	24.00	
10/15/CCYY	IV CATHETER	47136049	1	24.00	
10/15/CCYY	IV START KIT	47137195	1	36.00	
10/15/CCYY	IV TUBING EXTENSION SET	47137278	1	14.00	
10/15/CCYY	D5.OZ NS 500 ML	47138219	1	35.00	
10/15/CCYY	D5.OZ NS 500 ML	47138219	1	35.00	
10/16/CCYY	D5.OZ NS 500 ML	47138219	1	35.00	
10/16/CCYY	D5.OZ NS 500 ML	47138219	1	35.00	
	TOTAL IV THERAPY				**238.00**

Jersey Main Hospital
3333 Jager Blvd.
Jersey, NJ 08071

Patient Name	Patient No.	Sex	Admission Date	Discharge Date	Page No.
JANET JENNINGS	10075	F	10/15/CCYY	10/17/CCYY	3

Guarantor Name and Address
JACK JENNINGS
4738 JASMINE ROAD
JERSEY, NJ 08077

Insurance Company: WINTER INSURANCE CO.
Claim Number: DOCUMENT 141
Attending Physician: JENNA JACKSON, M.D.

Date of Service	Description of Hospital Services	Service Code	Qty.	Charges	Total Charges
	SUMMARY OF CHARGES				
	2 DAYS PED/WRD @ 395			790.00	
	PHARMACY			138.00	
	IV THERAPY			238.00	
	MED-SURG SUPPLIES			434.00	
	LABORATORY OR (LAB)			770.00	
	DX X-RAY			2,413.00	
	SUBTOTAL OF CHARGES				4,783.00
	PAYMENTS AND ADJUSTEMNTS			NONE	
	SUBTOTAL PAYMENTS/ADJ				NONE
	BALANCE				4,783.00
	BALANCE DUE				4,783.00

Hospital Claims Beginning Financials

FURY FAMILY

Insurance Plan	Rover Insurers, Inc.—Ninja Enterprises				
Patient:	**FRED**	**FAY**	**FERN**	**FORREST**	
C/O DEDUCTIBLE	0.00	0.00	0.00	0.00	
DEDUCTIBLE	0.00	23.87	0.00	37.27	
COINSURANCE	0.00	0.00	0.00	0.00	
ACCIDENT BENEFIT	0.00	0.00	0.00	0.00	
LIFETIME MAXIMUM	2,976.29	64,927.38	7,627.00	675.00	
M/N OFFICE VISITS					
OFFICE VISITS					
HOSPITAL VISITS					
DXL					
SURGERY					
ASSISTANT SURGERY					
ANESTHESIA					

Hospital Admission Form

Provider Information

Name:	Fashion Medical Center				
Address:	7900 Felton Street				
City:	Folley	State:	FL	Zip Code:	32202
Telephone#:		Fax#:			
Medicare ID#:	100022	UPIN#:			
Tax ID #:	22-8837444	Accepts Medicare Assignment:	☐		
Provider Rep:	*Betty Biller*		Date:	*C9/17/CCYY*	

Admission Information

Admission Date:	09/14/CCYY	Time:	6:00 AM
Discharge Date:	09/17/CCYY	Time:	3:00 PM
Attending Phy's ID#:	K65422	Date of Injury:	
Attending Physician:	Fritz Fuller, M.D.		

Guarantor Information

Name:	Fred Fury
Address:	5555 Fairlane Blvd.

Patient Information

Name:	Fay Fury				
Address:	5555 Fairlane Blvd.				
City:	Folley	State:	FL	Zip Code:	32208
Telephone#:	(407) 555-3220	Patient Control #:	10076		
Date of Birth:	09/30/CCYY-60	Gender:	Female		
Marital Status:	Married	Relationship to Guarantor:		Spouse	
Student Status:	☐ Full-time	☐ Part-time			
Insurance Type:	☒ Pvt ☐ M/care ☐ M/caid ☐ WC ☐ Other _____				

City:	Folley	State:	FL	Zip Code:	32208
Insurance ID #:	44-6666 NIN	SSN:	222-44-6666		
Insurance Name:	Rover Insurers, Inc.				
Insurance Group #:	21088				
Employer Name:	Ninja Enterprises				

Authorization

☒ Authorization to Release Information
☒ Authorization for Assignment of Benefits
☐ Authorization for Consent for Treatment
☐ My insurance will be billed but there may be a balance due.
Signature: _Fay Fury_   Date: _9/14/CCYY_

Clinical Information

Principal Diagnosis:	Uterine leiomyoma	
Other Diagnosis:		
Surgical Procedure:	Total abdominal hysterectomy	9/14/CCYY
Other Procedures:	Electrocardiogram	9/14/CCYY
Remarks:	Pre-Certification #979742826	Second Surgical Opinion Performed

Previous Balance:		Payment:		Copay:		Adjustment:			
Total Fee:	$9960.20	Cash ☐ Check ☐ Credit ☐		Cash ☐ Check ☐ Credit ☐		Remarks:		New Balance:	$9960.20

Fashion Medical Center
7900 Felton Street
Folley, FL 32202

Patient Name	Patient No.	Sex	Admission Date	Discharge Date	Page No.
FAY FURY	10076	F	09/14/CCYY	09/17/CCYY	1

Guarantor Name and Address
FRED FURY
5555 FAIRLANE BLVD.
FOLLEY, FL 32208

Insurance Company: ROVER INSURERS, INC.
Claim Number: DOCUMENT 143
Attending Physician: FRITZ FULLER, M.D.

Post Mo/Da	Svc. Mo/Da	Description of Hospital Services	Service Code	Qty.	Charges	Patient Amount
09/14	09/14	SEMI-PRIVA330A	2340002	1	445.00	445.00
09/15	09/15	SEMI-PRIVA330A	2340002	1	445.00	445.00
09/15	09/16	SEMI-PRIVA330A	2340002	1	445.00	445.00
09/17	09/16	00055 SURGERY 3 ½ HRS	3210014	1	2,636.00	2,636.00
09/16	09/14	00066 RECOVRY 1 HOUR	3223004	1	83.00	83.00
09/17	09/16	00088 ANES 3 ½ HR	3700014	1	680.00	680.00
09/16	09/15	00099 BELT SANITARY 1 +	4010060	1	9.00	9.00
09/15	09/15	00099 PACK PT. CARE +	4010364	1	9.00	9.00
09/16	09/15	00099 PAD PERI PKG 12 +	4010384	1	9.00	9.00
09/15	09/14	00099 BAND STKNG THGH	4010503	1	57.00	57.00
09/16	09/15	00099 KIT COL SPEC UR	4010659	1	12.50	12.50
09/15	09/14	00099 BEDPAN DISP	4010705	1	9.00	9.00
09/17	09/16	00099 DRES B/A 8X6	4010783	1	9.00	9.00
09/16	09/15	00099 UNDRPAD TIS FAC*	4010823	1	16.50	16.50
09/17	09/16	00099 LINER SUCTION	4011257	1	24.50	24.50
09/16	09/15	00099 SLIPPERS SKD DR	4011385	1	9.50	9.50
09/16	09/15	00099 BAND BINDER ABD	4011643	1	79.00	79.00
09/17	09/16	00099 PULSE OXIMETER	4013022	1	65.00	65.00
09/17	09/16	00099 TRAY CATH FD+BA	4020093	1	91.50	91.50
09/17	09/16	00099 TRAY SCRUB SKIN	4020210	3	124.50	124.50
09/17	09/16	00099 CAUT SURGERY	4030010	1	142.50	142.50
09/17	09/16	00099 MNTR B/P D	4030025	1	77.00	77.00
09/16	09/15	00099 PUMP IV MED SS	4030120	1	45.00	45.00
09/16	09/15	00099 PUMP IV MED D*	4030121	1	45.00	45.00
09/17	09/16	00099 PUMP IV MED D*	4030121	1	45.00	45.00
09/18	09/17	00099 PUMP IV MED D*	4030121	1	45.00	45.00
09/17	09/16	00099 MNTR CARD DIGIT	4030280	1	110.00	110.00
09/17	09/16	00099 PULSE OXIMETER	4033076	1	65.00	65.00
09/17	09/16	00099 ANES BREATH/CIR	4060001	1	56.00	56.00
09/17	09/16	00099 ANES MASK DISP	4050007	1	18.50	18.50
09/17	09/16	00099 SPONGE 4X4 TRI1	4060184	2	19.00	19.00
09/17	09/16	00099 PACK MAJOR	4060397	1	228.50	228.50
09/17	09/16	00099 SUTR PAK GUT	4060641	20	350.00	350.00
09/17	09/16	00099 TEMP-A-STRIP	4060781	1	16.50	16.50
09/17	09/16	00099 SPONGE LAP	4060910	1	27.00	27.00

Fashion Medical Center
7900 Felton Street
Folley, FL 32202

Patient Name	Patient No.	Sex	Admission Date	Discharge Date	Page No.
FAY FURY	10076	F	09/14/CCYY	09/17/CCYY	2

Guarantor Name and Address
FRED FURY
5555 FAIRLANE BLVD.
FOLLEY, FL 32208

Insurance Company: ROVER INSURERS, INC.
Claim Number: DOCUMENT 143
Attending Physician: FRITZ FULLER, M.D.

Post Mo/Da	Svc. Mo/Da	Description of Hospital Services		Service Code	Qty.	Charges	Patient Amount
09/17	09/16	00099	PACK GYN 1	4060919	2	137.00	137.00
09/17	09/16	00099	DRAPE GOWN LG	4090920	3	117.00	117.00
09/17	09/16	00099	PAD CAUTERY GRO	4050964	1	53.50	53.50
09/17	09/16	00099	KIT BASIN DBL S	4060997	1	66.50	66.50
09/16	09/15	00099	RT INCENT EXRCS	4070041	1	54.50	54.50
09/16	09/14	00099	RT MASK O2	4070083	1	17.50	17.50
09/17	09/16	00099	RT TUBE ENDTRAC	4070103	1	43.50	43.50
09/17	09/16	00099	RT AIRWAY ORAL	4070109	1	7.50	7.50
09/14	09/13	8100524	URIN, CHEM/QUAL	4101005	1	17.50	17.50
09/15	09/14	8100524	URIN, CHEM/QUAL	4101005	1	17.50	17.50
09/14	09/13	8101524	URIN, MICROSCOPIC	4101015	1	17.50	17.50
09/15	09/14	8101524	URIN, MICROSCOPIC	4101015	1	17.50	17.50
09/14	09/13	8500724	DIFF MANUAL	4105007	1	34.50	34.50
09/15	09/14	8500724	DIFF MANUAL	4105007	1	34.50	34.50
09/16	09/15	8500724	DIFF MANUAL	4105007	1	34.50	34.50
09/14	09/13	8502124	HEMOGRAM, AUTOMID	4105021	1	34.50	34.50
09/15	09/14	8502124	HEMOGRAM, AUTOMID	4105021	1	34.50	34.50
09/16	09/15	8502124	HEMOGRAM, AUTOMID	4105021	1	34.50	34.50
09/14	09/13	8561024	PROTHROM TIME	4105610	1	45.50	45.50
09/14	09/13	8573024	ACT PROTHM. TIME	4105730	1	45.50	45.50
09/15	09/14	8600624	PREGNANCY TEST	4106023	1	41.00	41.00
09/16	09/13	8606824	BLD, CRSSMCH, ANTI	4106074	1	53.00	53.00
09/14	09/13	8659224	VDRL, RPR, DRT, QL	4106592	1	35.50	35.50
09/16	09/15	8708624	CULT, URIN CNT	4109086	1	82.00	82.00
09/14	09/13	36415	VENIPUNCTURE	4209011	1	25.00	25.00
09/15	09/14	36415	VENIPUNCTURE	4209011	1	25.00	25.00
09/16	09/15	36415	VENIPUNCTURE	4209011	1	25.00	25.00
09/16	09/13	99058	LAB STAT CHG *	4209063	1	27.00	27.00
09/15	09/14	99058	LAB STAT CHG *	4209063	1	27.00	27.00
09/16	09/15	88308304	SPATH DIAG, SMALL	4308304	1	65.50	65.50
09/16	09/16	8830527	SPATH, DIAG, LG	4308305	1	83.00	83.00
09/16	09/16	8830727	SPATH DIAG COMPL	4308307	1	187.50	187.50
09/14	09/13	93005	EKG	4603000	1	100.00	100.00
09/14	09/13	8132027	CHEST TWO VIEW	4901023	1	118.00	118.00
09/15	09/15	00099	CIPRO 500 MG	5302776	1	5.30	5.30
09/15	09/15	00099	CIPRO 500 MG	5302776	2	10.60	10.60

Fashion Medical Center
7900 Felton Street
Folley, FL 32202

Patient Name	Patient No.	Sex	Admission Date	Discharge Date	Page No.
FAY FURY	10076	F	09/14/CCYY	09/17/CCYY	3

Guarantor Name and Address
FRED FURY
5555 FAIRLANE BLVD.
FOLLEY, FL 32208

Insurance Company: ROVER INSURERS, INC.
Claim Number: DOCUMENT 143
Attending Physician: FRITZ FULLER, M.D.

Post Mo/Da	Svc. Mo/Da	Description of Hospital Services		Service Code	Qty.	Charges	Total Charges
09/16	09/16	00099	CIPRO 500 MG	5302776	2	10.60	10.60
09/17	09/17	00099	CIPRO 500 MG	5302775	2	10.60	10.60
09/17	09/17	00099	CIPRO 500 MG	5302776	2	10.60	10.60
09/17	09/14	90799	TRACRIUM 50 MG/5	5318368	1	52.00	52.00
09/17	09/14	1450395	ATROPINE .4 MG/ML	5318374	1	16.40	16.40
09/17	09/14	0053395	MEFOXIN 2 GM	5319054	1	85.30	85.30
09/14	09/14	0053395	MEFOXIN 2 GM	5319054	2	170.60	170.60
09/17	09/14	0210295	NEDSTIGM 1:1000	5322805	1	16.40	16.40
09/16	09/16	0010695	PHENERGAN 50 MG/M	5323798	3	49.20	49.20
09/17	09/14	90799	DIPRIVAN0-20 ML	5323845	1	36.70	36.70
09/17	09/14	0250995	SUCCINYLOCHOLINE	5324405	1	24.00	24.00
09/17	09/14	0250195	TUBORURARINE INJ	5325010	1	39.40	39.40
09/16	09/16	0392095	SUBLIMAZE .1-2 ML	5327501	1	22.90	22.90
09/16	09/16	0392095	SUBLIMAZE .1-2 ML	5327501	1	22.90	22.90
09/15	09/15	0391495	MEPERIDINE 50 MG/M	5327629	1	23.70	23.70
09/16	09/16	0391495	MEPERIDINE 50 MG/M	5327629	1	23.70	23.70
09/16	09/16	0391495	MEPERIDINE 50 MG/M	5327629	1	23.70	23.70
09/16	09/16	0391495	MEPERIDINE 50 MG/M	5327629	1	23.70	23.70
09/17	09/17	00099	PERCODAN	5327852	1	3.60	3.60
09/17	09/17	00099	PERCODAN	5327852	1	3.60	3.60
09/18	09/18	00099	PERCODAN	5327852	2	7.20	7.20
09/17	09/14	00099	FORANE 0-100 ML	5339053	1	156.60	156.60
09/14	09/14	00099	PROCESSING IVPB	5349008	2	34.60	34.60
09/16	09/15	00099	DAILY PROFILE RE	5349052	1	5.40	5.40
09/17	09/16	00099	DAILY PROFILE RE	5349052	1	5.40	5.40
09/18	09/17	00099	DAILY PROFILE RE	5349052	1	5.40	5.40
09/15	09/14	00099	PROFILE INIT FEE	5349108	1	7.10	7.10
09/15	09/14	00099	MAR PREPARATION	5349586	1	3.20	3.20
09/16	09/15	00099	MAR PREPARATION	5349586	1	3.20	3.20
09/17	09/16	00099	MAR PREPARATION	5349586	1	3.20	3.20
09/15	09/14	00099	IV FLOW SHEET PR	5349588	1	3.20	3.20
09/16	09/15	00099	IV FLOW SHEET PR	5349588	1	3.20	3.20
09/17	09/16	00099	IV FLOW SHEET PR	5349588	1	3.20	3.20
09/14	09/14	00920	IV D5 UF 5C	5410008	2	78.00	78.00
09/16	09/15	00920	IV LR 1M	5410096	1	39.00	39.00
09/17	09/16	00920	IV LR 1M	5410096	1	39.00	39.00

Fashion Medical Center
7900 Felton Street
Folley, FL 32202

Patient Name	Patient No.	Sex	Admission Date	Discharge Date	Page No.
FAY FURY	10076	F	09/14/CCYY	09/17/CCYY	4

Guarantor Name and Address
FRED FURY
5555 FAIRLANE BLVD.
FOLLEY, FL 32208

Insurance Company: ROVER INSURERS, INC.
Claim Number: DOCUMENT 143
Attending Physician: FRITZ FULLER, M.D.

Post Mo/Da	Svc. Mo/Da	Description of Hospital Services		Service Code	Qty.	Charges	Total Charges
09/17	09/16	00920	IV LR 1M	5410096	1	39.00	39.00
09/15	09/14	00920	IV LR D5 1M	5410099	1	39.00	39.00
09/16	09/15	00920	IV LR D5 1M	5410099	1	39.00	39.00
09/16	09/15	00920	IV LR D5 1M	5410099	1	39.00	39.00
09/16	09/15	00920	IV LR D5 1M	5410099	1	39.00	39.00
09/17	09/16	00920	IV LR D5 1M	5410099	1	39.00	39.00
09/17	09/16	00920	IRR H2O STER 2M	5410205	2	76.00	76.00
09/17	09/16	00920	IRR NACL .9 1M	5400206	2	58.00	58.00
09/15	09/14	00920	SSET SECND IV	5420005	1	54.00	54.00
09/17	09/16	00920	SET EXTN IV 2SIT	5420081	1	15.00	15.00
09/15	09/14	00920	IV CATH PLAC UNT	5420123	1	18.50	18.50
09/15	09/14	00920	IV CATH PLAC UNT	5420123	1	18.50	18.50
09/15	09/14	00920	IV CATH PLAC UNT	5420123	1	18.50	18.50
09/17	09/16	00920	SET ADM IV	5420244	1	47.50	47.50
09/17	09/16	00920	IV CATH PLAC UNT	5420243	1	18.50	18.50
09/16	09/14	94799	02 HRS REC RM	5500723	1	32.00	32.00
		TOTALS				9,960.20	9,960.20

Fashion Medical Center
7900 Felton Street
Folley, FL 32202

Patient Name	Patient No.	Sex	Admission Date	Discharge Date	Page No.
FAY FURY	10076	F	09/14/CCYY	09/17/CCYY	5

Guarantor Name and Address
FRED FURY
5555 FAIRLANE BLVD.
FOLLEY, FL 32208

Insurance Company: ROVER INSURERS, INC.
Claim Number: DOCUMENT 143
Attending Physician: FRITZ FULLER, M.D.

Post Mo/Da	Svc. Mo/Da	Description of Hospital Services	Service Code	Qty.	Charges	Total Charges
		SUMMARY BY SERVICE				
		SEMI-PRIVATE ROOM				
		3 DAYS @ 445.00			1,335.00	
		OPERATING ROOM		1	2,636.00	
		ANESTHESIA-HOSPITAL FEE		1	680.00	
		RECOVERY ROOM		1	83.00	
		PHARMACY		22	274.60	
		RADIOLOGY		1	118.00	
		PHARMACY-INJECTIONS		18	630.60	
		LABORATORY-CLINICAL		21	708.50	
		LABORATORY-PATHOLOGY		3	336.00	
		STERILE SUPPLIES		31	979.00	
		EKG		1	100.00	
		CENTRAL SUPPLY		38	1,523.50	
		INHALATION		1	32.00	
		IV THERAPY		14	524.00	
		TOTAL			9,960.20	

This constitutes a medical decision only: it is not a confirmation of benefits
Contact the benefit payer for an explanation of coverage.

Utilization Review Certification

1. **PT./SUBS. NAME**: _____ Fay Fury/Fred Fury _____
2. **GROUP NAME/#**: _____ Ninja Enterprises _____ **I.D. #**: __ 44-6666 NIN ____ **Hospital Claim #**: 143 __
3. **HOSPITAL**: _____ Fashion Medical Center __ **ADMIT DATE**: _____ 9/14/CCYY _____
4. **DATE NOTIFIED**: _____ **WORK COMP EMPLOYER**: _____

5. THIS ADMISSION IS:

Preauthorized:	YES _____	NO __✓__
Elective:	YES __✓__	NO _____
Emergency/OB:	YES _____	NO __✓__

6. TYPE OF APPROVAL:

Total Approval: ____✓____
Partial Denial: _____
Total Denial: _____

7. MEDICALLY NECESSARY DAYS:

__3__ DAYS are certified as medically necessary.

FROM ___9/14/CCYY___ THRU _9/17/ CCYY_

FROM _____ THRU _____

8. DENIED DAYS OR SERVICES:

_____ DAYS are not certified as medically necessary.

FROM _____ THRU _____

FROM _____ THRU _____

SERVICES not certified are:

_____

9. GRACE/ADMIN. DAYS ARE AUTHORIZED:

FROM _____ THRU _____

10. DENIAL LETTER GIVEN ON _____

11. DENIAL OCCURRED DURING:

_____ Concurrent Review
_____ Retrospective Review
_____ Prior Authorization

12. SERVICES WERE PROVIDED FOR THE FOLLOWING REASONS:

_____ Psychiatric Care
_____ Alcohol Detox
_____ Alcohol Rehab
_____ Date Alc. Rehab Began
_____ Drug Detox
_____ Drug Rehab
_____ Date Drug Rehab Began
_____ Cosmetic Surgery

____ Pre-Cert #: 979742826 _____

Type of Surgery
Cosmetic Surg. Related to:

_____ Congenital Condition
_____ Previous Surgery
_____ Previous Injury
_____ Dental due to accidental injury

ADDITIONAL COMMENTS:

_____

_____ Fiala Faraman _____
REVIEWER SIGNATURE

_____ 09/14/ CCYY _____
DATE CERT. GIVEN

**PLEASE ATTACH THIS FORM TO
YOUR CLAIM TO EXPEDITE PAYMENT**

PAYER COPY

Hospital Admission Form

Provider Information

Name:	Folley Medical Center					
Address:	9900 Fire Blvd.					
City:	Folley	State:	FL	Zip Code:	32203	
Telephone#:		Fax#:				
Medicare ID#:	100023	UPIN#:				
Tax ID #:	22-8877788	Accepts Medicare Assignment:		☐		
Provider Rep:	*Betty Biller*		Date: *10/20/CCYY*			

Admission Information

Admission Date:	10/17/CCYY	Time:	8:00 PM
Discharge Date:	10/20/CCYY	Time:	3:00 PM
Attending Phy's ID#:	L65400	Date of Injury:	
Attending Physician:	Frank Flanders, M.D.		

Guarantor Information

Name:	Fred Fury			
Address:	5555 Fairlane Blvd.			
City:	Folley	State:	FL	Zip Code: 32208
Insurance ID #:	44-6666 NIN	SSN:	222-44-6666	
Insurance Name:	Rover Insurers, Inc.			
Insurance Group #:	21088			
Employer Name:	Ninja Enterprises			

Patient Information

Name:	Fay Fury				
Address:	5555 Fairlane Blvd.				
City:	Folley	State:	FL	Zip Code:	32208
Telephone#:	(407) 555-3220	Patient Control #:	10076		
Date of Birth:	09/30/CCYY-60	Gender:	Female		
Marital Status:	Married	Relationship to Guarantor:	Spouse		
Student Status:	☐ Full-time	☐ Part-time			
Insurance Type:	☒ Pvt ☐ M/care ☐ M/caid ☐ WC ☐ Other _____				

Authorization

☒ Authorization to Release Information
☒ Authorization for Assignment of Benefits
☐ Authorization for Consent for Treatment
☐ My insurance will be billed but there may be a balance due.

Signature: *Fay Fury*   Date: *10/17/CCYY*

Clinical Information

Principal Diagnosis:	Acute pylonephritis
Other Diagnosis:	Proteus infection
Surgical Procedure:	
Other Procedures:	
Remarks:	Pre-Certification #: 789546528

Previous Balance:	$9960.20	Payment:		Copay:		Adjustment:		
Total Fee:	$4385.80	Cash ☐ Check ☐ Credit ☐		Cash ☐ Check ☐ Credit ☐		Remarks:	New Balance:	$14346.00

Folley Medical Center
9900 Fire Blvd.
Folley, FL 32203

Patient Name	Patient No.	Sex		Admission Date	Discharge Date	Page No.
FAY FURY	10076	F		10/17/CCYY	10/20/CCYY	1

Guarantor Name and Address
FRED FURY
5555 FAIRLANE BLVD.
FOLLEY, FL 32208

Insurance Company: ROVER INSURERS, INC.
Claim Number: DOCUMENT 144
Attending Physician: FRANK FLANDERS, M.D.

Date of Service	Description of Hospital Services	Service Code	Qty.	Unit Price	Total Charges
10/17/CCYY	MED-SURG SEMI-PRIVATE	3080002	1	425.00	425.00
10/18/CCYY	MED/SURG SEMI-PRIVATE	3080002	1	425.00	425.00
10/19/CCYY	MED/SURG SEMI-PRIVATE	3080002	1	425.00	425.00
	ROOM BOARD/SEMI **SUBTOTAL**	** 120			1,275.00
10/17/CCYY	TYLENOL 5 GR PO	4170135	2	1.00	2.00
10/17/CCYY	ANCEF 1 GM VIAL	4170161	1	32.00	32.00
	PHARMACY **SUBTOTAL**	** 250			34.00
10/17/CCYY	D5.45 NS 500 ML	4171333	1	28.00	28.00
10/17/CCYY	D5W 50 ML	4174046	1	28.00	28.00
	IV SOLUTIONS **SUBTOTAL**	** 258			56.00
10/17/CCYY	I.V. SERVICE FEE	4172419	1	23.00	23.00
	I.V. THERAPY **SUBTOTAL**	** 260			23.00
10/17/CCYY	ANGIOCATH	4051000	2	12.00	24.00
10/18/CCYY	FOLEY CATH TRAY	4051011	1	48.00	48.00
10/18/CCYY	SANITARY PAD (DZ)	4051042	1	6.00	6.00
10/17/CCYY	MIDSTREAM KIT	4051052	1	9.00	9.00
10/18/CCYY	MIDSTREAM KIT	4051052	1	9.00	9.00
10/18/CCYY	ICE BAG	4051060	4	8.00	32.00
10/19/CCYY	ICE BAG	4051060	2	8.00	16.00
10/17/CCYY	IV START PAK	4051190	1	12.00	12.00
10/17/CCYY	SPECIPAN	4051255	1	5.00	5.00
10/18/CCYY	BREAST PUMP	4051500	2	35.00	70.00
10/17/CCYY	AEROBIC CULTURETTE	4051541	2	4.00	8.00
10/18/CCYY	AEROBIC CULTURETTE	4051541	2	4.00	8.00
10/18/CCYY	ANAAEROBIC CULTURETTE	4051544	1	14.00	14.00
10/19/CCYY	UNDERPAD PER SIX	4053319	1	10.00	10.00
10/17/CCYY	ADDITIVE SET, V1444	4053320	1	16.00	16.00
10/17/CCYY	SECONDARY IV V1903 T	4053325	1	21.00	21.00
10/18/CCYY	SECONDARY IV V1903 T	4053325	1	21.00	21.00
10/17/CCYY	DIAL A FLO	4053329	1	28.00	28.00
	MED/SURG SUPPLIES **SUBTOTAL**	** 270			357.00
10/18/CCYY	SMA-24 80019	4060070	1	270.00	270.00

Folley Medical Center
9900 Fire Blvd.
Folley, FL 32203

Patient Name	Patient No.	Sex	Admission Date	Discharge Date	Page No.
FAY FURY	10076	F	10/17/CCYY	10/20/CCYY	2

Guarantor Name and Address
FRED FURY
5555 FAIRLANE BLVD.
FOLLEY, FL 32208

Insurance Company: ROVER INSURERS, INC.
Claim Number: DOCUMENT 144
Attending Physician: FRANK FLANDERS, M.D.

Date of Service	Description of Hospital Services	Service Code	Qty.	Unit Price	Total Charges
10/17/CCYY	COMPLETE BLOOD COUNT 85023	4060117	1	53.00	53.00
10/19/CCYY	COMPLETE BLOOD COUNT 85023	4060117	1	53.00	53.00
10/17/CCYY	CREATININE SERUM 82565	4060120	1	46.00	46.00
10/17/CCYY	GLUCOSE 82947	4060148	1	46.00	46.00
10/17/CCYY	SED RATE [ESR] 85650	4060380	1	35.00	35.00
10/19/CCYY	SED RATE [ESR] 85650	4060380	1	35.00	35.00
10/17/CCYY	WET MOUNT 87210	4060484	1	35.00	35.00
10/17/CCYY	ROUTINE URINALYSIS 81000	4060487	1	46.00	138.00
10/18/CCYY	ROUTINE URINALYSIS 81000	4060487	3	46.00	46.00
10/17/CCYY	BUN [UREA NITROGEN] 84520	4060497	1	46.00	46.00
10/17/CCYY	R P R [VDRL] QUAL. 86592	4060507	1	42.00	42.00
10/18/CCYY	CULTURE BLOOD #1 87040	4060510	1	92.00	92.00
10/17/CCYY	G C CULTURE 87070	4062144	1	90.00	90.00
10/17/CCYY	CULTURE VAGINAL 87070	4062163	1	79.00	79.00
10/18/CCYY	CULTURE VAGINAL 87070	4062163	1	79.00	79.00
10/18/CCYY	CULTURE URINE 87086	4062168	1	79.00	79.00
10/18/CCYY	CULTURE BLOOD #2 87040	4062172	1	84.00	84.00
10/17/CCYY	PREGNANCY TEST SERUM 84703	4062173	1	65.00	65.00
10/17/CCYY	ELECTROLYTES PANEL 80004	4062177	1	171.00	171.00
	LABORATORY **SUBTOTAL**	** 300	1		1,584.00
10/17/CCYY	CHLAMYDIA DNA *SKL	4090164	1	82.80	82.80
	OTHER LAB **SUBTOTAL**	** 309			82.80
10/18/CCYY	CHEST 2 VIEWS EA 71010	4140063	1	105.00	105.00
10/18/CCYY	TECH CALL AFTER HOURS 99052	4140206	1	44.00	44.00
	DX X-RAY **SUBTOTAL**	** 320			149.00
10/18/CCYY	RENAL ULTRASOUND 76770	4150404	1	400.00	400.00
10/18/CCYY	PELVIC ULTRASOUND 76856	4152000	1	400.00	400.00
	ULTRASOUND **SUBTOTAL**	** 402			800.00
10/17/CCYY	PATIENT CARE KIT	4051081	1	25.00	25.00
	PT CONVENIENCE **SUBTOTAL**	** 990			25.00
	TOTAL				**4,385.80**

Folley Medical Center
9900 Fire Blvd.
Folley, FL 32203

Patient Name	Patient No.	Sex	Admission Date	Discharge Date	Page No.
FAY FURY	10076	F	10/17/CCYY	10/20/CCYY	3

Guarantor Name and Address
FRED FURY
5555 FAIRLANE BLVD.
FOLLEY, FL 32208

Insurance Company: ROVER INSURERS, INC.
Claim Number: DOCUMENT 144
Attending Physician: FRANK FLANDERS, M.D.

Date of Service	Description of Hospital Services	Service Code	Qty.	Unit Price	Total Charges
	SUMMARY OF CHARGES				
	ROOM BOARD/SEMI **SUBTOTAL**	** 120			1,275.00
	PHARMACY **SUBTOTAL**	** 250			34.00
	IV SOLUTIONS **SUBTOTAL**	** 258			56.00
	I.V. THERAPY **SUBTOTAL**	** 260			23.00
	MED/SURG SUPPLIES **SUBTOTAL**	** 270			357.00
	LABORATORY **SUBTOTAL**	** 300			1,584.00
	OTHER LAB **SUBTOTAL**	** 309			82.80
	DX X-RAY **SUBTOTAL**	** 320			149.00
	ULTRASOUND **SUBTOTAL**	** 402			800.00
	PT CONVENIENCE **SUBTOTAL**	** 990			25.00
	TOTAL				**4,385.80**
	PLEASE PAY THIS AMOUNT				4,385.80

This constitutes a medical decision only: it is not a confirmation of benefits
Contact the benefit payer for an explanation of coverage.

Utilization Review Certification

1. **PT./SUBS. NAME**: _____ Fay Fury/Fred Fury _____

2. **GROUP NAME/#:** _____ Ninja Enterprises _____ **I.D. #:** __44-6666 NIN_____ **Hospital Claim #:** 144

3. **HOSPITAL:** _____ Folley Medical Center _____ **ADMIT DATE:** _____ 10/17/CCYY _____

4. **DATE NOTIFIED:** _____ **WORK COMP EMPLOYER:** _____

5. **THIS ADMISSION IS:**

Preauthorized:	YES _____	NO ___✓___
Elective:	YES _____	NO ___✓___
Emergency/OB:	YES ___✓___	NO _____

6. **TYPE OF APPROVAL:**

Total Approval: _____✓_____
Partial Denial: _____
Total Denial: _____

7. **MEDICALLY NECESSARY DAYS:**

__3___ DAYS are certified as medically necessary.

FROM ___10/17/CCYY___ THRU __10/20/CCYY__

FROM _____ THRU _____

8. **DENIED DAYS OR SERVICES:**

_____ DAYS are not certified as medically necessary.

FROM _____ THRU _____

FROM _____ THRU _____

SERVICES not certified are:

_____

9. **GRACE/ADMIN. DAYS ARE AUTHORIZED:**

FROM _____ THRU _____

10. **DENIAL LETTER GIVEN ON** _____

11. **DENIAL OCCURRED DURING:**

_____ Concurrent Review
_____ Retrospective Review
_____ Prior Authorization

12. **SERVICES WERE PROVIDED FOR THE FOLLOWING REASONS:**

_____ Psychiatric Care
_____ Alcohol Detox
_____ Alcohol Rehab
_____ Date Alc. Rehab Began
_____ Drug Detox
_____ Drug Rehab
_____ Date Drug Rehab Began
_____ Cosmetic Surgery

_____ Pre-Cert #: 789546528 _____

Type of Surgery
Cosmetic Surg. Related to:

_____ Congenital Condition
_____ Previous Surgery
_____ Previous Injury
_____ Dental due to accidental injury

ADDITIONAL COMMENTS:

_____ Fiala Faraman _____
REVIEWER SIGNATURE

_____ 10/17/CCYY _____
DATE CERT. GIVEN

PLEASE ATTACH THIS FORM TO
YOUR CLAIM TO EXPEDITE PAYMENT

PAYER COPY

Hospital Admission Form

Provider Information					
Name:	Folley General Hospital				
Address:	5656 Farrell Drive				
City:	Folley	State:	FL	Zip Code:	32201
Telephone#:		Fax#:			
Medicare ID#:	100024	UPIN#:			
Tax ID #:	22-3374854	Accepts Medicare Assignment:	☐		
Provider Rep:	*Betty Biller*		Date:	*8/25/CCYY*	

Admission Information				
Admission Date:	08/23/CCYY	Time:		2:00 PM
Discharge Date:	08/25/CCYY	Time:		2:00 PM
Attending Phy's ID#:	M44218	Date of Injury:		
Attending Physician:	Felix Fries, M.D.			

Guarantor Information				
Name:	Fred Fury			
Address:	5555 Fairlane Blvd.			
City:	Folley	State:	FL	Zip Code:	32208
Insurance ID #:	44-6666 NIN	SSN:	222-44-6666	
Insurance Name:	Rover Insurers, Inc.			
Insurance Group #:	21088			
Employer Name:	Ninja Enterprises			

Patient Information					
Name:	Fred Fury				
Address:	5555 Fairlane Blvd.				
City:	Folley	State:	FL	Zip Code:	32208
Telephone#:	(407) 555-3220	Patient Control #:	10077		
Date of Birth:	11/07/CCYY-56	Gender:	Male		
Marital Status:	Married	Relationship to Guarantor:		Self	
Student Status:	☐ Full-time	☐ Part-time			
Insurance Type:	☒ Pvt ☐ M/care ☐ M/caid ☐ WC ☐ Other _____				

Authorization
☒ Authorization to Release Information
☒ Authorization for Assignment of Benefits
☐ Authorization for Consent for Treatment
☐ My insurance will be billed but there may be a balance due.
Signature: *Fred Fury*   Date: *8/23/CCYY*

Clinical Information	
Principal Diagnosis:	Pneumonia, organism
Other Diagnosis:	
Surgical Procedure:	Electrocardiogram 8/23/CCYY
Other Procedures:	
Remarks:	Pre-Certification #: 258965445

Previous Balance:		Payment:		Copay:		Adjustment:			
Total Fee:	$3420.25	Cash ☐ Check ☐ Credit ☐		Cash ☐ Check ☐ Credit ☐		Remarks:		New Balance:	$3420.25

Folley General Hospital
5656 Farrell Drive
Folley, FL 32201

Patient Name	Patient No.	Sex	Admission Date	Discharge Date	Page No.
FRED FURY	10077	M	08/23/CCYY	08/25/CCYY	1

Guarantor Name and Address
FRED FURY
5555 FAIRLANE BLVD.
FOLLEY, FL 32208

Insurance Company: ROVER INSURERS, INC.
Claim Number: DOCUMENT 145
Attending Physician: FELIX FRIES, M.D.

Date of Service	Description of Hospital Services	Service Code	Qty.	Charges	Total Charges
	DETAIL OF CURRENT CHARGES				
08/23/CCYY	ROOM & BOARD	99010902	1	395.00	
08/24/CCYY	ROOM & BOARD	99010902	1	395.00	
	TOTAL ROOM & BOARD				**790.00**
08/23/CCYY	ADMIT KITS	40503021	1	42.00	
08/23/CCYY	PILLOW DISP	40555252	1	12.25	
08/23/CCYY	PILLOW DISP	40555252	1	12.25	
08/25/CCYY	SYRINGE-INSULIN	40572059	1	1.25	
08/23/CCYY	SYRINGE 1 CC TO 10 CC W/NEEDLE	40572166	1	4.75	
08/23/CCYY	SYRINGE 1 CC TO 10 CC W/NEEDLE	40572166	1	4.75	
08/23/CCYY	URINE CUP STERILE	40580052	1	2.25	
08/23/CCYY	URINE CUP STERILE	40580052	1	2.25	
08/25/CCYY	IMED PUMP RENTAIL DAILY 01	40584393	3	174.00	
08/23/CCYY	IMED PRIMARY SET CS20	40584401	1	25.50	
	TOTAL CENTRAL SUPPLY				**281.25**
08/23/CCYY	CH-CREATININE BLD	40603151	1	42.00	
08/23/CCYY	SMA 12	40609505	1	166.00	
08/23/CCYY	CHEMA-SMA6	40609752	1	142.50	
08/23/CCYY	HEMA-CBC	40611600	1	45.00	
08/23/CCYY	HE-PLATELET COUNT	40612657	1	27.50	
08/23/CCYY	IM-COLD AGG TITRE	40614703	1	70.50	
08/23/CCYY	I-SKIN TEST, T.B.	40616757	1	36.00	
08/23/CCYY	MICRO-GRAM STAIN	40617854	1	33.00	
08/23/CCYY	MC-ROUTINE CULTUR	40618001	1	81.50	
08/23/CCYY	MIC SENSITIVITY	40618050	1	61.00	
08/23/CCYY	URIN-ROUTINE UA	40619355	1	31.00	
08/23/CCYY	VENI-PUNCTURE	40619611	1	18.00	
08/23/CCYY	VENI-PUNCTURE	40619611	1	18.00	
	TOTAL LAB CLINICAL				**772.00**
08/23/CCYY	EKG ROUNTINE	41100504	1	79.00	
	TOTAL EKG				**79.00**

Folley General Hospital
5656 Farrell Drive
Folley, FL 32201

Patient Name	Patient No.	Sex	Admission Date	Discharge Date	Page No.
FRED FURY	10077	M	08/23/CCYY	08/25/CCYY	2

Guarantor Name and Address
FRED FURY
5555 FAIRLANE BLVD.
FOLLEY, FL 32208

Insurance Company: ROVER INSURERS, INC.
Claim Number: DOCUMENT 145
Attending Physician: FELIX FRIES, M.D.

Date of Service	Description of Hospital Services	Service Code	Qty.	Charges	Total Charges
08/23/CCYY	IV ADDITIVE FEE	41705369	4	74.00	
08/24/CCYY	IV ADDITIVE FEE	41705369	3	55.50	
08/25/CCYY	IV ADDITIVE FEE	41705369	1	18.50	
08/23/CCYY	MED. PIGGY BACKS	41710047	4	114.00	
08/24/CCYY	MED. PIGGY BACKS	41710047	3	85.50	
08/25/CCYY	MED. PIGGY BACKS	41710047	1	28.50	
08/25/CCYY	TYLENOL 325 MG	41737701	4	2.00	
08/23/CCYY	ANCEF 1 GM IV/IM	41742750	4	190.00	
08/24/CCYY	ANCEF 1 GM IV/IM	41742750	3	142.50	
08/25/CCYY	ANCEF 1 GM IV/IM	41742750	1	47.50	
08/25/CCYY	PROFILE SERV CHRG	41763756	3	42.00	
08/23/CCYY	3 CC NS/ALUPNT.3CC	41774209	2	18.00	
08/24/CCYY	3 CC NS/ALUPNT.3CC	41774209	3	27.00	
08/25/CCYY	3 CC NS/ALUPNT.3CC	41774209	1	9.00	
	TOTAL PHARMACY				**854.00**
08/23/CCYY	H H N CIRCUIT	41800806	1	28.00	
08/24/CCYY	H H N CIRCUIT	41800806	1	28.00	
08/25/CCYY	H H N CIRCUIT	41800806	1	28.00	
08/23/CCYY	H H N TREATMENT	41800855	2	70.00	
08/24/CCYY	H H N TREATMENT	41800855	3	105.00	
08/25/CCYY	H H N TREATMENT	41800855	1	35.00	
	TOTAL INHALATION THERAPY				**294.00**

Folley General Hospital
5656 Farrell Drive
Folley, FL 32201

Patient Name	Patient No.	Sex	Admission Date	Discharge Date	Page No.
FRED FURY	10077	M	08/23/CCYY	08/25/CCYY	3

Guarantor Name and Address
FRED FURY
5555 FAIRLANE BLVD.
FOLLEY, FL 32208

Insurance Company: ROVER INSURERS, INC.
Claim Number: DOCUMENT 145
Attending Physician: FELIX FRIES, M.D.

Date of Service	Description of Hospital Services	Service Code	Qty.	Charges	Total Charges
08/23/CCYY	IV CATHETER	47136049	1	24.00	
08/23/CCYY	IV START KIT	47137195	1	36.00	
08/23/CCYY	IV TUBING EXTENSION SET	47138278	1	14.00	
08/23/CCYY	IV TUBING SECONDARY SET	47137567	1	35.00	
08/24/CCYY	IV TUBING SECONDARY SET	47137567	1	35.00	
08/23/CCYY	SOL D-5-0.9NS 1000 ML	47138110	1	40.00	
08/23/CCYY	SOL D-5-0.9NS 1000 ML	47138110	1	40.00	
08/23/CCYY	SOL D-5-0.9NS 1000 ML	47138110	1	40.00	
08/24/CCYY	SOL D-5-0.9NS 1000 ML	47138110	1	40.00	
08/24/CCYY	SOL D-5 LR 1000 ML	47138177	1	46.00	
	TOTAL IV THERAPY				**350.00**

Folley General Hospital
5656 Farrell Drive
Folley, FL 32201

Patient Name	Patient No.	Sex	Admission Date	Discharge Date	Page No.
FRED FURY	10077	M	08/23/CCYY	08/25/CCYY	4

Guarantor Name and Address
FRED FURY
5555 FAIRLANE BLVD.
FOLLEY, FL 32208

Insurance Company: ROVER INSURERS, INC.
Claim Number: DOCUMENT 145
Attending Physician: FELIX FRIES, M.D.

Date of Service	Description of Hospital Services	Service Code	Qty.	Charges	Total Charges
	SUMMARY OF CHARGES				
	2 DAYS MED/WRD @ 395			790.00	
	PHARMACY			854.00	
	IV THERAPY			350.00	
	MED-SUR SUPPLIES			281.25	
	LABORATORY OR (LAB)			772.00	
	RESPIRATORY SVC			294.00	
	EKG-ECG			79.00	
	SUBTOTAL OF CHARGES				3,420.25
	PAYMENTS AND ADJUSTMENTS			NONE	
	SUBTOTAL PAYMENTS/ADJ				NONE
	BALANCE				3,420.25
	BALANCE DUE				3,420.25

This constitutes a medical decision only: it is not a confirmation of benefits
Contact the benefit payer for an explanation of coverage.

Utilization Review Certification

1. **PT./SUBS. NAME**: _____Fred Fury/Fred Fury_____
2. **GROUP NAME/#**: _____Ninja Enterprises_____   **I.D. #**: __44-6666 NIN__   **Hospital Claim #**: _145_
3. **HOSPITAL**: _____Folley General_____   **ADMIT DATE**: _____8/23/CCYY_____
4. **DATE NOTIFIED**: _____   **WORK COMP EMPLOYER**: _____

5. THIS ADMISSION IS:

Preauthorized:	YES _____	NO __✓__
Elective:	YES _____	NO __✓__
Emergency/OB:	YES __✓__	NO _____

6. TYPE OF APPROVAL:

Total Approval: _____
Partial Denial: _____
Total Denial: __✓__

7. MEDICALLY NECESSARY DAYS:

__0__   DAYS are certified as medically necessary.

FROM _____   THRU _____

FROM _____   THRU _____

8. DENIED DAYS OR SERVICES:

__2__   DAYS are not certified as medically necessary.

FROM __8/23/CCYY__   THRU __8/25/CCYY__

FROM _____   THRU _____

SERVICES not certified are:

_____

9. GRACE/ADMIN. DAYS ARE AUTHORIZED:

FROM _____   THRU _____

10. DENIAL LETTER GIVEN ON ___9/25/CCYY___

11. DENIAL OCCURRED DURING:

_____ Concurrent Review
__✓__ Retrospective Review
_____ Prior Authorization

12. SERVICES WERE PROVIDED FOR THE FOLLOWING REASONS:

_____ Psychiatric Care
_____ Alcohol Detox
_____ Alcohol Rehab
_____ Date Alc. Rehab Began
_____ Drug Detox
_____ Drug Rehab
_____ Date Drug Rehab Began
_____ Cosmetic Surgery

__ Pre-Cert #: 258965445 _____

Type of Surgery
Cosmetic Surg. Related to:

_____ Congenital Condition
_____ Previous Surgery
_____ Previous Injury
_____ Dental due to accidental injury

ADDITIONAL COMMENTS:

_____

___Frieda Faraman_____
REVIEWER SIGNATURE

___8/23/CCYY_____
DATE CERT. GIVEN

PLEASE ATTACH THIS FORM TO YOUR CLAIM TO EXPEDITE PAYMENT

PAYER COPY

Hospital Admission Form

Provider Information

Name:	Franklin Medical Center
Address:	789 First Street

City:	Folley	State:	FL	Zip Code:	32204	
Telephone#:		Fax#:				
Medicare ID#:	100025	UPIN#:				
Tax ID #:	22-5984755	Accepts Medicare Assignment:	☐			
Provider Rep:	Betty Biller	Date: 9/2/CCYY				

Patient Information

Name:	Fern Fury
Address:	5555 Fairlane Blvd.

City:	Folley	State:	FL	Zip Code:	32208	
Telephone#:	(407) 555-3220	Patient Control #:	10078			
Date of Birth:	11/05/CCYY-17	Gender:	Female			
Marital Status:	Single	Relationship to Guarantor:		Child		
Student Status:	☒ Full-time	☐ Part-time				
Insurance Type:	☒ Pvt ☐ M/care ☐ M/caid ☐ WC ☐ Other _____					

Admission Information

Admission Date:	08/29/CCY	Time:	8:00 PM
Discharge Date:	09/02/CCY	Time:	2:00 PM
Attending Phy's ID#:	A02132	Date of Injury:	
Attending Physician:	Ford Fisher, M.D.		

Guarantor Information

Name:	Fred Fury				
Address:	5555 Fairlane Blvd.				
City:	Folley	State:	FL	Zip Code:	32208
Insurance ID #:	44-6666 NIN	SSN:	222-44-6666		
Insurance Name:	Rover Insurers, Inc.				
Insurance Group #:	21088				
Employer Name:	Ninja Enterprises				

Authorization

☒ Authorization to Release Information
☒ Authorization for Assignment of Benefits
☐ Authorization for Consent for Treatment
☐ My insurance will be billed but there may be a balance due.

Signature: _Fred Fury_   Date: 8/29/CCYY

Clinical Information

Principal Diagnosis:	Hyperplasia of appendix	
Other Diagnosis:	Abdominal pain	
Surgical Procedure:	Appendectomy	8/30/CCYY
Other Procedures:		
Remarks:	Pre-Certification #: 335668711	

Previous Balance:		Payment:		Copay:		Adjustment:			
Total Fee:	$10068.25	Cash ☐ Check ☐ Credit ☐		Cash ☐ Check ☐ Credit ☐		Remarks:		New Balance	$10068.25

Franklin Medical Center
789 First Street
Folley, FL 32204

Patient Name	Patient No.	Sex	Admission Date	Discharge Date	Page No.
FERN FURY	10078	F	08/29/CCYY	09/02/CCYY	1

Guarantor Name and Address
FRED FURY
5555 FAIRLANE BLVD.
FOLLEY, FL 32208

Insurance Company: ROVER INSURERS, INC.
Claim Number: DOCUMENT 146
Attending Physician: FORD FISHER, M.D.

Date of Service	Description of Hospital Services	Service Code	Qty.	Charges	Total Charges
08/29/CCYY	ROOM & BOARD	99010407	1	395.00	
08/30/CCYY	ROOM & BOARD	99010407	1	395.00	
08/31/CCYY	ROOM & BOARD	99010407	1	395.00	
09/01/CCYY	ROOM & BOARD	99010407	1	395.00	
	TOTAL ROOM & BOARD				**1,580.00**
08/30/CCYY	MAJ SURG TIME 1.25 HR	40200123	1	798.00	
08/30/CCYY	SURG-EMERGENCY FEE	40200727	1	158.00	
08/30/CCYY	SUR-MONITR EKG CHG	40200784	1	58.00	
08/30/CCYY	SURG-BOVIE	40200826	1	32.00	
08/30/CCYY	RECOV EMERG	40202384	1	236.00	
08/30/CCYY	MAJOR TRAY	40205015	1	809.00	
08/30/CCYY	PULSE OXIMETER	40205189	1	46.00	
08/30/CCYY	SUTURE MAJOR 1.5	40205437	1	63.00	
08/30/CCYY	SUR-MONITR B/P CHG	40205460	1	58.00	
	TOTAL SURGERY AND RECOVERY				**2,258.00**
08/30/CCYY	NITROUS 75 MIN	40404832	1	198.00	
08/30/CCYY	FORANE 75 MIN	40405128	1	195.00	
08/30/CCYY	OXYGEN 75 MIN	40405326	1	76.00	
08/30/CCYY	ANESTH UNIT	40405912	1	260.00	
08/30/CCYY	ANES O2/SENSOR	40405920	1	150.00	
	TOTAL ANESTHESIOLOGY				**879.00**
08/29/CCYY	ADMIT KITS	40503021	1	42.00	
08/30/CCYY	AIR WAY	40503062	1	8.50	
08/30/CCYY	PACK CUSTOM MRJ/OR	40505174	1	160.25	
08/30/CCYY	BED PAN	40511081	1	8.50	
08/30/CCYY	CATH FOLEY	40515348	1	26.75	
08/30/CCYY	DRSNG GZE 4X4(10)	40525289	1	5.75	
08/30/CCYY	DRS STRI STRP ½	40525834	1	7.00	
08/30/CCYY	SRS STRI STRP ½	40525834	1	7.00	
08/30/CCYY	DRESS-TELFA 3X4	40525909	1	1.25	

Franklin Medical Center
789 First Street
Folley, FL 32204

Patient Name	Patient No.	Sex	Admission Date	Discharge Date	Page No.
FERN FURY	10078	F	08/29/CCYY	09/02/CCYY	2

Guarantor Name and Address
FRED FURY
5555 FAIRLANE BLVD.
FOLLEY, FL 32208

Insurance Company: ROVER INSURERS, INC.
Claim Number: DOCUMENT 146
Attending Physician: FORD FISHER, M.D.

Date of Service	Description of Hospital Services	Service Code	Qty.	Charges	Total Charges
08/30/CCYY	ELECTRODE DISPERS (BOVIE PAD)	40528085	1	28.50	
08/30/CCYY	GLOVES SURG	40532053	1	2.25	
08/30/CCYY	GLOVES SURG	40532053	3	6.75	
08/30/CCYY	L-LOTION HAND	40544108	1	3.75	
08/30/CCYY	MISC CENTRAL SUPPLY POOL SUCT INSTRU	40545303	1	4.25	
08/31/CCYY	O2 MASK	40549412	1	20.50	
08/31/CCYY	O2 HUMIDIFIER	40549420	1	30.25	
08/29/CCYY	PILLOW DISP	40555252	1	12.25	
08/30/CCYY	PILLOW DISP	40555252	1	12.25	
08/30/CCYY	SOL-IRRIGT NS 2 L	40564197	1	11.50	
08/30/CCYY	SOL-IRRIGT NS 2 L	40564197	1	11.50	
08/30/CCYY	SUCTN LINER 2000	40569279	1	26.75	
08/30/CCYY	SUCTION YANKAUR HNDL	40569303	1	38.50	
08/30/CCYY	SYRINGE BULB	40572141	1	8.50	
08/30/CCYY	SYRINGE 1 CC TO 10 CC W/NEEDLE	40572166	1	4.75	
08/30/CCYY	SYRINGE 1 CC TO 10 CC W/NEEDLE	40572166	1	4.75	
08/31/CCYY	SYRINGE 1 CC TO 10 CC W/NEEDLE	40572166	1	4.75	
09/01/CCYY	SYRINGE 1 CC TO 10 CC W/NEEDLE	40572166	1	4.75	
09/01/CCYY	SYRINGE 1 CC TO 10 CC W/NEEDLE	40572166	1	4.75	
08/30/CCYY	SLIPPERS/PILLOW PAWS	40573149	1	4.00	
08/29/CCYY	SPECIPAN	40573156	1	14.00	
08/30/CCYY	SPECIPAN	40573156	1	14.00	
08/30/CCYY	TRAC ENDO TBE 3 TO 10 FR	40575011	1	25.50	
08/30/CCYY	TRAY FOLEY CATH	40577249	1	54.25	
08/30/CCYY	TRAY FOLEY CATH	40577249	1	54.25	
08/30/CCYY	TRAY-IRRIGATION	40577330	1	10.25	
08/30/CCYY	TRAY SKIN PREP W/PVP I	40577579	1	26.75	
08/30/CCYY	TUBE CULTURETTE	40579106	1	2.75	
08/30/CCYY	TUBE CULT ANEROBI	40579114	1	14.25	
08/30/CCYY	TBE CONNECTGN 120	40579189	1	14.00	
08/30/CCYY	PACK TOWEL (6)	40579039	1	14.00	
08/29/CCYY	URINE CUP STERILE	40580052	1	2.25	
08/30/CCYY	URINE CUP STERILE	40580052	1	2.25	
09/02/CCYY	IMED PUMP RENTAL DAILY 01	40584393	5	290.00	

Franklin Medical Center
789 First Street
Folley, FL 32204

Patient Name	Patient No.	Sex	Admission Date	Discharge Date	Page No.
FERN FURY	10078	F	08/29/CCYY	09/02/CCYY	3

Guarantor Name and Address
FRED FURY
5555 FAIRLANE BLVD.
FOLLEY, FL 32208

Insurance Company: ROVER INSURERS, INC.
Claim Number: DOCUMENT 146
Attending Physician: FORD FISHER, M.D.

Date of Service	Description of Hospital Services	Service Code	Qty.	Charges	Total Charges
08/29/CCYY	IMED PRIMARY SET CS20	40584401	1	25.50	
	TOTAL CENTRAL SUPPLY				**1,076.25**
08/29/CCYY	CH-CREATININE BLD	40603151	1	42.00	
08/31/CCYY	CH-CREATININE BLD	40603151	1	42.00	
08/29/CCYY	CHEM-SMA 6	40609752	1	142.50	
08/31/CCYY	CHEM-SMA 6	40609752	1	142.50	
08/29/CCYY	HEMA-CBC	40611600	1	45.00	
08/30/CCYY	HEMA-CBC	40611600	1	45.00	
08/31/CCYY	HEMA-CBC	40611600	1	45.00	
09/02/CCYY	HEMA-CBC	40611600	1	45.00	
08/29/CCYY	HEMA-DIFFERENTIAL	40611907	1	23.00	
08/29/CCYY	HE-PLATELET COUNT	40612657	1	27.50	
08/29/CCYY	H-PROTHROMBINTIME	40612756	1	40.50	
08/29/CCYY	HEMA-PTT	40612855	1	51.00	
08/29/CCYY	HE-SEDIMENTATION	40613150	1	27.00	
08/29/CCYY	IMMU-PREG TB TEST	40616120	1	54.00	
08/29/CCYY	URIN-ROUTINE UA	40619355	1	31.00	
08/29/CCYY	VENI-PUNCTURE	40619611	1	18.00	
08/30/CCYY	VENI-PUNCTURE	40619611	1	18.00	
08/31/CCYY	VENI-PUNCTURE	40619611	1	18.00	
09/02/CCYY	VENI-PUNCTURE	40619611	1	18.00	
	TOTAL LAB CLINICAL				**875.00**
08/30/CCYY	PATH DIAG, SM PART-A	40705105	1	70.00	
08/30/CCYY	PATH HANDLING PART-A	40705196	1	35.50	
	TOTAL LAB PATH				**105.50**
08/30/CCYY	ABDMN FLAT KUB 1V	41400557	1	85.00	
08/30/CCYY	BARIM ENEMA COLON	41401159	1	189.00	
08/30/CCYY	CHEST 2V AP & LAT	41401902	1	113.00	
08/30/CCYY	X-RAY EMRGNCY CAL	41410408	1	39.00	
	TOTAL RADIOLOGY				**426.00**
08/30/CCYY	IV ADDITIVE FEE	41705369	10	185.00	
08/31/CCYY	IV ADDITIVE FEE	41705369	3	55.50	

Franklin Medical Center
789 First Street
Folley, FL 32204

Patient Name	Patient No.	Sex	Admission Date	Discharge Date	Page No.
FERN FURY	10078	F	08/29/CCYY	09/02/CCYY	4

Guarantor Name and Address
FRED FURY
5555 FAIRLANE BLVD.
FOLLEY, FL 32208

Insurance Company: ROVER INSURERS, INC.
Claim Number: DOCUMENT 146
Attending Physician: FORD FISHER, M.D.

Date of Service	Description of Hospital Services	Service Code	Qty.	Charges	Total Charges
09/01/CCYY	IV ADDITIVE FEE	41705369	3	55.50	
09/02/CCYY	IV ADDITIVE FEE	41705369	1	18.50	
08/30/CCYY	MED. PIGGY BACKS	41710047	4	114.00	
08/31/CCYY	MED. PIGGY BACKS	41710047	3	85.50	
09/01/CCYY	MED. PIGGY BACKS	41410047	3	85.50	
09/02/CCYY	MED. PIGGY BACKS	41710047	1	28.50	
08/31/CCYY	TYLENOL W COD TAB	41718501	2	6.00	
08/30/CCYY	DEMEROL INJ	41746900	2	34.00	
09/02/CCYY	DEMEROL INJ	41746900	1	17.00	
08/30/CCYY	KCI INJ	41750910	3	42.00	
08/30/CCYY	MEFOXIN 1 GM IV/IM	41753054	4	226.00	
08/31/CCYY	MEFOXIN 1 GM IV/IM	41753054	3	169.50	
09/01/CCYY	MEFOXIN 1 GM IV/IM	41753054	3	169.50	
09/02/CCYY	MEFOXIN 1 GM IV/IM	41753054	1	56.50	
08/30/CCYY	MVI-12	41754151	3	48.00	
08/30/CCYY	PENTOTHAL SDM 1 GM	47156305	1	77.50	
08/30/CCYY	PROSTIGMN 1:1000	47457493	1	17.00	
08/30/CCYY	ROBUNIL 1 CC	41758103	1	16.50	
08/30/CCYY	ROBUNIL 1 CC	41758103	1	16.50	
08/30/CCYY	SUBLIMAZE 2 CC	41759804	1	21.50	
08/30/CCYY	TRACRIUM 50 MG AMP	41761669	1	70.00	
09/02/CCYY	VISTARIL INJ	41762501	1	16.50	
08/30/CCYY	PROFILE SERV CHRG	41763756	1	14.00	
08/31/CCYY	PROFILE SERV CHRG	41763756	1	14.00	
09/02/CCYY	PROFILE SERV CHRG	41763756	2	28.00	
09/02/CCYY	HEPARN 100UNT FLS	41769704	4	70.00	
08/30/CCYY	XYLOCAIN JELY 2%	41777301	1	20.50	
	TOTAL PHARMACY				**1,778.50**
08/30/CCYY	OXYGEN SET-UP	41801952	1	62.00	
08/30/CCYY	OXYGEN PER HOUR	41802208	1	11.00	
	TOTAL INHALATION THERAPY				**73.00**
08/30/CCYY	ULTRASND-PELVIS	42501403	1	475.00	
	TOTAL ULTRA SOUND				**475.00**

Franklin Medical Center
789 First Street
Folley, FL 32204

Patient Name	Patient No.	Sex	Admission Date	Discharge Date	Page No.
FERN FURY	10078	F	08/29/CCYY	09/02/CCYY	5

Guarantor Name and Address
FRED FURY
5555 FAIRLANE BLVD.
FOLLEY, FL 32208

Insurance Company: ROVER INSURERS, INC.
Claim Number: DOCUMENT 146
Attending Physician: FORD FISHER, M.D.

Date of Service	Description of Hospital Services	Service Code	Qty.	Charges	Total Charges
08/29/CCYY	IV CATHETER	47136049	1	24.00	
08/31/CCYY	IV CATHETER	47136049	1	24.00	
08/29/CCYY	IV START KIT	47137195	1	36.00	
08/29/CCYY	IV TUBING EXTENSION SET	47137278	1	14.00	
09/01/CCYY	IV TUBING EXTENSION SET	47137278	1	14.00	
08/30/CCYY	IV TUBING SECONDARY SET	47137567	1	35.00	
08/31/CCYY	IV TUBING SECONDARY SET	47137567	1	35.00	
09/01/CCYY	IV TUBING SECONDARY SET	47137567	1	35.00	
09/01/CCYY	IV INJECTION SITE	47137583	1	21.00	
08/29/CCYY	SOL D-5-0.45NS 1000 ML	47138136	1	44.00	
08/29/CCYY	SOL D-5-0.45NS 1000 ML	47138136	1	44.00	
08/31/CCYY	SOL D-5-0.45NS 1000 ML	47138136	1	44.00	
08/31/CCYY	SOL D-5-0.45NS 1000 ML	47138136	1	44.00	
09/01/CCYY	SOL D-5-0.45NS 1000 ML	47138136	1	44.00	
08/30/CCYY	SOL D-5-0.2NS 1000 ML	47138136	1	44.00	
08/30/CCYY	D5 W/NS & KCL 1000	47138409	1	40.00	
	TOTAL IV THERAPY				**542.00**

Franklin Medical Center
789 First Street
Folley, FL 32204

Patient Name	Patient No.	Sex	Admission Date	Discharge Date	Page No.
FERN FURY	10078	F	08/29/CCYY	09/02/CCYY	6

Guarantor Name and Address
FRED FURY
5555 FAIRLANE BLVD.
FOLLEY, FL 32208

Insurance Company: ROVER INSURERS, INC.
Claim Number: DOCUMENT 146
Attending Physician: FORD FISHER, M.D.

Date of Service	Description of Hospital Services	Service Code	Qty.	Charges	Total Charges
	SUMMARY OF CHARGES				
	4 DAYS MED/WRD @ 395			1,580.00	
	PHARMACY			1,778.50	
	IV THERAPY			542.00	
	MED-SUR SUPPLIES			2,142.25	
	LABORATORY OR (LAB)			875.00	
	PATHOLOGY LAB OR (PATH LAB)			105.50	
	DX- X-RAY			901.00	
	OR SERVICES			956.00	
	ANESTHESIA			879.00	
	RESPIRATORY SVC			73.00	
	RECOVERY ROOM			236.00	
	SUBTOTAL OF CHARGES				10,068.25
	PAYMENTS AND ADJUSTMENTS			NONE	
	SUBTOTAL AND ADJUSTMENTS				NONE
	BALANCE				10,068.25
	BALANCE DUE				10,068.25

This constitutes a medical decision only: it is not a confirmation of benefits
Contact the benefit payer for an explanation of coverage.

Utilization Review Certification

1. **PT./SUBS. NAME**: _____ Fern Fury/Fred Fury _____

2. **GROUP NAME/#**: ___ Ninja Enterprises ____   **I.D. #**: __ 44-6666NIN ____   **Hospital Claim #**: 146 __

3. **HOSPITAL**: _____ Franklin Medical Center ___   **ADMIT DATE**: _____ 8/29/CCYY _____

4. **DATE NOTIFIED**: _____   **WORK COMP EMPLOYER**: _____

5. THIS ADMISSION IS:

Preauthorized: YES _____   NO ___✓___

Elective: YES _____   NO ___✓___

Emergency/OB: YES ___✓___   NO _____

6. TYPE OF APPROVAL:

Total Approval: ___✓___

Partial Denial: _____

Total Denial: _____

7. MEDICALLY NECESSARY DAYS:

__4__   DAYS are certified as medically necessary.

FROM __8/29/CCYY__   THRU __9/02/CCYY__

FROM _____   THRU _____

8. DENIED DAYS OR SERVICES:

_____   DAYS are not certified as medically necessary.

FROM _____   THRU _____

FROM _____   THRU _____

SERVICES not certified are:

_____

9. GRACE/ADMIN. DAYS ARE AUTHORIZED:

FROM _____   THRU _____

10. DENIAL LETTER GIVEN ON _____

11. DENIAL OCCURRED DURING:

_____ Concurrent Review
_____ Retrospective Review
_____ Prior Authorization

12. SERVICES WERE PROVIDED FOR THE FOLLOWING REASONS:

_____ Psychiatric Care
_____ Alcohol Detox
_____ Alcohol Rehab
_____ Date Alc. Rehab Began
_____ Drug Detox
_____ Drug Rehab
_____ Date Drug Rehab Began
_____ Cosmetic Surgery

____ Pre-Cert #: 335668711 _____

Type of Surgery
Cosmetic Surg. Related to:

_____ Congenital Condition
_____ Previous Surgery
_____ Previous Injury
_____ Dental due to accidental injury

ADDITIONAL COMMENTS:

____ Flora Felton _____
REVIEWER SIGNATURE

____ 8/29/CCYY _____
DATE CERT. GIVEN

**PLEASE ATTACH THIS FORM TO
YOUR CLAIM TO EXPEDITE PAYMENT**

PAYER COPY

Hospital Admission Form

Provider Information

Name:	Farnham Memorial Hospital
Address:	9009 Foster Avenue
City:	Folley State: FL Zip Code: 32205
Telephone#:	Fax#:
Medicare ID#:	100026 UPIN#:
Tax ID #:	22-3388909 Accepts Medicare Assignment: ☐
Provider Rep:	*Betty Biller* Date: *10/18/CCYY*

Admission Information

Admission Date:	10/14/CCYY	Time:	6:00 PM
Discharge Date:	10/18/CCYY	Time:	3:00 PM
Attending Phy's ID#:	B02084	Date of Injury:	
Attending Physician:	Florence Faulk, M.D.		

Guarantor Information

Name:	Fred Fury
Address:	5555 Fairlane Blvd.
City:	Folley State: FL Zip Code: 32208
Insurance ID #:	44-6666 NIN SSN: 222-44-6666
Insurance Name:	Rover Insurers, Inc.
Insurance Group #:	21088
Employer Name:	Ninja Enterprises

Patient Information

Name:	Forrest Fury
Address:	5555 Fairlane Blvd.
City:	Folley State: FL Zip Code: 32208
Telephone#:	(407) 555-3220 Patient Control #: 10079
Date of Birth:	09/08/CCYY-18 Gender: Male
Marital Status:	Single Relationship to Guarantor: Child
Student Status:	☒ Full-time ☐ Part-time
Insurance Type:	☒ Pvt ☐ M/care ☐ M/caid ☐ WC ☐ Other _____

Authorization

☒ Authorization to Release Information
☒ Authorization for Assignment of Benefits
☐ Authorization for Consent for Treatment
☐ My insurance will be billed but there may be a balance due.
Signature: *Fred Fury* Date: *10/14/CCYY*

Clinical Information

Principal Diagnosis:	Non-infectious gastroenteritis
Other Diagnosis:	Hypovolemia
Surgical Procedure:	
Other Procedures:	
Remarks:	Pre-Certification #: 458854992

Previous Balance:		Payment:		Copay:		Adjustment:			
Total Fee:	$4243.50	Cash ☐ Check ☐ Credit ☐		Cash ☐ Check ☐ Credit ☐		Remarks:		New Balance:	$4243.50

Farnham Memorial Hospital
9009 Foster Avenue
Folley, FL 32205

Patient Name	Patient No.	Sex	Admission Date	Discharge Date	Page No.
FORREST FURY	10079	M	10/14/CCYY	10/18/CCYY	1

Guarantor Name and Address
FRED FURY
5555 FAIRLANE BLVD.
FOLLEY, FL 32208

Insurance Company: ROVER INSURERS, INC.
Claim Number: DOCUMENT 147
Attending Physician: FLORENCE FAULK, M.D.

Date of Service	Description of Hospital Services	Service Code	Qty.	Charges	Total Charges
	DETAIL OF CURRENT CHARGES				
10/14/CCYY	ROOM & BOARD	99020208	1	395.00	
10/15/CCYY	ROOM & BOARD	99020208	1	395.00	
10/16/CCYY	ROOM & BOARD	99020208	1	395.00	
10/17/CCYY	ROOM & BOARD	99020208	1	395.00	
	TOTAL ROOM & BOARD				**1,580.00**
10/14/CCYY	BED PAN	40511081	1	8.50	
10/14/CCYY	CUP SPECIMEN W/LID	40522294	1	2.25	
10/14/CCYY	PED ADMIT KIT CS 12	40525602	1	38.75	
10/14/CCYY	IV ARM SUPPORT	40539090	1	5.00	
10/17/CCYY	L-LOTION HAND	40544108	1	3.75	
10/14/CCYY	MISC CENTRAL SUPPLY ENSURE-IT DRESS	40545303	1	4.00	
10/17/CCYY	MISC CENTRAL SUPPLY ENSURE-IT DRESS	40545303	1	4.00	
10/14/CCYY	MISTREAM URINE COLLECTOR	40546178	1	8.25	
10/14/CCYY	PILLOW DISP	40555252	1	12.25	
10/14/CCYY	SYRINGE 1 CC TO 10 CC W/NEEDLE	40572166	1	4.75	
10/18/CCYY	SYRINGE 1 CC TO 10 CC W/NEEDLE	40572166	1	4.75	
10/14/CCYY	SLIPPERS/PILLOW PAWS	40573149	1	4.00	
10/15/CCYY	SLIPPERS/PILLOW PAWS	40573149	1	4.00	
10/17/CCYY	SLIPPERS/PILLOW PAWS	40573149	1	4.00	
10/17/CCYY	SLIPPERS/PILLOW PAWS	40573149	1	4.00	
10/17/CCYY	SLIPPERS/PILLOW PAWS	40573149	1	4.00	
10/14/CCYY	URINE CUP	40580037	1	2.25	
10/16/CCYY	URINE CUP	40580037	1	2.25	
10/14/CCYY	URINAL	40580060	1	5.00	
10/17/CCYY	URINAL	40580060	1	5.00	
10/17/CCYY	BTL SHAMPOO	40583205	1	3.75	
10/17/CCYY	BTL SHAMPOO	40583205	1	3.75	
10/18/CCYY	BTL SHAMPOO	40583205	1	3.75	
10/14/CCYY	IMED BURETROL SET 10	40584377	1	35.00	
10/18/CCYY	IMED PUMP RENTAL DAILY 01	40584393	5	290.00	
	TOTAL CENTRAL SUPPLY				**467.00**

Farnham Memorial Hospital
9009 Foster Avenue
Folley, FL 32205

Patient Name	Patient No.	Sex	Admission Date	Discharge Date	Page No.
FORREST FURY	10079	M	10/14/CCYY	10/18/CCYY	2

Guarantor Name and Address
FRED FURY
5555 FAIRLANE BLVD.
FOLLEY, FL 32208

Insurance Company: ROVER INSURERS, INC.
Claim Number: DOCUMENT 147
Attending Physician: FLORENCE FAULK, M.D.

Date of Service	Description of Hospital Services	Service Code	Qty.	Charges	Total Charges
10/14/CCYY	CH-CREATININE BLD	40603151	1	42.00	
10/14/CCYY	CHEM-SMA 6	40609752	1	142.50	
10/14/CCYY	HEMA-CBC	40611600	1	45.00	
10/14/CCYY	HEMA-DIFFERENTIAL	40611907	1	23.00	
10/14/CCYY	HE-PLATELET COUNT	40612657	1	27.50	
10/14/CCYY	HE-SEDIMENTATION	40613150	1	27.00	
10/18/CCYY	LAB-S.O HNDLING CH	40617201	1	27.50	
10/18/CCYY	REF LAB CHARGE STOOL CULT	40618217	1	12.50	
10/14/CCYY	URIN-ROUTINE UA	41619355	1	31.00	
10/14/CCYY	VENI-PUNCTURE	40619611	1	18.00	
	TOTAL LAB CLINICAL				**396.00**
10/15/CCYY	IV ADDITIVE FEE	41705369	8	148.00	
10/16/CCYY	IV ADDITIVE FEE	41705369	8	148.00	
10/17/CCYY	IV ADDITIVE FEE	41705369	6	111.00	
10/18/CCYY	IV ADDITIVE FEE	41705369	2	37.00	
10/16/CCYY	TYLENOL 325 MG	41737701	3	1.50	
10/15/CCYY	KCI INJ	41750910	4	56.00	
10/16/CCYY	KCI INJ	41750910	4	56.00	
10/17/CCYY	KCI INJ	41750910	3	42.00	
10/18/CCYY	KCI INJ	41750910	1	14.00	
10/15/CCYY	MVI-12	41754151	4	64.00	
10/16/CCYY	MVI-12	41754151	4	64.00	
10/17/CCYY	MVI-12	41754151	3	48.00	
10/18/CCYY	MVI-12	41754151	1	16.00	
10/16/CCYY	PROFILE SERV CHRG	41763756	3	42.00	
10/18/CCYY	PROFILE SERV CHRG	41763756	1	14.00	
10/16/CCYY	BACTRIM LIQ DOSE	41778101	8	24.00	
10/18/CCYY	BACTRIM LIQ DOSE	41778101	3	9.00	
10/16/CCYY	DONNAGEL LIQ DOSE	41778176	9	27.00	
10/18/CCYY	DONNAGEL LIQ DOSE	41778176	4	12.00	
	TOTAL PHARMACY				**933.50**

Farnham Memorial Hospital
9009 Foster Avenue
Folley, FL 32205

Patient Name	Patient No.	Sex	Admission Date	Discharge Date	Page No.
FORREST FURY	10079	M	10/14/CCYY	10/18/CCYY	3

Guarantor Name and Address
FRED FURY
5555 FAIRLANE BLVD.
FOLLEY, FL 32208

Insurance Company: ROVER INSURERS, INC.
Claim Number: DOCUMENT 147
Attending Physician: FLORENCE FAULK, M.D.

Date of Service	Description of Hospital Services	Service Code	Qty.	Charges	Total Charges
10/14/CCYY	IV CATHETER	47136049	1	24.00	
10/14/CCYY	IV CATHETER	47136049	1	24.00	
10/17/CCYY	IV CATHETER	47136049	1	24.00	
10/17/CCYY	IV CATHETER	47136049	1	24.00	
10/14/CCYY	NDL BUTTERFLY	47136098	1	12.00	
10/14/CCYY	IV START KIT	47137195	1	36.00	
10/14/CCYY	IV TUBING EXTENSION SET	47137278	1	14.00	
10/14/CCYY	IV TUBING SECONDARY SET	47137567	1	35.00	
10/16/CCYY	IV TUBING SECONDARY SET	47137567	1	35.00	
10/14/CCYY	SOL D-5-0.4NS 500 ML	47138128	1	35.00	
10/14/CCYY	SOL D-5-0.4NS 500 ML	47138128	1	35.00	
10/15/CCYY	SOL D-5-0.4NS 500 ML	47138128	1	35.00	
10/15/CCYY	SOL D-5-0.4NS 500 ML	47138128	1	35.00	
10/15/CCYY	SOL D-5-0.4NS 500 ML	47138128	1	35.00	
10/15/CCYY	SOL D-5-0.4NS 500 ML	47138128	1	35.00	
10/15/CCYY	SOL D-5-0.4NS 500 ML	47138128	1	35.00	
10/16/CCYY	SOL D-5-0.4NS 500 ML	47138128	1	35.00	
10/16/CCYY	SOL D-5-0.4NS 500 ML	47138128	1	35.00	
10/17/CCYY	SOL D-5-0.4NS 500 ML	47138128	1	35.00	
10/17/CCYY	SOL D-5-0.4NS 500 ML	47138128	1	35.00	
10/17/CCYY	SOL D-5-0.4NS 500 ML	47138128	1	35.00	
10/17/CCYY	SOL D-5-0.4NS 500 ML	47138128	1	35.00	
10/17/CCYY	SOL D-5-0.4NS 500 ML	47138128	1	35.00	
10/17/CCYY	SOL D-5-0.4NS 500 ML	47138128	1	35.00	
10/18/CCYY	SOL D-5-0.4NS 500 ML	47138128	1	35.00	
10/16/CCYY	SOL D-5 LR 500 ML	47138169	1	44.00	
10/16/CCYY	D5.OZ NS 500 ML	47138219	1	35.00	
	TOTAL IV THERAPY				**867.00**

Farnham Memorial Hospital
9009 Foster Avenue
Folley, FL 32205

Patient Name	Patient No.	Sex	Admission Date	Discharge Date	Page No.
FORREST FURY	10079	M	10/14/CCYY	10/18/CCYY	4

Guarantor Name and Address
FRED FURY
5555 FAIRLANE BLVD.
FOLLEY, FL 32208

Insurance Company: ROVER INSURERS, INC.
Claim Number: DOCUMENT 147
Attending Physician: FLORENCE FAULK, M.D.

Date of Service	Description of Hospital Services	Service Code	Qty.	Charges	Total Charges
	SUMMARY OF CHARGES				
	4 DAYS PED-WRD @ 395			1,580.00	
	PHARMACY			933.50	
	IV THERAPY			867.00	
	MED-SUR SUPPLIES			467.00	
	LABORATORY OR (LAB)			396.00	
	SUBTOTAL OF CHARGES				4,243.50
	PAYMENTS AND ADJUSTMENTS			NONE	
	SUBTOTAL PAYMENTS/ADJ				NONE
	BALANCE				4,243.50
	BALANCE DUE				4,243.50

This constitutes a medical decision only: it is not a confirmation of benefits
Contact the benefit payer for an explanation of coverage.

Utilization Review Certification

1. **PT./SUBS. NAME**: _____ Forrest Fury/Fred Fury _____
2. **GROUP NAME/#**: _____ Ninja Enterprises _____ **I.D. #**: _44-6666 NIN_____ **Hospital Claim #**: _147_
3. **HOSPITAL**: _____ Farnham Memorial _____ **ADMIT DATE**: _____ 10/14/CCYY _____
4. **DATE NOTIFIED**: _____ **WORK COMP EMPLOYER**: _____

5. THIS ADMISSION IS:

Preauthorized:	YES _____	NO __✓__
Elective:	YES _____	NO __✓__
Emergency/OB:	YES __✓__	NO _____

6. TYPE OF APPROVAL:

Total Approval: _____ ✓ _____
Partial Denial: _____
Total Denial: _____

7. MEDICALLY NECESSARY DAYS:

__4__ DAYS are certified as medically necessary.

FROM __10/14/CCYY__   THRU __10/18/CCYY__

FROM _____   THRU _____

8. DENIED DAYS OR SERVICES:

_____ DAYS are not certified as medically necessary.

FROM _____   THRU _____

FROM _____   THRU _____

SERVICES not certified are:

_____

9. GRACE/ADMIN. DAYS ARE AUTHORIZED:

FROM _____   THRU _____

10. DENIAL LETTER GIVEN ON _____

11. DENIAL OCCURRED DURING:

_____ Concurrent Review
_____ Retrospective Review
_____ Prior Authorization

12. SERVICES WERE PROVIDED FOR THE FOLLOWING REASONS:

_____ Psychiatric Care
_____ Alcohol Detox
_____ Alcohol Rehab
_____ Date Alc. Rehab Began
_____ Drug Detox
_____ Drug Rehab
_____ Date Drug Rehab Began
_____ Cosmetic Surgery

_____ Pre Cert #: 458854992 _____

Type of Surgery
Cosmetic Surg. Related to:

_____ Congenital Condition
_____ Previous Surgery
_____ Previous Injury
_____ Dental due to accidental injury

ADDITIONAL COMMENTS:

_____

_____ Flora Felton _____
REVIEWER SIGNATURE

_____ 10/14/CCYY _____
DATE CERT. GIVEN

**PLEASE ATTACH THIS FORM TO
YOUR CLAIM TO EXPEDITE PAYMENT**

PAYER COPY

Health Claims Examining Exercises

(**Instructor's Note:** Medical Billing exercises in the entire text should be completed prior to students starting Health Claims Examining Exercise 8–A. New files should be set up for the Health Claims Examining exercises.)

Exercise **8-A**

Directions: Complete an Insurance Coverage Form (located in the **Forms** chapter) and set up Family Files for all families in this chapter. Refer to the Family Data Tables (**Documents 112–116**) located in the beginning of this chapter, and the Contracts located in the **Contracts, UCR Conversion Factor Report, and Relative Value Study** chapter.

Exercise **8-B**

Directions: Complete a Payment Worksheet (located in the **Forms** chapter) for UB-92 claims (**Documents 118–122, 124–128, 130–134, 136–141, and 143–147**) using the guidelines contained in the **Introduction** chapter and using the UCR Conversion Factor Report, Relative Value Study, and Contracts located in the **Contracts, UCR Conversion Factor Report, and Relative Value Study** chapter.

When processing claims, the Beginning Financials (**Documents 117, 123, 129, 135, and 142**) should be incorporated as payment history and claim calculations should be adjusted accordingly. Any carryover deductible listed should be included in the current year deductible for that individual. Therefore, in figuring current year deductible, students should be instructed to subtract the carryover deductible from the current year's amount.

Upon completion of each claim complete or update the Family Benefits Tracking Sheet (located in the **Forms** chapter) by compiling all of the claims payment data for the family.

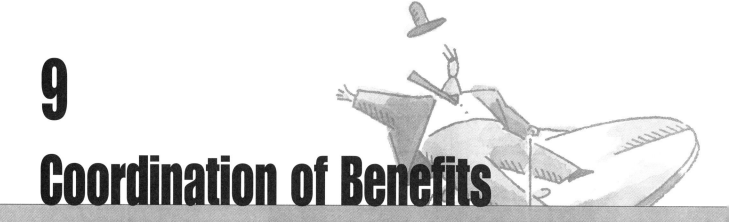

9
Coordination of Benefits

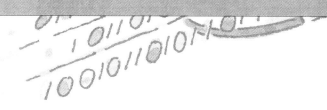

Medical Billing Exercises
Exercise 9-1

Directions: Complete Patient Information Sheets (leave **Assigned Provider** field blank), Ledger Cards, and Insurance Coverage Forms and set up patient charts for the following families using copies of the forms in the **Forms** chapter. Refer to the following Family Data Tables **(Documents 148–150)** for information.

   Individual folders with dividers may be used to store information for each family. One Patient Information Sheet and Insurance Coverage Form should be filled out for the entire family.

DOCUMENT 148

FAMILY DATA TABLE

BROWN FAMILY	INSURED'S INFORMATION	SPOUSE'S INFORMATION	CHILD #1	CHILD #2	CHILD #3
Name	Bernice Brown	Bobby Brown	Brenda Brown		
Address	4949 Backwoods Blvd. Baton Rouge, LA 70810	4949 Backwoods Blvd. Baton Rouge, LA 70810	4949 Backwoods Blvd. Baton Rouge, LA 70810		
Email Address	berniceb@brown.com				
TELEPHONE #					
Home:	(225) 555-7081	(225) 555-7081	(225) 555-7081		
Work:	(225) 555-7082	(225) 555-7085			
Cell:	(225) 555-7083				
Date of Birth	12/30/CCYY-55	12/01/CCYY-50	08/13/CCYY-18		
Social Security #	494-94-9494	494-94-9495	494-94-9496		
Marital Status/Gender	Married/Female	Married/Male	Single/Female		
Student Status			Full-time		
Patient Account #	10081	10080	10083		
Allergies/Medical Conditions	None	None	None		
PRIMARY INSURANCE CARRIERS					
Name Address	Rover Insurers, Inc. 5931 Rolling Road Ronson, CO 81369	Berkeley Insurance Group 4769 Baker Blvd. Berkeley, CA 94721	Berkeley Insurance Group 4769 Baker Blvd. Berkeley, CA 94721		
Effective Date	01/01/CCPY	01/01/CCPY	01/01/CCPY		
Member's ID #	94-9494 NIN	94-9495 BER	94-9495 BER		
Group Policy #	21088	73429	73429		
Policy/Employer	Ninja Enterprises 1234 Nockout Road Newton, NM 88012	Berkeley Institute 6923 Berdan Blvd. Berkeley, CA 94721			
OTHER INSURANCE CARRIER					
Name Address	Berkeley Insurance Group 4769 Baker Blvd. Berkeley, CA 94721	Rover Insurers, Inc. 5931 Rolling Road Ronson, CO 81369	Rover Insurers, Inc. 5931 Rolling Road Ronson, CO 81369		
Effective Date	01/01/CCPY	01/01/CCPY	01/01/CCPY		
Member's ID #	94-9495 BER	94-9494 NIN	94-9494 NIN		
Group Policy #	73429	21088	21088		
Policy/Employer					
Responsible Party	Self	Self	Insured		
EMERGENCY CONTACT					
Name	Bailey Becker	Bailey Becker	Bailey Becker		
Telephone #	(225) 555-7084	(225) 555-7084	(225) 555-7084		
Address	9494 Backwoods Blvd. Baton Rouge, LA 70810	9494 Backwoods Blvd. Baton Rouge, LA 70810	9494 Backwoods Blvd. Baton Rouge, LA 70810		

DOCUMENT 149

FAMILY DATA TABLE

ALLRED FAMILY	INSURED'S INFORMATION	SPOUSE'S INFORMATION	CHILD #1	CHILD #2	CHILD #3
Name	**Allen Allred**	**Allison Allred**	**Ann Allred**		
Address	6565 Apache Avenue Los Angeles, CA 90028	6565 Apache Avenue Los Angeles, CA 90028	6565 Apache Avenue Los Angeles, CA 90028		
Email Address	allena@allred.com				
TELEPHONE #					
Home: Work: Cell:	(323) 555-8200 (323) 555-8201 (323) 555-8202	(323) 555-8200 (323) 555-8204	(323) 555-8200		
Date of Birth	04/14/CCYY-51	01/15/CCYY-48	12/25/CCYY-16		
Social Security #	765-65-7654	765-65-7655	765-65-7656		
Marital Status/Gender	Married/Male	Married/Female	Single/Female		
Student Status			Full-time		
Patient Account #	10086	10085	10087		
Allergies/Medical Conditions	None	None	None		
PRIMARY INSURANCE CARRIER					
Name **Address**	Winter Insurance Company 9763 Western Way Whittier, CO 82963	Berkeley Insurance Group 4769 Baker Blvd. Berkeley, CA 94721	Berkeley Insurance Group 4769 Baker Blvd. Berkeley, CA 94721		
Effective Date	01/01/CCPY	01/01/CCPY	01/01/CCPY		
Member's ID #	65-7654 ABC	65-7655 BER	65-7655 BER		
Group Policy #	36928	73429	73429		
Policy/Employer	ABC Corporation 1234 Whitaker Lane Colter, CO 81222	Berkeley Institute 6923 Berdan Blvd. Berkeley, CA 94721			
OTHER INSURANCE CARRIER					
Name **Address**	Berkeley Insurance Group 4769 Baker Blvd. Berkeley, CA 94721	Winter Insurance Company 9763 Western Way Whittier, CO 82963	Winter Insurance Company 9763 Western Way Whittier, CO 82963		
Effective Date	01/01/CCPY	01/01/CCPY	01/01/CCPY		
Member's ID #	65-7655 BER	65-7654 ABC	65-7654 ABC		
Group Policy #	73429	36928	36928		
Policy/Employer					
Responsible Party	Self	Self	Insured		
EMERGENCY CONTACT					
Name **Telephone #** **Address**	Alfonso Arisco (323) 555-8203 5656 Apache Avenue Los Angeles, CA 90028	Alfonso Arisco (323) 555-8203 5656 Apache Avenue Los Angeles, CA 90028	Alfonso Arisco (323) 555-8203 5656 Apache Avenue Los Angeles, CA 90028		

FAMILY DATA TABLE

INNMAN FAMILY	INSURED'S INFORMATION	SPOUSE'S INFORMATION	CHILD #1	CHILD #2	CHILD #3
Name	Ike Innman	Ingrid Innman	Ian Innman		
Address	2100 Ink Street Ibarra, IL 61515	2100 Ink Street Ibarra, IL 61515	2100 Ink Street Ibarra, IL 61515		
Email Address	ikei@innman.com				
TELEPHONE #					
Home:	(708) 555-6151	(708) 555-6151	(708) 555-6151		
Work:	(708) 555-6152	(708) 555-6155			
Cell:	(708) 555-6153				
Date of Birth	03/07/CCYY-46	06/01/CCYY-47	10/25/CCYY-17		
Social Security #	333-44-5555	333-44-5556	333-44-5557		
Marital Status/Gender	Married/Male	Married/Female	Single/Male		
Student Status			Full-time		
Patient Account #	10054	10088	10089		
Allergies/Medical Conditions	None	None	None		
PRIMARY INSURANCE CARRIER					
Name Address	Ball Insurance Carriers 3895 Bubble Blvd. Ste. 283 Boxwood, CO 85926	Berkeley Insurance Group 4769 Baker Blvd. Berkeley, CA 94721	Ball Insurance Carriers 3895 Bubble Blvd. Ste. 283 Boxwood, CO 85926		
Effective Date	01/01/CCPY	01/01/CCPY	01/01/CCPY		
Member's ID #	44-5555 XYZ	44-5556 BER	44-5555 XYZ		
Group Policy #	62958	73429	62958		
Policy/Employer	XYZ Corporation 9817 Bobcat Blvd. Bastion, CO 81369	Berkeley Institute 6923 Berdan Blvd. Berkeley, CA 94721			
OTHER INSURANCE CARRIER					
Name Address	Berkeley Insurance Group 4769 Baker Blvd. Berkeley, CA 94721	Ball Insurance Carriers 3895 Bubble Blvd. Ste. 283 Boxwood, CO 85926	Ball Insurance Carriers 3895 Bubble Blvd. Ste. 283 Boxwood, CO 85926		
Effective Date	01/01/CCPY	01/01/CCPY	01/01/CCPY		
Member's ID #	44-5556 BER	44-5555 XYZ	44-5555 XYZ		
Group Policy #	73429	62958	62958		
Policy/Employer					
Responsible Party	Self	Self	Insured		
EMERGENCY CONTACT					
Name	Iriana Ingemar	Iriana Ingemar	Iriana Ingemar		
Telephone #	(708) 555-6154	(708) 555-6154	(708) 555-6154		
Address	12 Ink Street Ibarra, IL 61515	12 Ink Street Ibarra, IL 61515	12 Ink Street Ibarra, IL 61515		

Exercise **9-2**

Directions: Complete a CMS-1500 for each of the Encounter Forms (**Documents 152–154, 156, 158, 160–161, 163, 167, and 169**) and a UB-92 for each of the Hospital Admission Forms (**Documents 157, 162, 164, 166, and 170**) in this chapter. These forms may be provided by your instructor or purchased from a stationery store.

After completion of CMS-1500 and UB-92 forms, complete a Patient Receipt (if a payment was made), and post the transaction(s) to the patient Ledger Card/Statement of Account previously created.

Enter either **Inpt Hospital Svcs** or **Otpt Hospital Svcs**, in the **Description of Service** column on the Ledger Card/Statement of Account for hospital claims.

Exercise **9-3**

Directions: Upon completion of all of the activities in Exercise 9–2 complete a Bank Deposit Slip/Ticket (located in the **Forms** chapter) for all payments made on the patient's account in this chapter.

Exercise **9-4**

Directions: Using an Insurance Claims Register (located in the **Forms** chapter) list all claims that have been fully prepared and are ready for submission to the insurance carrier for payment. Enter the date that you created the CMS-1500 or UB-92 in the **Date Claim Filed** column.

Exercise **9-5**

Directions: Complete an Insurance Tracer Form (located in the **Forms** chapter) for the following claim. For additional information refer to the Family Data Table (**Document 43**), completed claim form or the Encounter Form.

Patient	Date Billed	Date of Service	Date of Illness	Diagnosis	Claim #
Guillermo Gates	10/31/CCYY	10/01/CCYY	10/01/CCYY	709.9	Document 45

Coordination of Benefits Claims Beginning Financials
BROWN FAMILY

Insurance Plan	Rover Insurers, Inc.—Ninja Enterprises				
Patient:	BERNICE	BOBBY	BRENDA		
C/O DEDUCTIBLE	0.00	0.00	0.00		
DEDUCTIBLE	75.15	0.00	5.00		
COINSURANCE	0.00	0.00	0.00		
ACCIDENT BENEFIT	0.00	0.00	0.00		
LIFETIME MAXIMUM	245.73	981.10	150.72		
M/N OFFICE VISITS					
OFFICE VISITS					
HOSPITAL VISITS					
DXL					
SURGERY					
ASSISTANT SURGERY					
ANESTHESIA					

Encounter Form

Provider Information

Name:	Brad Barstow, D.C.
Address:	4949 Beetlebrow
City:	Baton Rouge State: LA Zip Code: 70449
Telephone #:	Fax #:
Medicare ID#:	UPIN #: U02115
Tax ID #:	49-4949494 Accepts Medicare Assignment: ☐
Provider's Signature:	_Brad Barstow , DC_ Date: _1/5/CCYY_

Appointment Information

Appointment Date:		Time:
Next Appt. Date:		Time:
Date of First Visit:	01/02/CCYY	Date of Injury:
Referring Physician:		

Guarantor Information

Name:	Bobby Brown
Address:	4949 Backwoods Blvd.
City:	Baton Rouge State: LA Zip Code: 70810
Insurance ID #:	94-9495 BER/ 94-9494 NIN
Insurance Name:	Berkeley Ins. Group/ Rover Insurers, Inc.
Insurance Group #:	73429/ 21088
Employer Name:	Berkeley Institute/ Ninja Enterprises

Patient Information

Name:	Bobby Brown
Address:	4949 Backwoods Blvd.
City:	Baton Rouge State: LA Zip Code: 70810
Telephone #:	(225) 555-7081 Account #: 10080
Date of Birth:	12/01/CCYY-50 Gender: Male
Marital Status:	Married Relationship to Guarantor: Self
Student Status:	☐ Full-time ☐ Part-time
Insurance Type:	☒Pvt ☐ M/care ☐ M/caid ☐ WC ☒ Other ___ COB
Hospitalization Date:	
Hospital Information:	

Authorization

☒ Authorization to Release Information
☒ Authorization for Assignment of Benefits
☐ Authorization for Consent for Treatment
☐ My insurance will be billed but there may be a balance due.
Signature: _Bobby Brown_   Date: _1/5/CCYY_

Clinical Information

	DOS	POS	CPT®/HCPCS Description	ICD-9-CM (*Indicates diagnosis for all lines)	Amount
1	01/05/CCYY	Office	Diathermy	*Cervical Strain	$ 45.00
2	01/05/CCYY	Office	Manipulation	*	$ 30.00
3					
4					
5					
6					

Remarks:					
Previous Balance:		Payment: $44.00	Copay:	Adjustment:	
Total Fee:	$75.00	Cash ☒ Check ☐ Credit ☐	Cash ☐ Check ☐ Credit ☐	Remarks:	New Balance: $31.00

Berkeley Insurance Group   4769 Baker Blvd.   Berkeley, CA   94721

Bobby Brown
4949 Backwoods Blvd.
Baton Rouge, LA 70810

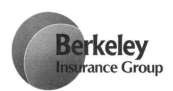

Date through which claims for these benefits were processed:	
January 30, CCYY	
Insurance ID #:	**94 9495 BER**
Insurance Group #:	**73429**
Claim #:	**D o c u m e n t 152**

THIS IS NOT A BILL
Please retain this Benefit Statement for your records.

Explanation of Medical Benefits	**Retain This Benefits Statement For Your Records.**
This statement reflects benefits for: Bobby Brown	
Your provider has also been sent an explanation of benefits statement relating to this claim	

Dear Bobby Brown,

We received a medical claim for you.

The information on this form presents an explanation of benefits due under your plan. This form should be saved for your tax records. Any additional information or questions should be directed to the customer service office.

TOTAL EXPENSES SUBMITTED ON THIS CLAIM $75.00
OUR PAYMENT ON YOUR CLAIM $44.00

Description of Service	Date of Service	Expenses Submitted	Expenses Excluded	Reason (see below)	Covered Balance	%	Payment Amount
OV W/DIATHERMY	01/05/CCYY	$45.00	$15.00	203	$30.00	80	$24.00
MANIPULATION	01/05/CCYY	$30.00	$5.00	203	$25.00	80	$20.00
		75.00	20.00		55.00		44.00
Brad Barstow, D.C.							

203 – EXPENSES EXCEED THE PLAN'S ALLOWED AMOUNT

Encounter Form

Provider Information					
Name:	Bart Bailey, M.D.				
Address:	449 Barstow Blvd				
City:	Baton Rouge	State:	LA	Zip Code:	70849
Telephone #:		Fax #:			
Medicare ID#:		UPIN #:	D02138		
Tax ID #:	49-9494949	Accepts Medicare Assignment:	☐		
Provider's Signature:	*Bart Bailey, MD*		Date: *5/13/CCYY*		

Appointment Information			
Appointment Date:		Time:	
Next Appt. Date:		Time:	
Date of First Visit:	08/13/CCYY	Date of Injury:	
Referring Physician:			

Guarantor Information

Name:	Bernice Brown
Address:	4949 Backwoods Blvd

City:	Baton Rouge	State:	LA	Zip Code:	70810
Insurance ID #:	94-9494 NIN/ 94-9495 BER				
Insurance Name:	Rover Insurers, Inc./ Berkeley Ins. Group				
Insurance Group #:	21088/ 73429				
Employer Name:	Ninja Enterprises/ Berkeley Institute				

Patient Information

Name:	Bernice Brown				
Address:	4949 Backwoods Blvd.				
City:	Baton Rouge	State:	LA	Zip Code:	70810
Telephone #:	(225) 555-7081	Account #:	10081		
Date of Birth:	12/30/CCYY-55	Gender:	Female		
Marital Status:	Married	Relationship to Guarantor:		Self	
Student Status:	☐ Full-time		☐ Part-time		
Insurance Type:	☒ Pvt ☐ M/care ☐ M/caid ☐ WC ☒ Other ___ COB				
Hospitalization Date:					
Hospital Information:					

Authorization

☒	Authorization to Release Information
☒	Authorization for Assignment of Benefits
☐	Authorization for Consent for Treatment
☐	My insurance will be billed but there may be a balance due.

Signature: *Bernice Brown*   Date: *5/13/CCYY*

Clinical Information

	DOS	POS	CPT® /HCPCS Description	ICD-9-CM (*Indicates diagnosis for all lines)	Amount
1	05/13/CCYY	Office	New pt, detailed hist & exam, low complexity	Chronic Rhinitis; Chronic Otitis External	$ 70.00
2					
3					
4					
5					
6					
Remarks:					
Previous Balance:		Payment:		Copay:	Adjustment:	
Total Fee:	$70.00	Cash ☐ Check ☐ Credit ☐	Cash ☐ Check ☐ Credit ☐	Remarks:	New Balance: $70.00

Berkeley Insurance Group 4769 Baker Blvd. Berkeley, CA 94721

Bobby Brown
4949 Backwoods Blvd.
Baton Rouge, LA 70810

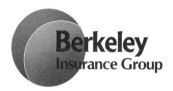

Date through which claims for these benefits were processed:	
August 31, CCYY	
Insurance ID #:	**94 9495 BER**
Insurance Group #:	**73429**
Claim #:	**Document 153**

THIS IS NOT A BILL
Please retain this Benefit Statement for your records.

Explanation of Medical Benefits	**Retain This Benefits**
This statement reflects benefits for: Bernice Brown	**Statement For Your Records.**
Your provider has also been sent an explanation of benefits statement relating to this claim	

Dear Bobby Brown,

We received a medical claim for you.

The information on this form presents an explanation of benefits due under your plan. This form should be saved for your tax records. Any additional information or questions should be directed to the customer service office.

TOTAL EXPENSES SUBMITTED ON THIS CLAIM $ 70.00
OUR PAYMENT ON YOUR CLAIM $ 56.00

Description of Service	Date of Service	Expenses Submitted	Expenses Excluded	Reason (see below)	Covered Balance	%	Payment Amount
DR'S VISIT – INTER EXAM
Bart Bailey, M.D.	08/13/CCYY	$70.00	0.00		$70.00	80	$56.00

Encounter Form

Provider Information

Name:	B.R. Health Care Medical Group
Address:	P.O. Box 4949
City:	Baton Rouge

City:	Baton Rouge	State:	LA	Zip Code:	70667

Telephone #:	Fax #:
Medicare ID#:	UPIN #: W00018
Tax ID #:	49-6001312	Accepts Medicare Assignment: ☐
Provider's Signature:	*Broward Baxter, MD* Date: *6/7/CCYY*

Patient Information

Name:	Bernice Brown
Address:	4949 Backwoods Blvd.

City:	Baton Rouge	State:	LA	Zip Code:	70810

Telephone #:	(225) 555-7081	Account #:	10081
Date of Birth:	12/30/CCYY-55	Gender:	Female
Marital Status:	Married	Relationship to Guarantor:	Self
Student Status:	☐ Full-time	☐ Part-time	
Insurance Type:	☒ Pvt ☐ M/care ☐ M/caid ☐ WC ☒ Other ___ COB		
Hospitalization Date:			
Hospital Information:			

Appointment Information

Appointment Date:		Time:	
Next Appt. Date:		Time:	
Date of First Visit:	06/07/CCYY	Date of Injury:	
Referring Physician:			

Guarantor Information

Name:	Bernice Brown
Address:	4949 Backwoods

City:	Baton Rouge	State:	LA	Zip Code:	70810

Insurance ID #:	94-9494 NIN/ 94-9495 BER
Insurance Name:	Rover Insurers, Inc./ Berkeley Ins. Group
Insurance Group #:	21088/ 73429
Employer Name:	Ninja Enterprises/ Berkeley Institute

Authorization

☒ Authorization to Release Information
☒ Authorization for Assignment of Benefits
☐ Authorization for Consent for Treatment
☐ My insurance will be billed but there may be a balance due.

Signature: *Bernice Brown*   Date: *6/7/CCYY*

Clinical Information

	DOS	POS	CPT® /HCPCS Description	ICD-9-CM (*Indicates diagnosis for all lines)	Amount
1	06/07/CCYY	Office	Alpha-fetoprotein; serum	Pregnancy	$ 49.00
2					
3					
4					
5					
6					

Remarks:	Services provided by Broward Baxter, M.D. UPIN #: E84020 at the office.				
Previous Balance:	$70.00	Payment: $39.20	Copay:	Adjustment:	New Balance: $79.80
Total Fee:	$49.00	Cash ☒ Check ☐ Credit ☐	Cash ☐ Check ☐ Credit ☐	Remarks:	

Berkeley Insurance Group   4769 Baker Blvd. Berkeley, CA 94721

Bobby Brown
4949 Backwoods Blvd.
Baton Rouge, LA 70810

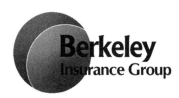

Date through which claims for these benefits were processed:	
August 31, CCYY	
Insurance ID #:	**94 9495 BER**
Insurance Group #:	**73429**
Claim #:	**Document 154**

THIS IS NOT A BILL
Please retain this Benefit Statement for your records.

Explanation of Medical Benefits

This statement reflects benefits for: Bernice Brown

Retain This Benefits Statement For Your Records.

Your provider has also been sent an explanation of benefits statement relating to this claim

Dear Bobby Brown,

We received a medical claim for you.

The information on this form presents an explanation of benefits due under your plan. This form should be saved for your tax records. Any additional information or questions should be directed to the customer service office.

TOTAL EXPENSES SUBMITTED ON THIS CLAIM $49.00
OUR PAYMENT ON YOUR CLAIM $39.20

Description of Service	Date of Service	Expenses Submitted	Expenses Excluded	Reason (see below)	Covered Balance	%	Payment Amount
APF TEST BR Health Care Medical Group	06/07/CCYY	$49.00	0.00		$49.00	80	$39.20

Patient Claim Form

Information must be printed or typewritten. Claim form must be completed and returned to us at the indicated address.

Medicare Patients: Submit this claim to Medicare FIRST! A copy of the Medicare Summary Notice or Medicare Remittance Advice must be submitted with this claim form.

TO BE COMPLETED BY MEMBER

1. Information Pertaining To Member

Name: Last, First, M.I. Brown, Bernice		Sex: F	Date Of Birth 12/30/CCYY-55	Member ID# 64-9494 NIN
Home Address: Street 4949 Backwoods Blvd.	City Baton Rouge	State LA	Zip 70810	Telephone Number (225) 555-7081
Marital Status Married	Name Of Spouse Bobby Brown		Spouse's Date Of Birth 12/01/CCYY-50	Member ID# 64-9495 BER
Is Spouse Employed? No	If Yes, Name And Address Of Employer			Employer Phone Number

2. Information Pertaining To Patient

Patient Name: Last, First, M.I. Brown, Bernice		Sex F	Date Of Birth 12/30/CCYY-55	Member ID# 64-6464 NIN
Home Address: Street 4949 Backwoods Blvd.	City Baton Rouge	State LA	Zip 70810	Telephone Number (225) 555-7081
Is Patient Employed? (Full-Time) Part Time No	Relationship To Employee? Self	If Dependent Child Over 19, Name Of School Where Full-time Student:		

3. Information Regarding Current Treatment

Related To Illness? Yes	Related To Pregnancy? Yes	Related To Work? No	Description Of Illness Or Injury Pregnancy, Chronic Rhinitis, Chronic Otitis External
Date Of Accident N/A	Where Happened? N/A	Describe Accident	

4. Information Regarding Insurance

Are You, Your Spouse, or Dependent Children Covered By Any Other Insurance? Yes	Name Of Insured Bernice Brown	
If Yes, Name And Address Of Insurance Berkeley Insurance Group 4769 Baker Blvd. Berkeley, CA 94721		Insurance Phone Number

Patient's Or Guardian's Signature

I certify that the above information is true and correct and I authorize the release of any medical information necessary to process this claim.

Signed: *Bernice Brown*   Date: 08/07/ccyy

Assignment of Benefits:

I assign payment of benefits to the following provider:

Address: Street	City	State	Zip	Telephone Number

Health Claims Examining Program ONLY

TO BE COMPLETED BY PHYSICIAN

Patient's Name: Last, First, M.I.

Brown, Bernice

Home Address: Street	City	State	Zip	Telephone Number
4949 Backwoods Blvd.	Baton Rouge	LA	70810	(225) 555-7081

Is Condition Due To Illness?	Injury?	Work Related?	Pregnancy?	If Yes, Date Of Last Menstrual Period
Yes	No	No	Yes	03/01/CCYY

Diagnosis Or Nature Of Illness Or Injuries. Give Description And ICD-9-CM Code.

Chronic Rhinitis,   Chronic Otitis External,   Pregnancy

Date Of Service	Place Of Service	Description Of Medical Services Or Supplies Provided	CPT® Code	ICD-9 Code	Charge
07/19/CCYY	Pharmacy	Prenatal Vit	RX		39.20
08/06/CCYY	Pharmacy	Coly-Mycin Otic	RX		20.60
08/07/CCYY	Pharmacy	E.E.S. 400 Film Tabs	RX		12.29
08/07/CCYY	Pharmacy	Acetaminophen w/Cod #3 Tabs	RX		5.39

Date Of First Symptoms	Date Of Accident	Date Patient First Seen		Total Charges	$77.48
Dates Patient Unable To Work From To:	If Still Disabled, Date Patient Should Return To Work			Amount Paid	$77.48
Patient Still Under Care For This Condition?	Date Of Same Or Similar Illness Or Condition		Does Patient Have Other Health Coverage?		

Under Section 6019 Of The Internal Revenue Code, Recipients Of Medical Payments Must Provide Identifying Numbers To Payors Who Must Report Such Payments To The Internal Revenue Service.   Taxpayer ID Number: _____ Social Security Number: _____

Physician's Name: _____   Signature: _____

Street Address   City   State   Zip

INFORMATION REGARDING THIS CLAIM FORM

A Separate Claim Must Be Filed For Each Different Injury Or Illness.

A Claim Must Be Filed Within 90 Days of The Date Of Service Or Claim Benefits May Be Reduced.

If Patient Is Medicare Eligible, Claim Must First Be Submitted To Medicare For Payment. We Cannot Process Claim Without Information Regarding Medicare's Payment.

THANK YOU FOR SHOPPING

RXpress Drugs

Bernice Brown
Reg 38   07/19/CCYY
Bailey, MD   Qty. 100
RX # 177-644

Prenatal Vit   39.20

Refills – 3

Total   39.20

THANK YOU FOR SHOPPING

RXpress Drugs

Bernice Brown
Reg 38   08/06/CCYY
Bailey, MD   Qty. 5
RX # 550943

Coly-Mycin Otic
Drops   20.60

Total   20.60

THANK YOU FOR SHOPPING

RXpress Drugs

Bernice Brown
Reg 38   08/07/CCYY
Bailey, MD   Qty. 30
RX # M007436

E.E.S. 400 Film-
Tabs   12.29

Refills – Call

Total   12.29

THANK YOU FOR SHOPPING

RXpress Drugs

Bernice Brown
Reg 38   08/07/CCYY
Bailey, MD   Qty. 12
RX # M007437

Acetaminophen
W/Cod #3 Tab   5.39

Refills – Call

Total   5.39

Berkeley Insurance Group 4769 Baker Blvd. Berkeley, CA 94721

Bobby Brown
4949 Backwoods Blvd.
Baton Rouge, LA 70810

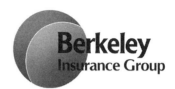

Date through which claims for these benefits were processed:	
August 31, CCYY	
Insurance ID #:	**94 9495 BER**
Insurance Group #:	**73429**
Claim #:	**Document 155**

THIS IS NOT A BILL
Please retain this Benefit Statement for your records.

Explanation of Medical Benefits	**Retain This Benefits Statement For Your Records.**
This statement reflects benefits for: Bernice Brown	
Your provider has also been sent an explanation of benefits statement relating to this claim	

Dear Bobby Brown,

We received a medical claim for you.

The information on this form presents an explanation of benefits due under your plan. This form should be saved for your tax records. Any additional information or questions should be directed to the customer service office.

TOTAL EXPENSES SUBMITTED ON THIS CLAIM	$77.48
OUR PAYMENT ON YOUR CLAIM	$61.98

Description of Service	Date of Service	Expenses Submitted	Expenses Excluded	Reason (see below)	Covered Balance	%	Payment Amount
PRESCRIPTION DRUGS	07/19/CCYY	$39.20	0.00		$39.20	80	$31.36
PRESCRIPTION DRUGS	08/07/CCYY	$5.39	0.00		$5.39	80	$4.31
PRESCRIPTION DRUGS	08/06/CCYY	$20.60	0.00		$20.60	80	$16.48
PRESCRIPTION DRUGS	08/07/CCYY	$12.29	0.00		$12.29	80	$9.83
		$77.48			$77.48		$61.98

Encounter Form

DOCUMENT 156

Provider Information					
Name:	Benita Bernstein, M.D.				
Address:	567 Banning Blvd.				
City:	Baton Rouge	State:	LA	Zip Code:	71046
Telephone #:		Fax #:			
Medicare ID#:		UPIN #:	F20884		
Tax ID #:	49-4466531	Accepts Medicare Assignment: ☐			
Provider's Signature:	*Benita Bernstein, MD*		Date: 3/29/CCYY		

Appointment Information			
Appointment Date:		Time:	
Next Appt. Date:		Time:	
Date of First Visit:	10/01/CCPY	Date of Injury:	
Referring Physician:			

Patient Information

Patient Information	
Name:	Brenda Brown
Address:	4949 Backwoods Blvd.

City:	Baton Rouge	State:	LA	Zip Code:	70810
Telephone #:	(225) 555-7081	Account #:	10083		
Date of Birth:	08/13/CCYY-18	Gender:	Female		
Marital Status:	Single	Relationship to Guarantor:		Child	
Student Status:	☒ Full-time	☐ Part-time			
Insurance Type:	☒ Pvt ☐ M/care ☐ M/caid ☐ WC ☒ Other COB				
Hospitalization Date:					
Hospital Information:					

Guarantor Information

Guarantor Information					
Name:	Bobby Brown				
Address:	4949 Backwoods Blvd.				
City:	Baton Rouge	State:	LA	Zip Code:	70810
Insurance ID #:	94-9495 BER/ 94-9494 NIN				
Insurance Name:	Berkeley Ins. Group/ Rover Insurers, Inc.				
Insurance Group #:	73429/ 21088				
Employer Name:	Berkeley Institute/ Ninja Enterprises				

Authorization

☒ Authorization to Release Information
☒ Authorization for Assignment of Benefits
☐ Authorization for Consent for Treatment
☐ My insurance will be billed but there may be a balance due.
Signature: *Bernice Brown* Date: 3/29/CCYY

Clinical Information

	DOS	POS	CPT® /HCPCS Description	ICD-9-CM (*Indicates diagnosis for all lines)	Amount
1	03/29/CCYY	Office	Est pt, comprehensive exam, high complexity	*Dysplasia of cervix	$ 75.00
2	03/29/CCYY	Office	Collection of venous blood by venipuncture	*	$ 20.00
3					
4					
5					
6					

Remarks:					
Previous Balance:		Payment:		Copay:	Adjustment:
Total Fee:	$95.00	Cash ☐ Check ☐ Credit ☐	Cash ☐ Check ☐ Credit ☐	Remarks:	New Balance: $95.00

Berkeley Insurance Group 4769 Baker Blvd. Berkeley, CA 94721

Bobby Brown
4949 Backwoods Blvd.
Baton Rouge, LA 70810

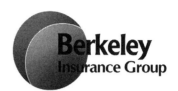

	Date through which claims for these benefits were processed:
	April 30, CCYY
Insurance ID #:	**94 9495 BER**
Insurance Group #:	**73429**
Claim #:	**D o c u m e n t 156**

THIS IS NOT A BILL
Please retain this Benefit Statement for your records.

Explanation of Medical Benefits		**Retain This Benefits Statement For Your Records.**
This statement reflects benefits for:	Brenda Brown	
Your provider has also been sent an explanation of benefits statement relating to this claim		

Dear Bobby Brown,

We received a medical claim for you.

The information on this form presents an explanation of benefits due under your plan. This form should be saved for your tax records. Any additional information or questions should be directed to the customer service office.

TOTAL EXPENSES SUBMITTED ON THIS CLAIM $95.00
OUR PAYMENT ON YOUR CLAIM $76.00

Description of Service	Date of Service	Expenses Submitted	Expenses Excluded	Reason (see below)	Covered Balance	%	Payment Amount
PHYSICIAN	03/29/CCYY	$75.00	0.00		$75.00	80	$60.00
LABORATORY	03/29/CCYY	$20.00	0.00		$20.00	80	$16.00
		$95.00			$95.00		$76.00
Benita Bernstein, M.D.							

Hospital Admission Form

Provider Information

Name:	Baton Rouge General Hospital
Address:	P.O. Box 8593

City:	Baton Rouge	State:	LA	Zip Code:	70478	

Telephone#:		Fax#:	
Medicare ID#:	190027	UPIN#:	
Tax ID #:	49-6859486	Accepts Medicare Assignment:	☐
Provider Rep:	*Betty Biller*	Date: *8/28/CCYY*	

Patient Information

Name:	Bobby Brown
Address:	4949 Backwoods Blvd.

City:	Baton Rouge	State:	LA	Zip Code:	70810	

Telephone#:	(225) 555-7081	Patient Control #:	10084
Date of Birth:	12/01/CCYY-50	Gender:	Male
Marital Status:	Married	Relationship to Guarantor:	Self
Student Status:	☐ Full-time	☐ Part-time	
Insurance Type:	☒ Pvt ☐ M/care ☐ M/caid ☐ WC ☒ Other ___ COB		

Admission Information

Admission Date:	08/27/CCYY	Time:	11:00 AM
Discharge Date:	08/28/CCYY	Time:	9:00 AM
Attending Phy's ID#:	G05440	Date of Injury:	
Attending Physician:	Burton Barsheda, M.D.		

Guarantor Information

Name:	Bobby Brown
Address:	4949 Backwoods Blvd.

City:	Baton Rouge	State:	LA	Zip Code:	70810	

Insurance ID #:	94-9595 BER	SSN:	494-94-9494
Insurance Name:	Berkeley Ins. Group/ Rover Insurers, Inc.		
Insurance Group #:	73429/ 21088		
Employer Name:	Berkeley Institute/ Ninja Enterprises		

Authorization

☒ Authorization to Release Information
☒ Authorization for Assignment of Benefits
☐ Authorization for Consent for Treatment
☐ My insurance will be billed but there may be a balance due.

Signature: *Bobby Brown*   Date: *8/27/CCYY*

Clinical Information

Principal Diagnosis:	Calculus of Uterer
Other Diagnosis:	
Surgical Procedure:	
Other Procedures:	
Remarks:	

Previous Balance:	$31.00	Payment:		Copay:		Adjustment:			
Total Fee:	$2432.80	Cash ☐ Check ☐ Credit ☐		Cash ☐ Check ☐ Credit ☐		Remarks:		New Balance:	$2463.80

Garberville General Hospital
1234 Gary Lane
Garberville, GA 30014

Patient Name	Patient No.	Sex	Admission Date	Discharge Date	Page No.
BOBBY BROWN	10084	M	08/27/CCYY	08/28/CCYY	1

Guarantor Name and Address
BOBBY BROWN
4949 BACKWOODS BLVD.
BATON ROUGE, LA 70810

Insurance Company: BER INS GRP/ROVERS INS, INC
Claim Number: DOCUMENT 157
Attending Physician: BURTON BARSHEDA, M.D.

Date of Service	Description of Hospital Services	Service Code	Qty.	Charges	Total Charges
	SUMMARY OF CHARGES				
	ROOM-BOARD/SEMI		1	622.00	
	PHARMACY		1	48.00	
	MED-SURG SUPPLIES		10	572.00	
	LABORATORY OR (LAB)		12	785.80	
	PATHOLOGY LAB		2	54.00	
	DX X-RAY		1	341.00	
	PERSONAL ITEMS		1	10.00	
	SUBTOTAL OF CHARGES				$2432.80
	PAYMENTS AND ADJUSTMENTS			NONE	
	SUBTOTAL PAYMENTS/ADJ				NONE
	BALANCE				$2432.80
	BALANCE DUE				$2432.80

Berkeley Insurance Group 4769 Baker Blvd. Berkeley, CA 94721

Bobby Brown
4949 Backwoods Blvd.
Baton Rouge, LA 70810

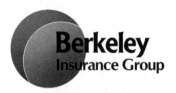

Date through which claims for these benefits were processed:	
September 9, CCYY	
Insurance ID #:	**94 9495 BER**
Insurance Group #:	**73429**
Claim #:	**Document 157**

THIS IS NOT A BILL
Please retain this Benefit Statement for your records.

Explanation of Medical Benefits   **Retain This Benefits Statement For Your Records.**

This statement reflects benefits for: Bobby Brown

Your provider has also been sent an explanation of benefits statement relating to this claim

Dear Bobby Brown,

We received a medical claim for you.

The information on this form presents an explanation of benefits due under your plan. This form should be saved for your tax records. Any additional information or questions should be directed to the customer service office.

TOTAL EXPENSES SUBMITTED ON THIS CLAIM $2432.00
OUR PAYMENT ON YOUR CLAIM $902.00

Description of Service	Date of Service	Expenses Submitted	Expenses Excluded	Reason (see below)	Covered Balance	%	Payment Amount
SEMI-PRIV/WARD	08/27/CCYY	$622.00	$359.94	A	$262.06	80	$209.65
DRUGS	08/27/CCYY	$48.00	$27.78	A	$20.22	80	$16.18
SUPPLIES	08/27/CCYY	$330.00	$190.96	A	$139.04	80	$111.23
LABORATORY	08/27/CCYY	$785.80	$454.72	A	$192.50	80	$154.00
					$138.58	100	$138.58
LABORATORY	08/27/CCYY	$54.00	$31.25	A	$22.75	100	$22.75
X-RAY	08/27/CCYY	$341.00	$197.33	A	$143.67	100	$143.67
ANCILLARY CHARGE	08/27/CCYY	$252.00	$145.82	A	$106.18	100	$106.18
		$2432.80	$1407.80		$1025.00		$902.24
Baton Rouge General Hospital							

A – THE AMOUNT CHARGED HAS BEEN REDUCED BY CONTRACT WITH YOUR PROVIDER.

Encounter Form

Provider Information

Name:	Bay Gastroenterology Medical Group
Address:	2334 Bay View Blvd.
City:	Baton Rouge	State: LA	Zip Code: 70489
Telephone #:		Fax #:
Medicare ID#:		UPIN #: W00019
Tax ID #:	44-4456733	Accepts Medicare Assignment: ☐
Provider's Signature:	Bryant Brown, MD	Date: 11/22/CCYY

Appointment Information

Appointment Date:		Time:	
Next Appt. Date:		Time:	
Date of First Visit:	11/05/CCYY	Date of Injury:	
Referring Physician:			

Guarantor Information

Name:	Bobby Brown
Address:	4949 Backwoods Blvd.
City: Baton Rouge	State: LA	Zip Code: 70810
Insurance ID #:	94-9495 BER/ 94-9494 NIN
Insurance Name:	Berkeley Ins. Group/ Rover Insurers, Inc.
Insurance Group #:	73429/ 21088
Employer Name:	Berkeley Institute/ Ninja Enterprises

Patient Information

Name:	Bobby Brown
Address:	4949 Backwoods Blvd.
City:	Baton Rouge	State: LA	Zip Code: 70810
Telephone #:	(225) 555-7081	Account #: 10084
Date of Birth:	12/01/CCYY-50	Gender: Male
Marital Status:	Married	Relationship to Guarantor: Self
Student Status:	☐ Full-time ☐ Part-time
Insurance Type:	☒ Pvt ☐ M/care ☐ M/caid ☐ WC ☒ Other ____ COB
Hospitalization Date:	
Hospital Information:	Baton Rouge General Hospital, P.O. Box 600, Baton Rouge, LA 70489.

Authorization

☒ Authorization to Release Information
☒ Authorization for Assignment of Benefits
☐ Authorization for Consent for Treatment
☐ My insurance will be billed but there may be a balance due.

Signature: _Bobby Brown_   Date: 11/22/CCYY

Clinical Information

	DOS	POS	CPT® /HCPCS Description	ICD-9-CM (*Indicates diagnosis for all lines)	Amount
1	11/05/CCYY	Office	New pt, comprehensive hist & exam, high complexity	*Intestinal Blockage	$225.00
2	11/22/CCYY	Otpt Hosp	Diag, colonoscopy, flex, proximal to splenic flexure	*	$750.00
3					
4					
5					
6					

Remarks:	Services provided by Bryant Brown, M.D. UPIN #: H56540			
Previous Balance:	$2463.80	Payment:	Copay:	Adjustment:
Total Fee:	$975.00	Cash ☐ Check ☐ Credit ☐	Cash ☐ Check ☐ Credit ☐	Remarks:	New Balance: $3438.80

Berkeley Insurance Group   4769 Baker Blvd.   Berkeley, CA   94721

Bobby Brown
4949 Backwoods Blvd.
Baton Rouge, LA 70810

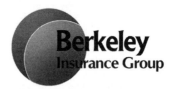

Date through which claims for these benefits were processed:
December 15, CCYY

Insurance ID #:	**94 9495 BER**
Insurance Group #:	**73429**
Claim #:	**D o c u m e n t 158**

THIS IS NOT A BILL
Please retain this Benefit Statement for your records.

Explanation of Medical Benefits   Retain This
                                                                                                                        Benefits
This statement reflects benefits for: Bobby Brown   Statement For
                                                                                                                        Your Records.

Your provider has also been sent an explanation of benefits statement relating to this claim

Dear Bobby Brown,

We received a medical claim for you.

The information on this form presents an explanation of benefits due under your plan. This form should be saved for your tax records. Any additional information or questions should be directed to the customer service office.

TOTAL EXPENSES SUBMITTED ON THIS CLAIM	$225.00
OUR PAYMENT ON YOUR CLAIM	$111.70

Description of Service	Date of Service	Expenses Submitted	Expenses Excluded	Reason (see below)	Covered Balance	%	Payment Amount
DR'S VISIT Bay Gastroenterology Medical Group	11/05/CCYY	$225.00	$10.00/$103.30	426/406	$111.70	100	$111.70

406 – THE EXCLUDED AMOUNT IS OVER THE PROVIDER'S CONTRACTED FEE. YOU ARE NOT RESPONSIBLE FOR THIS AMOUNT

426 – THIS EXCLUDED AMOUNT IS THE PORTION PAYABLE BY THE PATIENT, WHICH IS CALLED THE CO-PAYMENT

Berkeley Insurance Group 4769 Baker Blvd. Berkeley, CA 94721

Bobby Brown
4949 Backwoods Blvd.
Baton Rouge, LA 70810

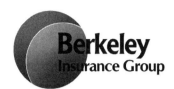

Date through which claims for these benefits were processed:
December 15, CCYY

Insurance ID #:	**94 9495 BER**
Insurance Group #:	**73429**
Claim #:	**Document 158**

THIS IS NOT A BILL
Please retain this Benefit Statement for your records.

Explanation of Medical Benefits	**Retain This Benefits Statement For Your Records.**
This statement reflects benefits for: Bobby Brown	
Your provider has also been sent an explanation of benefits statement relating to this claim	

Dear Bobby Brown,

We received a medical claim for you.

The information on this form presents an explanation of benefits due under your plan. This form should be saved for your tax records. Any additional information or questions should be directed to the customer service office.

TOTAL EXPENSES SUBMITTED ON THIS CLAIM $750.00
OUR PAYMENT ON YOUR CLAIM $592.92

Description of Service	Date of Service	Expenses Submitted	Expenses Excluded	Reason (see below)	Covered Balance	%	Payment Amount
SURGERY	11/22/CCYY	$750.00	$157.08	406	$592.92	100	$592.92
Bay Gastroenterology Medical Group							

406 – THE EXCLUDED AMOUNT IS OVER THE PROVIDER'S CONTRACTED FEE. YOU ARE NOT RESPONSIBLE FOR THIS AMOUNT

Coordination of Benefits Claims Beginning Financials

ALLRED FAMILY

Insurance Plan	Winter Insurance Company—ABC Corporation				
Patient:	**ALLEN**	**ALLISON**	**ANN**		
C/O DEDUCTIBLE	0.00	0.00	0.00		
DEDUCTIBLE	100.00	20.40	0.00		
COINSURANCE	0.00	0.00	0.00		
ACCIDENT BENEFIT	0.00	0.00	0.00		
LIFETIME MAXIMUM	1,426.32	5,276.00	2,162.42		
M/N OFFICE VISITS					
OFFICE VISITS					
HOSPITAL VISITS					
DXL					
SURGERY					
ASSISTANT SURGERY					
ANESTHESIA					

Encounter Form

Provider Information

Name:	Amanda Angel, M.D.
Address:	P.O. Box 721
City:	Los Angeles State: CA Zip Code: 90048
Telephone #:	Fax #:
Medicare ID#:	UPIN #: I33320
Tax ID #:	95-2233445 Accepts Medicare Assignment: ☐
Provider's Signature:	*Amanda Angel, MD* Date: 3/30/CCYY

Appointment Information

Appointment Date:		Time:
Next Appt. Date:		Time:
Date of First Visit:	03/30/CCYY	Date of Injury:
Referring Physician:		

Guarantor Information

Name:	Allison Allred
Address:	6565 Apache Avenue
City:	Los Angeles State: CA Zip Code: 90028
Insurance ID #:	65-7655 BER/ 65-7654 ABC
Insurance Name:	Berkeley Ins. Group/ Winter Ins. Company
Insurance Group #:	73429/ 36928
Employer Name:	Berkeley Institute/ ABC Corporation

Patient Information

Name:	Allison Allred
Address:	6565 Apache Avenue
City:	Los Angeles State: CA Zip Code: 90028
Telephone #:	(323) 555-8200 Account #: 10085
Date of Birth:	01/15/CCYY-48 Gender: Female
Marital Status:	Married Relationship to Guarantor: Self
Student Status:	☐ Full-time ☐ Part-time
Insurance Type:	☒ Pvt ☐ M/care ☐ M/caid ☐ WC ☒ Other ___COB___
Hospitalization Date:	
Hospital Information:	

Authorization

☒ Authorization to Release Information
☐ Authorization for Assignment of Benefits
☐ Authorization for Consent for Treatment
☐ My insurance will be billed but there may be a balance due.

Signature: *Allison Allred* Date: 3/30/CCYY

Clinical Information

	DOS	POS	CPT® /HCPCS Description	ICD-9-CM (*Indicates diagnosis for all lines)	Amount
1	03/30/CCYY	Office	Urinalysis; non-automated, with microscopy	*Pregnancy	$ 25.00
2	03/30/CCYY	Office	Hepatitis B surface antigen	*	$ 30.00
3	03/30/CCYY	Office	Obstetric panel	*	$ 16.00
4					
5					
6					

Remarks:				
Previous Balance:		Payment:	Copay:	Adjustment:
Total Fee: $71.00	Cash ☐ Check ☐ Credit ☐	Cash ☐ Check ☐ Credit ☐	Remarks:	New Balance: $71.00

Berkeley Insurance Group   4769 Baker Blvd.   Berkeley, CA   94721

Allison Allred
6565 Apache Avenue
Los Angeles, CA 90028

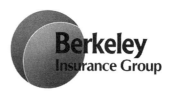

Date through which claims for these benefits were processed:	
December 30, CCYY	
Insurance ID #:	**65 7655 BER**
Insurance Group #:	**73429**
Claim #:	**Document 160**

THIS IS NOT A BILL
Please retain this Benefit Statement for your records.

Explanation of Medical Benefits	Retain This Benefits Statement For Your Records.
This statement reflects benefits for: Allison Allred	
Your provider has also been sent an explanation of benefits statement relating to this claim	

Dear Allison Allred,

We received a medical claim for you.

The information on this form presents an explanation of benefits due under your plan. This form should be saved for your tax records. Any additional information or questions should be directed to the customer service office.

TOTAL EXPENSES SUBMITTED ON THIS CLAIM $71.00
OUR PAYMENT ON YOUR CLAIM $56.80

Description of Service	Date of Service	Expenses Submitted	Expenses Excluded	Reason (see below)	Covered Balance	%	Payment Amount
LABORATORY	03/30/CCYY	$71.00			$71.00	80	$56.80
Amanda Angel, M.D.							

YOU MAY REQUEST AN APPEAL TO ANY DENIAL IN WRITING WITHIN 60 DAYS OF RECEIVING THIS FORM. PLEASE GIVE SPECIFIC REASONS FOR YOUR APPEAL AND SEND YOUR LETTER TO THE "APPEALS DIVISION."

Encounter Form

Provider Information

Name:	Amanda Angel, M.D.
Address:	P.O. Box 721

City:	Los Angeles	State:	CA	Zip Code:	90048

Telephone #:		Fax #:	
Medicare ID#:		UPIN #:	I33320
Tax ID #:	95-2233445	Accepts Medicare Assignment:	☐
Provider's Signature:	*Amanda Angel, MD*	Date: *9/9/CCYY*	

Appointment Information

Appointment Date:		Time:	
Next Appt. Date:		Time:	
Date of First Visit:	09/09/CCYY	Date of Injury:	
Referring Physician:			

Guarantor Information

Name:	Allison Allred
Address:	6565 Apache Avenue

City:	Los Angeles	State:	CA	Zip Code:	90028

Patient Information

Name:	Allison Allred
Address:	6565 Apache Avenue

City:	Los Angeles	State:	CA	Zip Code:	90028
Telephone #:	(323) 555-8200	Account #:	10085		

Insurance ID #:	65-7655 BER/ 65-7654 ABC		
Insurance Name:	Berkeley Ins. Group/ Winter Ins. Company		
Insurance Group #:	73429/ 36928		
Employer Name:	Berkeley Institute/ ABC Corporation		

Date of Birth:	01/15/CCYY-48	Gender:	Female
Marital Status:	Married	Relationship to Guarantor:	Self
Student Status:	☐ Full-time	☐ Part-time	
Insurance Type:	☒ Pvt ☐ M/care ☐ M/caid ☐ WC ☒ Other ___ COB		
Hospitalization Date:			
Hospital Information:			

Authorization

☒ Authorization to Release Information
☐ Authorization for Assignment of Benefits
☐ Authorization for Consent for Treatment
☐ My insurance will be billed but there may be a balance due.

Signature: *Allison Allred*　　　　Date: *9/9/CCYY*

Clinical Information

	DOS	POS	CPT® /HCPCS Description	ICD-9-CM (*Indicates diagnosis for all lines)	Amount
1	09/09/CCYY	Office	Est pt, comprehensive exam, high complexity	Hypercholesterolemia	$100.00
2					
3					
4					
5					
6					

Remarks:	Patient lab results indicate that patient has elevated cholesterol level.

Previous Balance:	$71.00	Payment:	$10.00	Copay:		Adjustment:
Total Fee:	$100.00	Cash ☒ Check ☐ Credit ☐		Cash ☐ Check ☐ Credit ☐	Remarks:	New Balance: $161.00

Berkeley Insurance Group 4769 Baker Blvd. Berkeley, CA 94721

Allison Allred
6565 Apache Avenue
Los Angeles, CA 90028

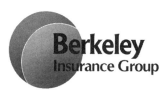

Date through which claims for these benefits were processed:	
December 30, CCYY	
Insurance ID #:	**65 7655 BER**
Insurance Group #:	**73429**
Claim #:	**Document 161**

THIS IS NOT A BILL
Please retain this Benefit Statement for your records.

Explanation of Medical Benefits	**Retain This Benefits Statement For Your Records.**
This statement reflects benefits for: Allison Allred	
Your provider has also been sent an explanation of benefits statement relating to this claim	

Dear Allison Allred,

We received a medical claim for you.

The information on this form presents an explanation of benefits due under your plan. This form should be saved for your tax records. Any additional information or questions should be directed to the customer service office.

TOTAL EXPENSES SUBMITTED ON THIS CLAIM $100.00
OUR PAYMENT ON YOUR CLAIM $78.51

Description of Service	Date of Service	Expenses Submitted	Expenses Excluded	Reason (see below)	Covered Balance	%	Payment Amount
PHYSICAL EXAM	09/09/CCYY	$100.00	21.49	426	$78.51	100	$78.51
Amanda Angel, M.D.							

426 – THIS EXCLUDED AMOUNT IS THE PORTION PAYABLE BY THE PATIENT, WHICH IS CALLED THE "CO-PAYMENT."

Hospital Admission Form

Provider Information

Name:	Anchors Aweigh Hospital
Address:	0987 Awasn Avenue

City:	Los Angeles	State:	CA	Zip Code:	90503

Telephone#:		Fax#:	
Medicare ID#:	050028	UPIN#:	

Tax ID #:	95-8495837	Accepts Medicare Assignment:	☐
Provider Rep:	_Betty Biller_	Date: _11/22/CCYY_	

Patient Information

Name:	Allen Allred
Address:	6565 Apache Avenue

City:	Los Angeles	State:	CA	Zip Code:	90028

Telephone#:	(323) 555-8200	Patient Control #:	10086
Date of Birth:	04/14/CCYY-51	Gender:	Male

Marital Status:	Married	Relationship to Guarantor:	Self
Student Status:	☐ Full-time	☐ Part-time	
Insurance Type:	☒ Pvt ☐ M/care ☐ M/caid ☐ WC ☒ Other ___COB___		

Admission Information

Admission Date:	11/22/CCYY	Time:	11:00 AM
Discharge Date:	11/22/CCYY	Time:	2:00 PM
Attending Phy's ID#:	K45001	Date of Injury:	
Attending Physician:	Andrea Arnold, M.D.		

Guarantor Information

Name:	Allen Allred
Address:	6565 Apache Avenue

City:	Los Angeles	State:	CA	Zip Code:	90028

Insurance ID #:	65-7654 ABC	SSN:	765-65-7654
Insurance Name:	Winter Ins. Company/ Berkeley Ins. Group		
Insurance Group #:	36928/ 73429		
Employer Name:	ABC Corporation/ Berkeley Institute		

Authorization

☒ Authorization to Release Information
☒ Authorization for Assignment of Benefits
☐ Authorization for Consent for Treatment
☐ My insurance will be billed but there may be a balance due.

Signature: _Allen Allred_   Date: _11/22/CCYY_

Clinical Information

Principal Diagnosis:	Colon Polyps
Other Diagnosis:	
Surgical Procedure:	Colonoscopy 11/22/CCYY
Other Procedures:	
Remarks:	

Previous Balance:		Payment:		Copay:		Adjustment:	
Total Fee:	$720.00	Cash ☐ Check ☐ Credit ☐	Cash ☐ Check ☐ Credit ☐	Remarks:		New Balance: $720.00

Anchors Aweigh Hospital
0987 Awasn Avenue
Los Angeles, CA 90503

Patient Name	Patient No.	Sex	Admission Date	Discharge Date	Page No.
ALLEN ALLRED	10086	M	11/22/CCYY	11/22/CCYY	1

Guarantor Name and Address
ALLEN ALLRED
6565 APACHE AVENUE
LOS ANGELES, CA 90028

Insurance Company: WINTER INS CO/ BERKELEY INS GRP
Claim Number: DOCUMENT 162
Attending Physician: ANDREA ARNOLD, M.D.

Date of Service	Description of Hospital Services	Service Code	Qty.	Charges	Total Charges
	SUMMARY OF CHARGES				
	CAMERA POLAROID		1	$43.50	
	PROCTO/GI TIME-1ST 30 MIN		1	$152.00	
	PROCTO/GI TIME-ADDL 15 MIN		6	$204.00	
	PACK, COLONOSCOPY		1	$65.00	
	COLONOSCOPY		1	$220.00	
	** TOTAL GI LAB **			$684.50	
	IV START KIT		1	$14.50	
	BUTTERFLY NEEDLE		1	$9.00	
	SODIUM CHLORIDE 0.9% BACT		1	$12.00	
	** TOTAL PHARMACY **			$35.50	
	SUBTOTAL OF CHARGES				$720.00
	PAYMENTS AND ADJUSTMENTS			NONE	
	SUBTOTAL PAYMENTS/ADJ				NONE
	BALANCE				$720.00
	BALANCE DUE				$720.00

Berkeley Insurance Group 4769 Baker Blvd. Berkeley, CA 94721

Allison Allred
6565 Apache Avenue
Los Angeles, CA 90028

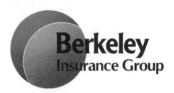

Date through which claims for these benefits were processed:	
December 30, CCYY	
Insurance ID #:	**65 7655 BER**
Insurance Group #:	**73429**
Claim #:	**Document 162**

THIS IS NOT A BILL
Please retain this Benefit Statement for your records.

Explanation of Medical Benefits

This statement reflects benefits for: Allen Allred

Retain This Benefits Statement For Your Records.

Your provider has also been sent an explanation of benefits statement relating to this claim

Dear Allison Allred,

We received a medical claim for you.

The information on this form presents an explanation of benefits due under your plan. This form should be saved for your tax records. Any additional information or questions should be directed to the customer service office.

TOTAL EXPENSES SUBMITTED ON THIS CLAIM $720.00
OUR PAYMENT ON YOUR CLAIM $576.00

Description of Service	Date of Service	Expenses Submitted	Expenses Excluded	Reason (see below)	Covered Balance	%	Payment Amount
PRESCRIPTION DRUGS	11/22/CCYY	$35.50	$7.10	406	$28.40	100	$28.40
OUTPATIENT SERVICE	11/22/CCYY	$108.50	$21.70	406	$86.80	100	$86.80
OUTPATIENT SERVICE	11/22/CCYY	$576.00	$115.20	406	$460.80	100	$460.80
		$720.00	$144.00		$576.00		$576.00
Anchors Aweigh Hospital							

406 – THE EXCLUDED AMOUNT IS OVER THE PROVIDER'S CONTRACTED FEE. YOU ARE NOT RESPONSIBLE FOR THIS AMOUNT.

Encounter Form

Provider Information

Name:	Anders Aumansen, M.D.
Address:	P.O. Box 428
City:	Los Angeles State: CA Zip Code: 90021
Telephone #:	Fax #:
Medicare ID#:	UPIN #: L12088
Tax ID #:	95-1122334 Accepts Medicare Assignment: ☐
Provider's Signature:	*Anders Aumansen, MD* Date: *12/23/CCYY*

Appointment Information

Appointment Date:	Time:
Next Appt. Date:	Time:
Date of First Visit: 12/23/CCYY	Date of Injury:
Referring Physician:	

Guarantor Information

Name:	Allison Allred
Address:	6565 Apache Avenue
City: Los Angeles	State: CA Zip Code: 90028
Insurance ID #:	65-7655 BER/ 65-7654 ABC
Insurance Name:	Berkeley Ins. Group/ Winter Ins. Company
Insurance Group #:	73429/ 36928
Employer Name:	Berkeley Institute/ ABC Corporation

Patient Information

Name:	Ann Allred
Address:	6565 Apache Avenue
City:	Los Angeles State: CA Zip Code: 90028
Telephone #:	(323) 555-8200 Account #: 10087
Date of Birth:	12/25/CCYY-16 Gender: Female
Marital Status:	Single Relationship to Guarantor: Child
Student Status:	☒ Full-time ☐ Part-time
Insurance Type:	☒ Pvt ☐ M/care ☐ M/caid ☐ WC ☒ Other COB
Hospitalization Date:	
Hospital Information:	

Authorization

☒ Authorization to Release Information
☒ Authorization for Assignment of Benefits
☐ Authorization for Consent for Treatment
☐ My insurance will be billed but there may be a balance due.

Signature: *Allen Allred*   Date: *12/23/CCYY*

Clinical Information

	DOS	POS	CPT® /HCPCS Description	ICD-9-CM (*Indicates diagnosis for all lines)	Amount
1	12/23/CCYY	Office	Est pt, comprehensive exam, high complexity	Borderline Glaucoma; Ocular Hypertension	$ 55.00
2					
3					
4					
5					
6					
Remarks:					

Previous Balance:		Payment:		Copay:		Adjustment:		
Total Fee:	$55.00	Cash ☐ Check ☐ Credit ☐		Cash ☐ Check ☐ Credit ☐		Remarks:	New Balance:	$55.00

Berkeley Insurance Group 4769 Baker Blvd. Berkeley, CA 94721

Allison Allred
6565 Apache Avenue
Los Angeles, CA 90028

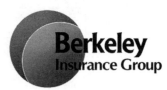

Date through which claims for these benefits were processed: **December 30, CCYY**	
Insurance ID #:	**65 7655 BER**
Insurance Group #:	**73429**
Claim #:	**D o c u m e n t 163**

THIS IS NOT A BILL
Please retain this Benefit Statement for your records.

Explanation of Medical Benefits		**Retain This Benefits Statement For Your Records.**
This statement reflects benefits for:	Ann Allred	
Patient Responsibility:	10.00	
Your provider has also been sent an explanation of benefits statement relating to this claim		

Dear Allison Allred,

We received a medical claim for you.

The information on this form presents an explanation of benefits due under your plan. This form should be saved for your tax records. Any additional information or questions should be directed to the customer service office.

TOTAL EXPENSES SUBMITTED ON THIS CLAIM $55.00
OUR PAYMENT ON YOUR CLAIM $45.00

Description of Service	Date of Service	Expenses Submitted	Expenses Excluded	Reason (see below)	Covered Balance	%	Payment Amount
OUTPATIENT SERVICE Anders Aumansen, M.D.	12/23/CCYY	$55.00	$10.00	426	$45.00	100	$45.00

426 – THIS EXCLUDED AMOUNT IS THE PORTION PAYABLE BY THE PATIENT, WHICH IS CALLED THE "CO-PAYMENT."

Hospital Admission Form

DOCUMENT *164*

Provider Information

Name:	All Saints Hospital				
Address:	9374 Anonda Way				
City:	Los Angeles	State:	CA	Zip Code:	90084
Telephone#:		Fax#:			
Medicare ID#:	050029	UPIN#:			
Tax ID #:	95-0928593	Accepts Medicare Assignment:	☐		
Provider Rep:	*Betty Biller*		Date: *11/21/CCYY*		

Admission Information

Admission Date:	11/19/CCYY	Time:	8:00 PM
Discharge Date:	11/21/CCYY	Time:	11:00 AM
Attending Phy's ID#:	I33320	Date of Injury:	
Attending Physician:	Amanda Angel, M.D.		

Patient Information

Name:	Allison Allred				
Address:	6565 Apache Avenue				
City:	Los Angeles	State:	CA	Zip Code:	90028
Telephone#:	(323) 555-8200	Patient Control #:	10085		
Date of Birth:	12/15/CCYY-48	Gender:	Female		
Marital Status:	Married	Relationship to Guarantor:		Self	
Student Status:	☐Full-time	☐ Part-time			
Insurance Type:	☒ Pvt ☐ M/care ☐ M/caid ☐ WC ☒ Other ___ COB				

Guarantor Information

Name:	Allison Allred				
Address:	6565 Apache Avenue				
City:	Los Angeles	State:	CA	Zip Code:	90028
Insurance ID #:	65-7655 BER	SSN:	765-65-7654		
Insurance Name:	Berkeley Ins. Group/ Winter Ins. Company				
Insurance Group #:	73429/ 36928				
Employer Name:	Berkeley Institute/ ABC Corporation				

Authorization

☒ Authorization to Release Information
☒ Authorization for Assignment of Benefits
☐ Authorization for Consent for Treatment
☐ My insurance will be billed but there may be a balance due.

Signature: *Allison Allred*   Date: *11/19/CCYY*

Clinical Information

Principal Diagnosis:	Normal Delivery; Delivery Single Liveborn	
Other Diagnosis:		
Surgical Procedure:	Manual Assist Spontaneous Delivery	11/20/CCYY
Other Procedures:	Episiotomy	11/20/CCYY
Remarks:		

Previous Balance:	$161.00	Payment:		Copay:		Adjustment:			
Total Fee:	$4055.19	Cash ☐ Check ☐ Credit ☐		Cash ☐ Check ☐ Credit ☐		Remarks:		New Balance:	$4216.19

All Saints Hospital
9374 Anonda Way
Los Angeles, CA 90084

Patient Name	Patient No.	Sex	Date of Birth	Admission Date	Discharge Date	Page No.
ALLISON ALLRED	10085	F	12/15/CCYY-48	11/19/CCYY	11/21/CCYY	1

Guarantor Name and Address
ALLISON ALLRED
6565 APACHE AVENUE
LOS ANGELES, CA 90028

Insurance Company: BERKELEY INS GRP/ WINTER INS CO
Claim Number: DOCUMENT 164
Attending Physician: AMANDA ANGEL, M.D.

Date of Service	Description of Hospital Services	Service Code	Qty.	Charges	Total Charges
	SUMMARY OF CHARGES				
	ROOM AND BOARD PRIVATE		1	$598.00	
	ROOM AND BOARD PRIVATE		1	$598.00	
	PHARMACY		22	$483.69	
	CENTRAL SERVICE		27	$699.50	
	LABORATORY CLINICAL		4	$91.50	
	BLOOD BANK		2	$135.50	
	LABOR AND DELIVERY		15	$1449.00	
	SUBTOTAL OF CHARGES				$4055.19
	PAYMENTS AND ADJUSTMENTS			NONE	
	SUBTOTAL PAYMENTS/ADJ				NONE
	BALANCE				$4055.19
	BALANCE DUE				$4055.19

Berkeley Insurance Group 4769 Baker Blvd. Berkeley, CA 94721

Allison Allred
6565 Apache Avenue
Los Angeles, CA 90028

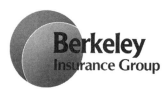

Date through which claims for these benefits were processed:	
December 30, CCYY	
Insurance ID #:	**65 7655 BER**
Insurance Group #:	**73429**
Claim #:	**D o c u m e n t 164**

THIS IS NOT A BILL
Please retain this Benefit Statement for your records.

Explanation of Medical Benefits	**Retain This Benefits Statement For Your Records.**
This statement reflects benefits for: Allison Allred	
Your provider has also been sent an explanation of benefits statement relating to this claim	

Dear Allison Allred,

Below is an explanation of plan benefits.

Date of Service	Type of Service	DRG/PDM #	DRG/PDM Amount
11/19/–11/20/CCYY	PER DIEM TOTAL BILLED DRG/PDM AMOUNT PATIENT LIABILITY BENEFIT AMOUNT	0028	$1000.00 $4055.19 $1000.00 0.00 $1000.00
All Saints Hospital			

REMARKS:

THIS PATIENT SHOULD NOT BE BILLED FURTHER CHARGES FOR THIS CONFINEMENT EXCEPT FOR PERSONAL ITEMS AND THE AMOUNT SHOWN AS PATIENT LIABILITY.

PLEASE KEEP THIS EXPLANATION OF BENEFITS STATEMENT FOR YOUR RECORDS. IF YOU HAVE ANY QUESTIONS REGARDING THIS CLAIM, PLEASE INCLUDE THE ABOVE REFERENCE NUMBER ON YOUR INQUIRY.

Coordination of Benefits Claims Beginning Financials

INNMAN FAMILY

Insurance Plan	Ball Insurance Carriers—XYZ Corporation				
Patient:	IKE*	INGRID	IAN		
C/O DEDUCTIBLE	0.00	0.00	0.00		
DEDUCTIBLE	0.00	50.00	27.00		
COINSURANCE	0.00	0.00	0.00		
ACCIDENT BENEFIT	0.00	0.00	0.00		
LIFETIME MAXIMUM	4,621.00	27,224.00	3,940.00		
M/N OFFICE VISITS					
OFFICE VISITS					
HOSPITAL VISITS					
DXL					
SURGERY					
ASSISTANT SURGERY					
ANESTHESIA					

Hospital Admission Form

Provider Information

Name:	Ibarra General Hospital
Address:	P.O. Box 84759K
City: Ibarra	State: IL	Zip Code: 61523
Telephone#:	Fax#:
Medicare ID#:	140030	UPIN#:
Tax ID #:	00-8574957	Accepts Medicare Assignment: ☐
Provider Rep: Betty Biller	Date: 8/1/CCYY

Admission Information

Admission Date:	07/29/CCYY	Time:	3:00 PM
Discharge Date:	08/01/CCYY	Time:	11:00 AM
Attending Phy's ID#:	B69956	Date of Injury:	
Attending Physician:	Ivan Isner, M.D.		

Guarantor Information

Name:	Ingrid Innman
Address:	2100 Ink Street
City: Ibarra	State: IL	Zip Code: 61515
Insurance ID #:	44-5556 BER	SSN: 333-44-5555
Insurance Name:	Berkeley Ins. Group/ Ball Ins Carriers
Insurance Group #:	73429/ 62958
Employer Name:	Berkeley Institute/ XYZ Corporation

Patient Information

Name:	Ingrid Innman
Address:	2100 Ink Street
City: Ibarra	State: IL	Zip Code: 61515
Telephone#:	(708) 555-6151	Patient Control #: 10088
Date of Birth:	06/01/CCYY-47	Gender: Female
Marital Status:	Married	Relationship to Guarantor: Self
Student Status:	☐ Full-time	☐ Part-time
Insurance Type:	☒ Pvt ☐ M/care ☐ M/caid ☐ WC ☒ Other COB

Authorization

☒ Authorization to Release Information
☒ Authorization for Assignment of Benefits
☐ Authorization for Consent for Treatment
☐ My insurance will be billed but there may be a balance due.

Signature: Ingrid Innman Date: 7/29/CCYY

Clinical Information

Principal Diagnosis:	Unspecified epilepsy	
Other Diagnosis:		
Surgical Procedure:	Spinal Tap	07/30/CCYY
Other Procedures:	Cat Scan of Head	07/30/CCYY
Remarks:		

Previous Balance:		Payment:		Copay:		Adjustment:		
Total Fee:	$4323.15	Cash ☐ Check ☐ Credit ☐		Cash ☐ Check ☐ Credit ☐		Remarks:	New Balance:	$4323.15

Ibarra General Hospital
P.O. Box 84759K
Ibarra, IL 61523

Patient Name	Patient No.	Sex	Date of Birth	Admission Date	Discharge Date	Page No.
INGRID INNMAN	10088	F	07/01/CCYY-47	07/29/CCYY	08/01/CCYY	1

Guarantor Name and Address
INGRID INNMAN
2100 INK STREET
IBARRA, IL 61515

Insurance Company: BERKELEY INS GRP/ BALL INS CRS
Claim Number: DOCUMENT 166
Attending Physician: IVAN ISNER, M.D.

Date of Service	Description of Hospital Services	Service Code	Qty.	Charges	Total Charges
	SUMMARY OF CHARGES				
	ROOM-BOARD PVT		1	$494.00	
	ICU/SURGICAL		1	$1104.00	
	PHARMACY		18	$131.00	
	MED-SURG SUPPLIES		22	$569.70	
	LABORATORY		13	$695.65	
	CT SCAN/HEAD		1	$485.80	
	RESPIRATORY SVC		21	$196.50	
	EMERG ROOM		6	$493.80	
	EEG		1	$152.70	
	SUBTOTAL OF CHARGES				$4323.15
	PAYMENTS AND ADJUSTMENTS			NONE	
	SUBTOTAL PAYMENTS/ADJ				NONE
	BALANCE DUE				$4323.15

Berkeley Insurance Group 4769 Baker Blvd. Berkeley, CA 94721

Ingrid Innman
2100 Ink Street
Ibarra, IL 61515

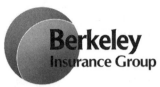

Date through which claims for these benefits were processed:	
August 30, CCYY	
Insurance ID #:	**44 5556 BER**
Insurance Group #:	**73429**
Claim #:	**D o c u m e n t 166**

THIS IS NOT A BILL
Please retain this Benefit Statement for your records.

Explanation of Medical Benefits	Retain This Benefits Statement For Your Records.
This statement reflects benefits for: Ingrid Innman	
Your provider has also been sent an explanation of benefits statement relating to this claim	

Dear Ingrid Innman,

We received a medical claim for you.

The information on this form presents an explanation of benefits due under your plan. This form should be saved for your tax records. Any additional information or questions should be directed to the customer service office.

TOTAL EXPENSES SUBMITTED ON THIS CLAIM $4323.15
OUR PAYMENT ON YOUR CLAIM $3454.76

Description of Service	Date of Service	Expenses Submitted	Expenses Excluded	Reason (see below)	Covered Balance	%	Payment Amount
ROOM AND BOARD	08/01/CCYY	$1598.00			$1598.00	80	$1278.40
HOSPITAL EXTRAS	08/01/CCYY	$2725.15	$4.70	A	$2720.45	80	$2176.36
		$4323.15	$4.70		$4318.45		$3454.76
Ibarra General Hospital							

A – CONVENIENCE ITEMS ARE NOT COVERED BY YOUR PLAN.

Encounter Form

Provider Information						Appointment Information			
Name:	Isaac Isenberg, M.D.					Appointment Date:		Time:	
Address:	2121 Independence Street					Next Appt. Date:		Time:	
City:	Ibarra	State:	IL	Zip Code:	61552	Date of First Visit:	07/01/CCYY	Date of Injury:	
Telephone #:		Fax #:				Referring Physician:			
Medicare ID#:		UPIN #:	C56565			**Guarantor Information**			
Tax ID #:	00-4859494	Accepts Medicare Assignment:	☐			Name:	Ingrid Innman		
Provider's Signature:	*Isaac Isenberg, MD* Date: 8/1/CCYY					Address:	2100 Ink Street		

Patient Information						Guarantor Information (cont.)			
						City:	Ibarra	State: IL	Zip Code: 61515
Name:	Ingrid Innman					Insurance ID #:	44-5556 BER/ 44-5555 XYZ		
Address:	2100 Ink Street					Insurance Name:	Berkeley Ins. Group/ Ball Ins. Carriers		
City:	Ibarra	State:	IL	Zip Code:	61515	Insurance Group #:	73429/ 62958		
Telephone #:	(708) 555-6151	Account #:	10088			Employer Name:	Berkeley Institute/ XYZ Corporation		
Date of Birth:	06/01/CCYY-47	Gender:	Female			**Authorization**			
Marital Status:	Married	Relationship to Guarantor:	Self			☒ Authorization to Release Information			
Student Status:	☐ Full-time	☐ Part-time				☒ Authorization for Assignment of Benefits			
Insurance Type:	☒ Pvt ☐ M/care ☐ M/caid ☐ WC ☒ Other ___ COB					☐ Authorization for Consent for Treatment			
						☐ My insurance will be billed but there may be a balance due.			
Hospitalization Date:	From: 07/29/CCYY To: 08/02/CCYY					Signature: *Ingrid Innman* Date: 8/1/CCYY			
Hospital Information:	Ibarra General Hospital, P.O. Box 84759K, Ibarra, IL 61523								

Clinical Information					
	DOS	POS	CPT® /HCPCS Description	ICD-9-CM (*Indicates diagnosis for all lines)	Amount
1	07/30/CCYY	Inpt Hosp	Sub hosp care, expand prob focused exam, mod comp	*Epilepsy	$ 55.00
2	08/01/CCYY	Inpt Hosp	Sub hosp care, expand prob focused exam, mod comp	*	$ 55.00
3					
4					
5					
6					
Remarks:					
Previous Balance:	$4323.15	Payment:		Copay:		Adjustment:		
Total Fee:	$110.00	Cash ☐ Check ☐ Credit ☐	Cash ☐ Check ☐ Credit ☐	Remarks:	New Balance: $4433.15

Berkeley Insurance Group 4769 Baker Blvd. Berkeley, CA 94721

Ingrid Innman
2100 Ink Street
Ibarra, IL 61515

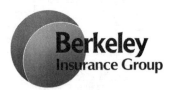

Date through which claims for these benefits were processed:	
August 30, CCYY	
Insurance ID #:	**44 5556 BER**
Insurance Group #:	**73429**
Claim #:	**Document 167**

THIS IS NOT A BILL
Please retain this Benefit Statement for your records.

Explanation of Medical Benefits   **Retain This Benefits Statement For Your Records.**

This statement reflects benefits for: Ingrid Innman

Your provider has also been sent an explanation of benefits statement relating to this claim

Dear Ingrid Innman,

We received a medical claim for you.

The information on this form presents an explanation of benefits due under your plan. This form should be saved for your tax records. Any additional information or questions should be directed to the customer service office.

TOTAL EXPENSES SUBMITTED ON THIS CLAIM $110.00
OUR PAYMENT ON YOUR CLAIM $88.00

Description of Service	Date of Service	Expenses Submitted	Expenses Excluded	Reason (see below)	Covered Balance	%	Payment Amount
7/30 HOSP VISIT	07/30/CCYY	$55.00			$55.00	80	$44.00
8/01 HOSP VISIT	08/01/CCYY	$55.00			$55.00	80	$44.00
		$110.00			$110.00		$88.00
Isaac Isenberg, M.D.							

Patient Claim Form

Information must be printed or typewritten. Claim form must be completed and returned to us at the indicated address.

Medicare Patients: Submit this claim to Medicare FIRST! A copy of the Medicare Summary Notice or Medicare Remittance Advice must be submitted with this claim form.

TO BE COMPLETED BY MEMBER

1. Information Pertaining To Member

Name: Last, First, M.I. Innman, Ike		Sex: M	Date Of Birth 03/07/CCYY-46	Member ID# 44-5555 XYZ

Home Address: Street 2100 Ink Street.	City Ibarra	State IL	Zip 61515	Telephone Number (708) 555-6151

Marital Status Married	Name Of Spouse Ingrid Innman		Spouse's Date Of Birth 06/01/CCYY-47	Member ID# 44-5556 BER

Is Spouse Employed? Yes	If Yes, Name And Address Of Employer Berkeley Institute 6923 Berdan Blvd. Berkeley, CA 94721	Employer Phone Number (708) 555-6155

2. Information Pertaining To Patient

Patient Name: Last, First, M.I. Innman, Ingrid		Sex F	Date Of Birth 06/01/CCYY-47	Member ID# 44-5555 XYZ

Home Address: Street 4949 Backwoods Blvd.	City Baton Rouge	State LA	Zip 70810	Telephone Number (708) 555-6151

Is Patient Employed? (Full-Time) Part Time No	Relationship To Employee? Spouse	If Dependent Child Over 19, Name Of School Where Full-time Student:

3. Information Regarding Current Treatment

Related To Illness? Yes	Related To Pregnancy? No	Related To Work? No	Description Of Illness Or Injury Epilepsy

Date Of Accident N/A	Where Happened? N/A	Describe Accident

4. Information Regarding Insurance

Are You, Your Spouse, or Dependent Children Covered By Any Other Insurance? Yes	Name Of Insured Ingrid Innman	

If Yes, Name And Address Of Insurance Berkeley Insurance Group 4769 Baker Blvd. Berkeley, CA 94721		Insurance Phone Number

Patient's Or Guardian's Signature

I certify that the above information is true and correct and I authorize the release of any medical information necessary to process this claim.

Signed: *Ingrid Innman*   Date: *08/31/CCYY*

Assignment of Benefits:

I assign payment of benefits to the following provider:

Address: Street	City	State Zip	Telephone Number

Health Claims Examining Program ONLY

TO BE COMPLETED BY PHYSICIAN

Patient's Name: Last, First, M.I.

Innman, Ingrid

Home Address: Street	City	State	Zip	Telephone Number
2100 Ink Street.	Ibarra	IL	61515	(708) 555-6151

Is Condition Due To Illness?	Injury?	Work Related?	Pregnancy?	If Yes, Date Of Last Menstrual Period
Yes	No	No	No	

Diagnosis Or Nature Of Illness Or Injuries. Give Description And ICD-9-CM Code.

_____ Epilepsy _____

_____

Date Of Service	Place Of Service	Description Of Medical Services Or Supplies Provided	CPT® Code	ICD-9 Code	Charge
08/31/CCYY	Pharmacy	Valium 50 mg	RX		92.60
08/31/CCYY	Pharmacy	Dilantin 20 mg	RX		74.52

Date Of First Symptoms	Date Of Accident	Date Patient First Seen		Total Charges	$167.12
Dates Patient Unable To Work From: To:		If Still Disabled, Date Patient Should Return To Work		Amount Paid	$167.12
Patient Still Under Care For This Condition?		Date Of Same Or Similar Illness Or Condition		Does Patient Have Other Health Coverage?	

Under Section 6019 Of The Internal Revenue Code, Recipients Of Medical Payments Must Provide Identifying Numbers To Payors Who Must Report Such Payments To The Internal Revenue Service. Taxpayer ID Number: _____ Social Security Number: _____

Physician's Name: _____ Signature: _____

_____

Street Address	City	State	Zip

INFORMATION REGARDING THIS CLAIM FORM

A Separate Claim Must Be Filed For Each Different Injury Or Illness.

A Claim Must Be Filed Within 90 Days of The Date Of Service Or Claim Benefits May Be Reduced.

If Patient Is Medicare Eligible, Claim Must First Be Submitted To Medicare For Payment. We Cannot Process Claim Without Information Regarding Medicare's Payment.

SafeAid thanks you!
SafeAid Pharmacy

Ingrid Innman
Reg 38   08/31/CCYY
Isenberg, MD   100
RX # 45721
Valium 50 mg   85.20

Subtotal   85.20
Tax   7.40
Total   92.60
Amount Tndd   95.00
Change   2.40

Refills–Call

SafeAid thanks you!
SafeAid Pharmacy

Ingrid Innman
Reg 38   08/31/CCYY
Isenberg, MD
RX # 44762
Dilantin 20 mg   70.31
Subtotal   70.31
Tax   4.21
Total   74.52

Amount Tndd   75.00
Change   .48

Refills–Call

Berkeley Insurance Group 4769 Baker Blvd. Berkeley, CA 94721

Ingrid Innman
2100 Ink Street
Ibarra, IL 61515

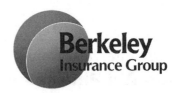

Date through which claims for these benefits were processed:
August 30, CCYY

Insurance ID #:	**44 5556 BER**
Insurance Group #:	**73429**
Claim #:	**D o c u m e n t 168**

THIS IS NOT A BILL
Please retain this Benefit Statement for your records.

Explanation of Medical Benefits   Retain This Benefits Statement For Your Records.

This statement reflects benefits for: Ingrid Innman

Your provider has also been sent an explanation of benefits statement relating to this claim

Dear Ingrid Innman,

We received a medical claim for you.

The information on this form presents an explanation of benefits due under your plan. This form should be saved for your tax records. Any additional information or questions should be directed to the customer service office.

TOTAL EXPENSES SUBMITTED ON THIS CLAIM $167.12
OUR PAYMENT ON YOUR CLAIM $133.69

Description of Service	Date of Service	Expenses Submitted	Expenses Excluded	Reason (see below)	Covered Balance	%	Payment Amount
PRESCRIPTIONS	08/31/CCYY	$167.12			$167.12	80	$133.69

Encounter Form

DOCUMENT 169

Provider Information

Name:	Ibrahim Innes, M.D.
Address:	427 East Imperial Drive

City:	Ibarra	State:	IL	Zip Code:	61589

Telephone #:		Fax #:	

Medicare ID#:		UPIN #:	E20036

Tax ID #:	00-4843158	Accepts Medicare Assignment:	☐

Provider's Signature:	Ibrahim Innes, MD	Date: 12/13/CCYY

Appointment Information

Appointment Date:		Time:	
Next Appt. Date:		Time:	
Date of First Visit:	12/01/CCYY	Date of Injury:	
Referring Physician:	Benita Bernstein, M.D.		

Guarantor Information

Name:	Ike Innman
Address:	2100 Ink Street

City:	Ibarra	State:	IL	Zip Code:	61515

Insurance ID #:	44-5555 XYZ/ 44-5556 BER
Insurance Name:	Ball Ins. Carriers/ Berkeley Ins. Group
Insurance Group #:	62958/ 73429
Employer Name:	XYZ Corporation/ Berkeley Institute

Patient Information

Name:	Ian Innman
Address:	2100 Ink Street

City:	Ibarra	State:	IL	Zip Code:	61515

Telephone #:	(708) 555-6151	Account #:	10089

Date of Birth:	10/25/CCYY-17	Gender:	Male

Marital Status:	Single	Relationship to Guarantor:	Child

Student Status:	☒ Full-time	☐ Part-time

Insurance Type:	☒ Pvt ☐ M/care ☐ M/caid ☐ WC ☒ Other ___ COB ___

Hospitalization Date:	From: 12/11/CCYY To: 12/14/CCYY

Hospital Information:	Ibarra General Hospital, P.O. Box 84759K, Ibarra, IL 61523

Authorization

☒ Authorization to Release Information
☒ Authorization for Assignment of Benefits
☐ Authorization for Consent for Treatment
☐ My insurance will be billed but there may be a balance due.

Signature: Ike Innman   Date: 12/13/CCYY

Clinical Information

	DOS	POS	CPT® /HCPCS Description	ICD-9-CM (*Indicates diagnosis for all lines)	Amount
1	12/11/CCYY	Inpt Hosp	Initial consult, prob foc hist & exam, straightforward	*Hypvolemia; *1 Hypertrophy of tonsils	$120.00
2	12/12/CCYY	Inpt Hosp	Sub hosp care, expand prob foc exam, moderate comp	*, *1	$ 75.00
3	12/13/CCYY	Inpt Hosp	Sub hosp care, expand prob foc exam, moderate comp	*, *1	$ 75.00
4					
5					
6					

Remarks:	Referring Physician: Benita Bernstein, M.D. UPIN #: F20884			

Previous Balance:		Payment:		Copay:		Adjustment:			
Total Fee:	$270.00	Cash ☐ Check ☐ Credit ☐		Cash ☐ Check ☐ Credit ☐		Remarks:		New Balance:	$270.00

Berkeley Insurance Group 4769 Baker Blvd. Berkeley, CA 94721

Ingrid Innman
2100 Ink Street
Ibarra, IL 61515

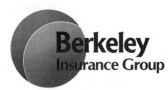

Date through which claims for these benefits were processed:	
December 30, CCYY	
Insurance ID #:	**44 5556 BER**
Insurance Group #:	73429
Claim #:	**Document 169**

THIS IS NOT A BILL
Please retain this Benefit Statement for your records.

Explanation of Medical Benefits

This statement reflects benefits for: Ian Innman

Retain This Benefits Statement For Your Records.

Your provider has also been sent an explanation of benefits statement relating to this claim

Dear Ingrid Innman,

We received a medical claim for you.

The information on this form presents an explanation of benefits due under your plan. This form should be saved for your tax records. Any additional information or questions should be directed to the customer service office.

TOTAL EXPENSES SUBMITTED ON THIS CLAIM $270.00
OUR PAYMENT ON YOUR CLAIM $216.00

Description of Service	Date of Service	Expenses Submitted	Expenses Excluded	Reason (see below)	Covered Balance	%	Payment Amount
HOSPITAL CONSULT	12/11/CCYY	$120.00			$120.00	80	$96.00
HOSPITAL VISIT	12/12/CCYY	$75.00			$75.00	80	$60.00
HOSPITAL VISIT	12/13/CCYY	$75.00			$75.00	80	$60.00
		$270.00			$270.00		$216.00
Ibrahim Innes, M.D.							

Hospital Admission Form

DOCUMENT *170*

Provider Information

Name:	Ibarra Main Hospital				
Address:	7492 Istanser Lane				
City:	Ibarra	State:	IL	Zip Code:	61529
Telephone#:		Fax#:			
Medicare ID#:	140031	UPIN#:			
Tax ID #:	00-8593487	Accepts Medicare Assignment:	☐		
Provider Rep:	*Betty Biller*		Date:	*12/14/CCYY*	

Admission Information

Admission Date:	12/11/CCYY	Time:	12:00 Noon
Discharge Date:	12/14/CCYY	Time:	12:00 Noon
Attending Phy's ID#:	D45455	Date of Injury:	
Attending Physician:	Isabel Ischer, M.D.		

Guarantor Information

Name:	Ike Innman				
Address:	2100 Ink Street				
City:	Ibarra	State:	IL	Zip Code:	61515
Insurance ID #:	44-5555 XYZ	SSN:	333-44-5555		
Insurance Name:	Ball Ins. Carriers/ Berkeley Ins. Group				
Insurance Group #:	62958/ 73429				
Employer Name:	XYZ Corporation/ Berkeley Institute				

Patient Information

Name:	Ian Innman				
Address:	2100 Ink Street				
City:	Ibarra	State:	IL	Zip Code:	61515
Telephone#:	(708) 555-6151	Patient Control #:	10089		
Date of Birth:	10/25/CCYY-17	Gender:	Male		
Marital Status:	Single	Relationship to Guarantor:		Child	
Student Status:	☒ Full-time	☐ Part-time			
Insurance Type:	☒ Pvt ☐ M/care ☐ M/caid ☐ WC ☒ Other ___ COB				

Authorization

☒ Authorization to Release Information
☒ Authorization for Assignment of Benefits
☐ Authorization for Consent for Treatment
☐ My insurance will be billed but there may be a balance due.

Signature: *Ike Innman*   Date: *12/11/CCYY*

Clinical Information

Principal Diagnosis:	Hypovolemia
Other Diagnosis:	Hypertrophy tonsils
Surgical Procedure:	
Other Procedures:	
Remarks:	

Previous Balance:	$270.00	Payment:		Copay:		Adjustment:
Total Fee:	$3192.00	Cash ☐ Check ☐ Credit ☐	Cash ☐ Check ☐ Credit ☐	Remarks:	New Balance:	$3462.00

Ibarra Main Hospital
7492 Istanser Lane
Ibarra, IL 61529

Patient Name	Patient No.	Sex	Date of Birth	Admission Date	Discharge Date	Page No.
IAN INNMAN	10089	M	10/25/CCYY-21	12/11/CCYY	12/14/CCYY	1

Guarantor Name and Address
IKE INNMAN
2100 INK STREET
IBARRA, IL 61515

Insurance Company: BALL INS CRS/ BERKELEY INS GRP
Claim Number: DOCUMENT 170
Attending Physician: ISABEL ISCHER, M.D.

Date of Service	Description of Hospital Services	Service Code	Qty.	Charges	Total Charges
	SUMMARY OF CHARGES				
	PEDS/WARD		3	$1356.00	
	PHARMACY		47	$1045.60	
	MED-SURG SUPPLIES & DEVCS		14	$207.20	
	LABORATORY		15	$583.20	
	SUBTOTAL OF CHARGES				$3192.00
	PAYMENTS AND ADJUSTMENTS			NONE	
	SUBTOTAL PAYMENTS/ADJ				NONE
	BALANCE DUE				$3192.00

Berkeley Insurance Group 4769 Baker Blvd. Berkeley, CA 94721

Ingrid Innman
2100 Ink Street
Ibarra, IL 61515

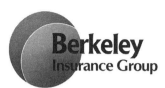

Date through which claims for these benefits were processed:	
December 31, CCYY	
Insurance ID #:	**44 5556 BER**
Insurance Group #:	**73429**
Claim #:	**Document 170**

THIS IS NOT A BILL
Please retain this Benefit Statement for your records.

Explanation of Medical Benefits	Retain This Benefits Statement For Your Records.
This statement reflects benefits for: Ian Innman	
Your provider has also been sent an explanation of benefits statement relating to this claim	

Dear Ingrid Innman,

We received a medical claim for you.

The information on this form presents an explanation of benefits due under your plan. This form should be saved for your tax records. Any additional information or questions should be directed to the customer service office.

TOTAL EXPENSES SUBMITTED ON THIS CLAIM $3192.00
OUR PAYMENT ON YOUR CLAIM $2553.60

Description of Service	Date of Service	Expenses Submitted	Expenses Excluded	Reason (see below)	Covered Balance	%	Payment Amount
ROOM AND BOARD	12/14/CCYY	$1356.00			$1356.00	80	$1084.80
HOSPITAL EXTRAS	12/14/CCYY	$1836.00			$1836.00	80	$1468.80
		$3192.00			$3192.00		$2553.60
Ibarra Main Hospital							

Health Claims Examining Exercises

(**Instructor's Note:** Medical Billing exercises in the entire text should be completed prior to students starting Health Claims Examining Exercise 9–A. New files should be set up for the Health Claims Examining exercises.)

Exercise **9–A**

Directions: Complete an Insurance Coverage Form (located in the **Forms** chapter) and set up Family Files for all families in this chapter. Refer to the Family Data Tables **(Documents 148–150)** located in the beginning of this chapter, and the Contracts located in the **Contracts, UCR Conversion Factor Report, and Relative Value Study** chapter.

Exercise **9–B**

Directions: Complete a Payment Worksheet (located in the **Forms** chapter) for CMS-1500s **(Documents 152–154, 156, 158, 160–161, 163, 167, and 169)** and UB-92s **(Documents 157, 162, 164, 166, and 170)** claims, and Patient Claim Forms **(Documents 155 and 168)**. Use the guidelines contained in the **Introduction** chapter and the UCR Conversion Factor Report, Relative Value Study, and Contracts located in the **Contracts, UCR Conversion Factor Report, and Relative Value Study** chapter. Also, complete a Coordination of Benefits Calculation Worksheet (located in the **Forms** chapter) for applicable claims. The applicable Explanation of Benefits should be referred to for claims payments and coordination of benefits information.

When processing claims, the Beginning Financials **(Documents 151, 159, and 165)** should be incorporated as payment history and claim calculations should be adjusted accordingly. Any carryover deductible listed should be included in the current year deductible for that individual. Therefore, in figuring current year deductible, students should be instructed to subtract the carryover deductible from the current year's amount.

Upon completion of each claim complete or update the Family Benefits Tracking Sheet (located in the **Forms** chapter) by compiling all of the claims payment data for the family.

10
Medicare
and Medicaid Services

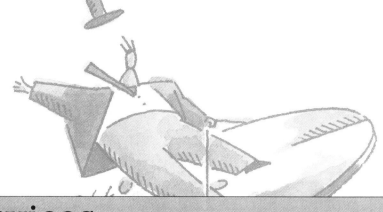

Medical Billing Exercises

Exercise 10-1

Directions: Complete Patient Information Sheets (leave **Assigned Provider** field blank), Ledger Cards, and Insurance Coverage Forms and set up patient charts for the following families using copies of the forms in the **Forms** chapter. Refer to the following Family Data Tables **(Documents 171–173)** for information.

Individual folders with dividers may be used to store information for each family. One Patient Information Sheet and Insurance Coverage Form should be filled out for the entire family.

FAMILY DATA TABLE

VAUGHN FAMILY	INSURED'S INFORMATION	SPOUSE'S INFORMATION	CHILD #1	CHILD #2	CHILD #3
Name	Vernon Vaughn	Vicki Vaughn			
Address	1234 Victory Blvd. Valley Vista, VT 05777	1234 Victory Blvd. Valley Vista, VT 05777			
Email Address	vernonv@vaughn.com				
TELEPHONE #					
Home: Work: Cell:	(802) 555-0577 (802) 555-0578 (802) 555-0579	(802) 555-0577			
Date of Birth	11/09/CCYY-71	10/08/CCYY-70			
Social Security #	777-77-0000	777-77-0001			
Marital Status/Gender	Married/Male	Married/Female			
Student Status					
Patient Account #	10090	10091			
Allergies/Medical Conditions	None	None			
PRIMARY INSURANCE CARRIER					
Name	Medicare	Medicare			
Address	567 Medicare Lane Anytown, USA 12345	567 Medicare Lane Anytown, USA 12345			
Effective Date	11/01/Age 65	10/01/Age 65			
Member's ID #	777-77-0000A	777-77-0000B			
Group Policy #					
Policy/Employer					
OTHER INSURANCE CARRIER					
Name	Winter Insurance Company	Winter Insurance Company			
Address	9763 Western Way Whittier, CO 82963	9763 Western Way Whittier, CO 82963			
Effective Date	01/01/CCPY	01/01/CCPY			
Member's ID #	77-0000 ABC	77-0000 ABC			
Group Policy #	36928	36928			
Employer/Retiree	ABC Corporation 1234 Whitaker Lane Colter, CO 81222				
Responsible Party	Self	Self			
EMERGENCY CONTACT					
Name	Victor Valone	Victor Valone			
Telephone #	(802) 555-0570	(802) 555-0570			
Address	4321 Victory Blvd. Valley Vista, VT 05777	4321 Victory Blvd. Valley Vista, VT 05777			

FAMILY DATA TABLE

CONNERS FAMILY	INSURED'S INFORMATION	SPOUSE'S INFORMATION	CHILD #1	CHILD #2	CHILD #3
Name	Chris Conners	Clara Conners			
Address	9009 Camelia Court Collins, CO 81221	9009 Camelia Court Collins, CO 81221			
Email Address	chrisc@conners.com				
TELEPHONE #					
Home:	(970) 555-8122	(970) 555-8122			
Work:	(970) 555-8123				
Cell:	(970) 555-8124				
Date of Birth	06/24/CCYY-78	11/13/CCYY-76			
Social Security #	444-55-4444	444-55-4445			
Marital Status/Gender	Married/Male	Married/Female			
Student Status					
Patient Account #	10092	10093			
Allergies/Medical Conditions	None	None			
PRIMARY INSURANCE CARRIER					
Name	Medicare	Medicare			
Address	567 Medicare Lane Anytown, USA 12345	567 Medicare Lane Anytown, USA 12345			
Effective Date	06/01/Age 65	11/01/Age 65			
Member's ID #	444-55-4444A	444-55-4444B			
Group Policy #					
Policy/Employer					
OTHER INSURANCE CARRIER					
Name	Ball Insurance Carriers	Ball Insurance Carriers			
Address	3895 Bubble Blvd. Ste. 283 Boxwood, CO 85926	3895 Bubble Blvd. Ste. 283 Boxwood, CO 85926			
Effective Date	01/01/CCPY	01/01/CCPY			
Member's ID #	55-4444 XYZ	55-4444 XYZ			
Group Policy #	62958	62958			
Employer/Retiree	XYZ Corporation 9817 Bobcat Blvd. Bastion, CO 81319				
Responsible Party	Self	Self			
EMERGENCY CONTACT					
Name	Ciara Conway	Ciara Conway			
Telephone #	(970) 555-8125	(907) 555-8125			
Address	5005 Camelia Court Collins, CO 81221	5005 Camelia Court Collins, CO 81221			

FAMILY DATA TABLE

HANAKA FAMILY	INSURED'S INFORMATION	SPOUSE'S INFORMATION	CHILD #1	CHILD #2	CHILD #3
Name	Hiro Hanaka	Holly Hanaka			
Address	293 Hornea Street Hilo, HI 96823	293 Hornea Street Hilo, HI 96823			
Email Address	hirih@hanaka.com				
TELEPHONE #					
Home:	(808) 555-9682	(808) 555-9682			
Work:	(808) 555-9683				
Cell:	(808) 555-9684				
Date of Birth	01/15/CCYY-75	12/18/CCYY-73			
Social Security #	666-77-8901	666-77-8902			
Marital Status/Gender	Married/Male	Married/Female			
Student Status					
Patient Account #	10094	10095			
Allergies/Medical Conditions	None	None			
PRIMARY INSURANCE CARRIER					
Name	Medicare	Medicare			
Address	567 Medicare Lane Anytown, USA 12345	567 Medicare Lane Anytown, USA 12345			
Effective Date	01/01/Age 65	12/01/Age 65			
Member's ID #	666-77-8901A	666-77-8901B			
Group Policy #					
Policy/Employer					
OTHER INSURANCE CARRIER					
Name	Rover Insurers, Inc.	Rover Insurers, Inc.			
Address	5931 Rolling Road Ronson, CO 81369	5931 Rolling Road Ronson, CO 81369			
Effective Date	01/01/CCPY	01/01/CCPY			
Member's ID #	77-8901 NIN	77-8901 NIN			
Group Policy #	21088	21088			
Employer/Retiree	Ninja Enterprises 1234 Nockout Road Newton, NM 88012				
Responsible Party	Self	Self			
EMERGENCY CONTACT					
Name	Hubert Halawaki	Hubert Halawaki			
Telephone #	(808) 555-9685	(808) 555-9685			
Address	392 Hornea Street Hilo, HI 96823	392 Hornea Street Hilo, HI 96823			

Exercise **10-2**

Directions: Complete a CMS-1500 for each of the Encounter Forms (**Documents 175–179, 181–183, 187–189, and 191**) and a UB-92 for each of the Hospital Admission Forms (**Documents 184–185 and 190**) in this chapter. These forms may be provided by your instructor or purchased from a stationery store.

After completion of CMS-1500 and UB-92 forms, complete a Patient Receipt (if a payment was made), and post the transaction(s) to the patient Ledger Card/Statement of Account previously created.

Enter either **Inpt Hospital Svcs** or **Otpt Hospital Svcs** in the **Description of Service** column on the Ledger Card/Statement of Account for hospital claims.

Exercise **10-3**

Directions: Upon completion of all of the activities in Exercise 10–2 complete a Bank Deposit Slip/Ticket (located in the **Forms** chapter) for all payments made on the patient's account in this chapter.

Exercise **10-4**

Directions: Using an Insurance Claims Register (located in the **Forms** chapter) list all claims that have been fully prepared and are ready for submission to the insurance carrier for payment. Enter the date that you created the CMS-1500 or UB-92 in the **Date Claim Filed** column.

Exercise **10-5**

Directions: Complete a Charge Slip and Treatment Authorization Request for the following scenario.

1. Verbal Control—8769
2. Type of Service Requested—Other
3. Is Request Retroactive?—Yes
4. Is Patient Medicare Eligible?—No
5. Provider Phone Number—(678) 555-1717
6. Patient's Authorized Representative (If Any) Enter Name and Address—Kiley King, 236 Kane Court, Klamath, KS 71717
7. Provider Name and Address—Kevin Key M.D., 298 Kasey Street, Klamath, KS 71717
8. Provider Number—KA5926K
9. For State Use—Leave Blank
10. Name and Address of Patient—Keisha King, 236 Kane Court, Klamath, KS 71717
11. Medicaid Identification Number—5729123
12. Sex—Female
13. Age—2
14. Date of Birth—08/07/CCYY-2
15. Patient Status—Acute
16. Patient's Phone Number—(678) 555-0912

17. Diagnosis Description—Urinary Tract Infection

18. ICD-9-CM Diagnosis Code—599.0

19. Medical Justification—Martin Luther King Medical Center, 9789 Kayla Avenue, Klamath, KS 71717

20. Authorized—Leave Blank

21. Approved Units—Leave Blank

22. Specific Services Requested—Straightforward Detailed Exam Inpatient Hospital

23. Units of Service—1

24. NDC/UPC or Procedure—99221

25. Quantity—1

26. Charges—$175.00

27. Authorization is Valid for Services Provided—Leave Blank

28. Account/ID Number—S29467

29. Provider Tax Identification Number—99-9901921

30. Date of Service—09/14/CCYY

31. No Prior Balance

32. Payment Made—$0

33. Signature of Physician or Provider—Student should sign and date the form and indicate their title as medical biller.

Exercise 10-6

Directions: Complete a Charge Slip and Treatment Authorization Request for the following scenario.

1. Verbal Control—1562

2. Type of Service Requested—Other

3. Is Request Retroactive?—Yes

4. Is Patient Medicare Eligible?—No

5. Provider Phone Number—(555) 456-7890

6. Patient's Authorized Representative (If Any) Enter Name and Address—N/A

7. Provider Name and Address—Sal Shakum MD, 123 N. Shell Street, Salem, SC 01010

8. Provider Number—S96170S

9. For State Use—Leave Blank

10. Name and Address of Patient—Shida Sears, 456 N. Sacred Street, Salem, SC 01010

11. Medicaid Identification Number—467321

12. Sex—Female

13. Age—32

14. Date of Birth—10/10/CCYY-32

15. Patient Status—SNF/ICF

16. Patient's Phone Number—(555) 456-1212

17. Diagnosis Description—Epilepsy

18. ICD-9-CM Diagnosis Code—345

19. Medical Justification—Shadow Stevens Rest Home, 789 Shelly Street, Salem, SC 01010

20. Authorized—Leave Blank

21. Approved Units—Leave Blank

22. Specific Services Requested—Straightforward Detailed History & Exam Nursing Home

23. Units of Service—1

24. NDC/UPC or Procedure—99301

25. Quantity—1

26. Charges—$150.00

27. Authorization is Valid for Services Provided—Leave Blank

28. Account/ID Number—182749

29. Provider Tax Identification Number—27-4936021

30. Date of Service—05/07/CCYY

31. No Prior Balance

32. Payment Made—$150.00

33. Signature of Physician or Provider—Student should sign and date the form and indicate their title as medical biller.

Exercise **10-7**

Directions: Complete an Insurance Tracer Form (located in the **Forms** chapter) for the following claim. For additional information refer to the Family Data Table (**Document 64**), completed claim form or the Encounter Form.

Patient	Date Billed	Date of Service	Date of Illness	Diagnoses	Claim #
Tony Thompson	08/31/CCYY	08/22/CCYY	08/22/CCYY	726.73, 728.71	Document 70

Medicare and Medicaid Claims Beginning Financials
VAUGHN FAMILY

Insurance Plan	Winter Insurance Company—ABC Corporation			
Patient:	**VERNON**	**VICKI**		
C/O DEDUCTIBLE	0.00	0.00		
DEDUCTIBLE	0.00	27.50		
COINSURANCE	0.00	0.00		
ACCIDENT BENEFIT	0.00	0.00		
LIFETIME MAXIMUM	142,327.00	257,600.00		
M/N OFFICE VISITS				
OFFICE VISITS				
HOSPITAL VISITS				
DXL				
SURGERY				
ASSISTANT SURGERY				
ANESTHESIA				

Encounter Form

Provider Information

Name:	Vera Vega, M.D.				
Address:	333 Verdugo Blvd.				
City:	Valley Vista	State:	VT	Zip Code:	05778
Telephone #:		Fax #:			
Medicare ID#:		UPIN #:	F15982		
Tax ID #:	55-4052798	Accepts Medicare Assignment:	☒		
Provider's Signature:	*Vera Vega, MD*		Date: *6/26/CCYY*		

Appointment Information

Appointment Date:		Time:	
Next Appt. Date:		Time:	
Date of First Visit:	06/26/CCYY	Date of Injury:	
Referring Physician:			

Guarantor Information

Name:	Vernon Vaughn				
Address:	1234 Victory Blvd.				
City:	Valley Vista	State:	VT	Zip Code:	05777
Insurance ID #:	777-77-0000A/ 77-0000 ABC				
Insurance Name:	Medicare/ Winter Insurance Company				
Insurance Group #:	36928				
Employer Name:	ABC Corporation				

Patient Information

Name:	Vernon Vaughn				
Address:	1234 Victory Blvd.				
City:	Valley Vista	State:	VT	Zip Code:	05777
Telephone #:	(802) 555-0577	Account #:	10090		
Date of Birth:	11/09/CCYY-71	Gender:	Male		
Marital Status:	Married	Relationship to Guarantor:		Self	
Student Status:	☐ Full-time	☐ Part-time			
Insurance Type:	☒ Pvt ☒ M/care ☐ M/caid ☐ WC ☐ Other		COB		
Hospitalization Date:					
Hospital Information:					

Authorization

☒ Authorization to Release Information
☒ Authorization for Assignment of Benefits
☐ Authorization for Consent for Treatment
☐ My insurance will be billed but there may be a balance due.

Signature: *Vernon Vaughn*   Date: *6/26/CCYY*

Clinical Information

	DOS	POS	CPT® /HCPCS Description	ICD-9-CM (*Indicates diagnosis for all lines)	Amount
1	06/26/CCYY	Office	Dilation of urethral structure by passage of filiform; initial	*Cancer of Prostate	$100.00
2	06/26/CCYY	Office	Injection of lidocaine, intramuscular	*	$ 35.00
3	06/26/CCYY	Office	Urinalysis; non-automated, w/ microscopy	*	$ 20.00
4	06/26/CCYY	Office	Injection, tobramycin sulfate, up to 80 mg	*	$ 25.00
5	06/26/CCYY	Office	Smear; with interp Giesma stain for bacteria	*	$ 20.00
6	06/26/CCYY	Office	Surgical tray	*	$ 35.00

Remarks:							
Previous Balance:		Payment:		Copay:		Adjustment:	
Total Fee:	$235.00	Cash ☐ Check ☐ Credit ☐		Cash ☐ Check ☐ Credit ☐		Remarks:	New Balance: $235.00

Encounter Form

Provider Information

Name:	Vera Vega, M.D.				
Address:	333 Verdugo Blvd.				
City:	Valley Vista	State:	VT	Zip Code:	05778
Telephone #:		Fax #:			
Medicare ID#:		UPIN #:	F15982		
Tax ID #:	55-4052798	Accepts Medicare Assignment:	☒		
Provider's Signature:	Vera Vega, MD		Date: 7/10/CCYY		

Appointment Information

Appointment Date:		Time:	
Next Appt. Date:		Time:	
Date of First Visit:	07/10/CCYY	Date of Injury:	
Referring Physician:			

Guarantor Information

Name:	Vernon Vaughn				
Address:	1234 Victory Blvd.				
City:	Valley Vista	State:	VT	Zip Code:	05777
Insurance ID #:	777-77-0000A/ 77-0000 ABC				
Insurance Name:	Medicare/ Winter Insurance Company				
Insurance Group #:	36928				
Employer Name:	ABC Corporation				

Patient Information

Name:	Vernon Vaughn				
Address:	1234. Victory Blvd.				
City:	Valley Vista	State:	VT	Zip Code:	05777
Telephone #:	(802) 555-0577	Account #:	10090		
Date of Birth:	11/09/CCYY-71	Gender:	Male		
Marital Status:	Married	Relationship to Guarantor:		Self	
Student Status:	☐ Full-time	☐ Part-time			
Insurance Type:	☒ Pvt ☒ M/care ☐ M/caid ☐ WC ☐ Other	COB			
Hospitalization Date:					
Hospital Information:					

Authorization

☒	Authorization to Release Information
☒	Authorization for Assignment of Benefits
☐	Authorization for Consent for Treatment
☐	My insurance will be billed but there may be a balance due.

Signature: Vernon Vaughn   Date: 7/10/CCYY

Clinical Information

	DOS	POS	CPT® /HCPCS Description	ICD-9-CM (*Indicates diagnosis for all lines)	Amount
1	07/10/CCYY	Office	Cystourethroscopy, w/calibration of urethral stricture	*Cancer of Prostate	$375.00
2	07/10/CCYY	Office	Urinalysis; non-automated, w/microscopy	*	$ 20.00
3	07/10/CCYY	Office	Injection, tobramycin sulfate, up to 80 mg	*	$ 25.00
4	07/10/CCYY	Office	Injection of lidocaine, intramuscular	*	$ 35.00
5	07/10/CCYY	Office	Smear; with interp Giemsa stain for bacteria	*	$ 20.00
6	07/10/CCYY	Office	Est pt, detailed exam, moderate complexity	*	$ 75.00
7	07/10/CCYY	Office	Surgical tray	*	$ 35.00
Remarks:					

Previous Balance:	$235.00	Payment:		Copay:		Adjustment:			
Total Fee:	$585.00	Cash ☐ Check ☐ Credit ☐		Cash ☐ Check ☐ Credit ☐		Remarks:		New Balance:	$820.00

Encounter Form

Provider Information

Name:	Vera Vega, M.D.				
Address:	333 Verdugo Blvd.				
City:	Valley Vista	State:	VT	Zip Code:	05778
Telephone #:		Fax #:			
Medicare ID#:		UPIN #:	F15982		
Tax ID #:	55-4052798	Accepts Medicare Assignment:	☒		
Provider's Signature:	Vera Vega, MD		Date: 7/29/CCYY		

Appointment Information

Appointment Date:		Time:	
Next Appt. Date:		Time:	
Date of First Visit:	06/26/CCYY	Date of Injury:	
Referring Physician:			

Guarantor Information

Name:	Vernon Vaughn				
Address:	1234 Victory Blvd.				
City:	Valley Vista	State:	VT	Zip Code:	05777
Insurance ID #:	777-77-0000A/ 77-0000 ABC				
Insurance Name:	Medicare/ Winter Insurance Company				
Insurance Group #:	36928				
Employer Name:	ABC Corporation				

Patient Information

Name:	Vernon Vaughn				
Address:	1234 Victory Blvd.				
City:	Valley Vista	State:	VT	Zip Code:	05777
Telephone #:	(802) 555-0577	Account #:	10090		
Date of Birth:	11/09/CCYY-71	Gender:	Male		
Marital Status:	Married	Relationship to Guarantor:		Self	
Student Status:	☐ Full-time	☐ Part-time			
Insurance Type:	☒ Pvt ☒ M/care ☐ M/caid ☐ WC ☐ Other	COB			
Hospitalization Date:					
Hospital Information:					

Authorization

☒	Authorization to Release Information
☒	Authorization for Assignment of Benefits
☐	Authorization for Consent for Treatment
☐	My insurance will be billed but there may be a balance due.

Signature: Vernon Vaughn   Date: 7/29/CCYY

Clinical Information

	DOS	POS	CPT® /HCPCS Description	ICD-9-CM (*Indicates diagnosis for all lines)	Amount
1	07/29/CCYY	Office	Injection of lidocaine, intramuscular	*Cancer of Prostate	$ 35.00
2	07/29/CCYY	Office	Dilation of urethral stricture by passage of sound; initial	*	$ 55.00
3	07/29/CCYY	Office	Surgical tray	*	$ 35.00
4					
5					
6					
Remarks:					

Previous Balance:	$820.00	Payment:		Copay:		Adjustment:			
Total Fee:	$125.00	Cash ☐ Check ☐ Credit ☐		Cash ☐ Check ☐ Credit ☐		Remarks:		New Balance:	$945.00

Encounter Form

Provider Information

Name:	Virginia Voss, M.D.
Address:	607 Venus Avenue
City:	Valley Vista State: VT Zip Code: 05779
Telephone #:	Fax #:
Medicare ID#:	UPIN #: I46220
Tax ID #:	55-0090088 Accepts Medicare Assignment: ☒
Provider's Signature:	*Virginia Voss, MD* Date: *6/10/CCYY*

Appointment Information

Appointment Date:	Time:
Next Appt. Date:	Time:
Date of First Visit:	06/01/CCYY Date of Injury:
Referring Physician:	

Guarantor Information

Name:	Vicki Vaughn
Address:	1234 Victory Blvd.
City:	Valley Vista State: VT Zip Code: 05777
Insurance ID #:	777-77-0000A/ 77-0000 ABC
Insurance Name:	Medicare/ Winter Insurance Company
Insurance Group #:	36928
Employer Name:	ABC Corporation

Patient Information

Name:	Vicki Vaughn
Address:	1234 Victory Blvd.
City:	Valley Vista State: VT Zip Code: 05777
Telephone #:	(802) 555-0577 Account #: 10091
Date of Birth:	10/08/CCYY-70 Gender: Female
Marital Status:	Married Relationship to Guarantor: Self
Student Status:	☐ Full-time ☐ Part-time
Insurance Type:	☒ Pvt ☒ M/care ☐ M/caid ☐ WC ☐ Other ___ COB ___
Hospitalization Date:	
Hospital Information:	

Authorization

☒ Authorization to Release Information
☒ Authorization for Assignment of Benefits
☐ Authorization for Consent for Treatment
☐ My insurance will be billed but there may be a balance due.

Signature: *Vernon Vaughn* Date: *6/10/CCYY*

Clinical Information

	DOS	POS	CPT® /HCPCS Description	ICD-9-CM (*Indicates diagnosis for all lines)	Amount
1	06/01/CCYY	Office	Est pt, detailed exam, moderate complexity	*Cellulitis; *1Thigh	$ 50.00
2	06/10/CCYY	Office	Est pt, expanded problem focused exam, low comp	*; *1	$ 50.00
3	06/10/CCYY	Office	Biopsy of skin, unless otherwise listed; single lesion	*; *1	$ 75.00
4	06/10/CCYY	Office	Level IV-surgical pathology, gross and micro, exam	*; *1	$ 45.00
5	06/10/CCYY	Office	Surgical tray	*; *1	$ 20.00
6					

Remarks:				
Previous Balance:	Payment:	Copay:	Adjustment:	
Total Fee: $240.00	Cash ☐ Check ☐ Credit ☐	Cash ☐ Check ☐ Credit ☐	Remarks:	New Balance: $240.00

Encounter Form

Provider Information

Name:	Valenzuela Vogue, M.D.
Address:	818 Ventura Street
City:	Valley Vista State: VT Zip Code: 05773
Telephone #:	Fax #:
Medicare ID#:	UPIN #: J78546
Tax ID #:	55-1098888 Accepts Medicare Assignment: ☒
Provider's Signature:	*Valenzuela Vogue, MD* Date: *8/14/CCYY*

Appointment Information

Appointment Date:	Time:
Next Appt. Date:	Time:
Date of First Visit:	08/13/CCYY Date of Injury:
Referring Physician:	

Guarantor Information

Name:	Vicki Vaughn
Address:	1234 Victory Blvd.
City:	Valley Vista State: VT Zip Code: 05777
Insurance ID #:	777-77-0000A/ 77-0000 ABC
Insurance Name:	Medicare/ Winter Insurance Company
Insurance Group #:	36928
Employer Name:	ABC Corporation

Patient Information

Name:	Vicki Vaughn
Address:	1234 Victory Blvd.
City:	Valley Vista State: VT Zip Code: 05777
Telephone #:	(802) 555-0577 Account #: 10091
Date of Birth:	10/08/CCYY-70 Gender: Female
Marital Status:	Married Relationship to Guarantor: Self
Student Status:	☐ Full-time ☐ Part-time
Insurance Type:	☒ Pvt ☒ M/care ☐ M/caid ☐ WC ☐ Other ___ COB ___
Hospitalization Date:	
Hospital Information:	

Authorization

☒ Authorization to Release Information
☒ Authorization for Assignment of Benefits
☐ Authorization for Consent for Treatment
☐ My insurance will be billed but there may be a balance due.

Signature: *Vicki Vaughn* Date: *8/14/CCYY*

Clinical Information

	DOS	POS	CPT® /HCPCS Description	ICD-9-CM (*Indicates diagnosis for all lines)	Amount
1	08/13/CCYY	Office	Visual field, extended examination, with interp & rpt	*Cataract Nuclear sclerosis; *1Drug Allergy	$175.00
2	08/14/CCYY	Office	Opth exam & eval w/ init of diag trmnt, comp	*; *1	$ 95.00
3					
4					
5					
6					

Remarks:				
Previous Balance: $240.00	Payment:	Copay:	Adjustment:	
Total Fee: $270.00	Cash ☐ Check ☐ Credit ☐	Cash ☐ Check ☐ Credit ☐	Remarks:	New Balance: $510.00

Medicare and Medicaid Claims Beginning Financials
CONNERS FAMILY

Insurance Plan	Ball Insurance Carriers—XYZ Corporation				
Patient:	**CHRIS**	**CLARA**			
C/O DEDUCTIBLE	0.00	0.00			
DEDUCTIBLE	27.27	76.52			
COINSURANCE	0.00	0.00			
ACCIDENT BENEFIT	0.00	0.00			
LIFETIME MAXIMUM	5,611.24	4,727.77			
M/N OFFICE VISITS					
OFFICE VISITS					
HOSPITAL VISITS					
DXL					
SURGERY					
ASSISTANT SURGERY					
ANESTHESIA					

Encounter Form

Provider Information

Name:	Cathy Collins, M.D.
Address:	611 Clinton Avenue
City:	Collins	State: CO	Zip Code: 81222
Telephone #:	Fax #:
Medicare ID#:	UPIN #: K45123
Tax ID #:	40-3896529	Accepts Medicare Assignment: ☒
Provider's Signature:	*Cathy Collins, MD* Date: *6/26/CCYY*

Appointment Information

Appointment Date:		Time:
Next Appt. Date:		Time:
Date of First Visit:	06/26/CCYY	Date of Injury:
Referring Physician:		

Guarantor Information

Name:	Chris Conners
Address:	9009 Camelia Court
City: Collins	State: CO	Zip Code: 81221

Patient Information

Name:	Chris Conners
Address:	9009 Camelia Court
City:	Collins	State: CO	Zip Code: 81221
Telephone #:	(970) 555-8122	Account #: 10092
Date of Birth:	06/24/CCYY-75	Gender: Male
Marital Status:	Married	Relationship to Guarantor: Self
Student Status:	☐ Full-time	☐ Part-time
Insurance Type:	☒ Pvt ☒ M/care ☐ M/caid ☐ WC ☐ Other ___ COB
Hospitalization Date:	
Hospital Information:	

Insurance ID #:	444-55-4444A/ 55-4444 XYZ
Insurance Name:	Medicare/ Ball Insurance Carriers
Insurance Group #:	62958
Employer Name:	XYZ Corporation

Authorization

☒ Authorization to Release Information
☒ Authorization for Assignment of Benefits
☐ Authorization for Consent for Treatment
☐ My insurance will be billed but there may be a balance due.
Signature: *Chris Conners*   Date: *6/26/CCYY*

Clinical Information

	DOS	POS	CPT® /HCPCS Description	ICD-9-CM (*Indicates diagnosis for all lines)	Amount
1	06/26/CCYY	Office	Est pt, detailed examination, moderate comp	Bilateral Below Knee Amputations	$ 50.00
2					
3					
4					
5					
6					
Remarks:					

Previous Balance:		Payment:		Copay:		Adjustment:		
Total Fee:	$50.00	Cash ☐ Check ☐ Credit ☐		Cash ☐ Check ☐ Credit ☐		Remarks:	New Balance:	$50.00

Encounter Form

Provider Information

Name:	Collins County Medical Group
Address:	499 Coffee Street
City:	Collins State: CO Zip Code: 81223
Telephone #:	Fax #:
Medicare ID#:	UPIN #: W00020
Tax ID #:	55-222-111 Accepts Medicare Assignment: ☒
Provider's Signature:	Cara Culver, MD Date: 9/5/CCYY

Patient Information

Name:	Clara Conners
Address:	9009 Camelia Court
City:	Collins State: CO Zip Code: 81221
Telephone #:	(970) 555-8122 Account #: 10093
Date of Birth:	11/13/CCYY-73 Gender: Female
Marital Status:	Married Relationship to Guarantor: Self
Student Status:	☐ Full-time ☐ Part-time
Insurance Type:	☒ Pvt ☒ M/care ☐ M/caid ☐ WC ☐ Other ___ COB
Hospitalization Date:	From: 09/04/CCYY To: 09/07/CCYY
Hospital Information:	Collins County Medical Center, P.O. Box 800, Collins, CO 81223

Appointment Information

Appointment Date:		Time:	
Next Appt. Date:		Time:	
Date of First Visit:	09/04/CCYY	Date of Injury:	
Referring Physician:			

Guarantor Information

Name:	Clara Conners
Address:	9009 Camelia Court
City: Collins	State: CO Zip Code: 81221
Insurance ID #:	444-55-4444B/ 55-4444 XYZ
Insurance Name:	Medicare/ Ball Insurance Carriers
Insurance Group #:	62958
Employer Name:	XYZ Corporation

Authorization

☒ Authorization to Release Information
☒ Authorization for Assignment of Benefits
☐ Authorization for Consent for Treatment
☐ My insurance will be billed but there may be a balance due.

Signature: Clara Conners   Date: 9/5/CCYY

Clinical Information

	DOS	POS	CPT® /HCPCS Description	ICD-9-CM (*Indicates diagnosis for all lines)		Amount
1	09/04/CCYY	Otpt Hosp	Init consult, comp hist & exam, high complexity	*Closed Fx Femoral Shaft;		$ 175.00
2	09/05/CCYY	Otpt Hosp	Radical resection of tumor femur	* 1Bone and Articular Cartilage		$2860.00
3	09/05/CCYY	Otpt Hosp	Open treatment of femoral shaft fracture, w/implant	*; *1		$3750.00
4	09/05/CCYY	Otpt Hosp	Radical resection of tumor femur	*; *1	(Assistant Surgeon)	$ 715.00
5	09/05/CCYY	Otpt Hosp	Open treatment of femoral shaft fracture, w/implant	*; *1	(Assistant Surgeon)	$ 937.50
6						

Remarks:	Surgical services performed by Cara Culver, M.D. UPIN #: H33372 and assistant surgeon Carl Coffin, M.D. UPIN #: I33382			
Previous Balance:		Payment:	Copay:	Adjustment:
Total Fee:	$8437.50	Cash ☐ Check ☐ Credit ☐	Cash ☐ Check ☐ Credit ☐	Remarks: New Balance: $8437.50

Encounter Form

Provider Information

Name:	Collins Surgical Supplies
Address:	818 Calvin Blvd.
City:	Collins State: CO Zip Code: 81224
Telephone #:	Fax #:
Medicare ID#:	UPIN #:
Tax ID #:	55-9993333 Accepts Medicare Assignment: ☒
Provider's Signature:	Betty Biller Date: 12/7/CCYY

Patient Information

Name:	Clara Conners
Address:	9009 Camelia Court
City:	Collins State: CO Zip Code: 81221
Telephone #:	(970) 555-8122 Account #: 10093
Date of Birth:	11/13/CCYY-73 Gender: Female
Marital Status:	Married Relationship to Guarantor: Self
Student Status:	☐ Full-time ☐ Part-time
Insurance Type:	☒ Pvt ☒ M/care ☐ M/caid ☐ WC ☐ Other ___ COB
Hospitalization Date:	
Hospital Information:	

Appointment Information

Appointment Date:		Time:	
Next Appt. Date:		Time:	
Date of First Visit:	07/07/CCYY	Date of Injury:	
Referring Physician:	Carlos Cruz, M.D.		

Guarantor Information

Name:	Clara Conners
Address:	9009 Camelia Court
City: Collins	State: CO Zip Code: 81221
Insurance ID #:	444-55-4444B/ 55-4444 XYZ
Insurance Name:	Medicare/ Ball Insurance Carriers
Insurance Group #:	62958
Employer Name:	XYZ Corporation

Authorization

☒ Authorization to Release Information
☒ Authorization for Assignment of Benefits
☐ Authorization for Consent for Treatment
☐ My insurance will be billed but there may be a balance due.

Signature: Clara Conners   Date: 12/7/CCYY

Clinical Information

	DOS	POS	CPT® /HCPCS Description	ICD-9-CM (*Indicates diagnosis for all lines)	Amount
1	10/7-11/6/CCYY	Home	Volume ventilator, stationary w/ back-up rate	*Emphysema; *1Resp Failure	$1000.00
2	11/7-12/6/CCYY	Home	Volume ventilator, stationary w/ back-up rate	*; *1	$1000.00
3					
4					
5					
6					

Remarks:	Carlos Cruz, M.D. UPIN #: M48620 prescribed a volume ventilator, secondary unit for the patient.			
Previous Balance:	$8437.50	Payment:	Copay:	Adjustment:
Total Fee:	$2000.00	Cash ☐ Check ☐ Credit ☐	Cash ☐ Check ☐ Credit ☐	Remarks: New Balance: $10437.50

Hospital Admission Form
DOCUMENT 184

Provider Information

Name:	Castle Memorial Medical Center
Address:	P.O. Box 79364

City:	Collins	State:	CO	Zip Code:	81234

Telephone#:		Fax#:	

Medicare ID#:	060032	UPIN#:	

Tax ID #:	40-7583047	Accepts Medicare Assignment:	☒

Provider Rep:	*Betty Biller*	Date: *7/28/CCYY*

Admission Information

Admission Date:	07/28/CCYY	Time:	2:00 PM
Discharge Date:	07/28/CCYY	Time:	7:00 PM
Attending Phy's ID#:	A12385	Date of Injury:	
Attending Physician:	Carol Cancer, M.D.		

Guarantor Information

Name:	Chris Conners
Address:	9009 Camelia Court

City:	Collins	State:	CO	Zip Code:	81221

Insurance ID #:	444-55-4444A	SSN:	444-55-4444
Insurance Name:	Medicare/ Ball Insurance Carriers		
Insurance Group #:	62958		
Employer Name:	XYZ Corporation		

Patient Information

Name:	Chris Conners
Address:	9009 Camelia Court

City:	Collins	State:	CO	Zip Code:	81221

Telephone#:	(970) 555-8122	Patient Control #:	10092
Date of Birth:	06/24/CCYY-75	Gender:	Male
Marital Status:	Married	Relationship to Guarantor:	Self

Student Status:	☐ Full-time	☐ Part-time

Insurance Type:	☒ Pvt ☒ M/care ☐ M/caid ☐ WC ☐ Other ___COB___

Authorization

☒ Authorization to Release Information
☒ Authorization for Assignment of Benefits
☐ Authorization for Consent for Treatment
☐ My insurance will be billed but there may be a balance due.

Signature: *Chris Conners*   Date: *7/28/CCYY*

Clinical Information

Principal Diagnosis:	Chronic Renal Failure
Other Diagnosis:	
Surgical Procedure:	Hemodialysis 7/28/CCYY
Other Procedures:	
Remarks:	ESRD diagnosed 8/21 three year prior

Previous Balance:	$50.00	Payment:		Copay:		Adjustment:			
Total Fee:	$3000.00	Cash ☐ Check ☐ Credit ☐		Cash ☐ Check ☐ Credit ☐		Remarks:		New Balance:	$3050.00

Castle Memorial Medical Center
P.O. Box 79364
Collins, CO 81234

Patient Name	Patient No.	Sex	Date of Birth	Admission Date	Discharge Date	Page No.
CHRIS CONNERS	10092	M	06/24/CCYY-75	07/28/CCYY	07/28/CCYY	1

Guarantor Name and Address
CHRIS CONNERS
9009 CAMELIA COURT
COLLINS, CO 81221

Insurance Company: MEDICARE/ BALL INS CARRIERS
Claim Number: DOCUMENT 184
Attending Physician: CAROL CANCER, M.D.

Date of Service	Description of Hospital Services	Service Code	Qty.	Charges	Total Charges
	SUMMARY OF CHARGES				
	TREATMENT ROOM		1	$350.00	
	PHARMACY		8	$297.00	
	LABORATORY		16	$468.00	
	MED-SURG SUPPLIES		23	$643.00	
	DIALYSIS TREATMENT		1	$1242.00	
	SUBTOTAL OF CHARGES				$3000.00
	PAYMENTS AND ADJUSTMENTS			NONE	
	SUBTOTAL PAYMENTS/ADJ				NONE
	BALANCE DUE				$3000.00

Hospital Admission Form

Provider Information

Name:	Castle Memorial Medical Center
Address:	P.O. Box 79364

City:	Collins	State:	CO	Zip Code:	81234

Telephone#:		Fax#:	

Medicare ID#:	060032	UPIN#:		
Tax ID #:	40-7583047	Accepts Medicare Assignment:	☒	
Provider Rep:	_Betty Biller_		Date: _11/21/CCYY_	

Patient Information

Name:	Chris Conners
Address:	9009 Camelia Court

City:	Collins	State:	CO	Zip Code:	81221
Telephone#:	(970) 555-8122	Patient Control #:	10092		

Date of Birth:	06/24/CCYY-75	Gender:	Male
Marital Status:	Married	Relationship to Guarantor:	Self

Student Status:	☐ Full-time ☐ Part-time
Insurance Type:	☒ Pvt ☒ M/care ☐ M/caid ☐ WC ☐ Other ___COB___

Admission Information

Admission Date:	11/19/CCYY	Time:	3:00 PM
Discharge Date:	11/21/CCYY	Time:	10:00 AM
Attending Phy's ID#:	A12385	Date of Injury:	
Attending Physician:	Carol Cancer, M.D.		

Guarantor Information

Name:	Chris Conners
Address:	9009 Camelia Court

City:	Collins	State:	CO	Zip Code:	81221
Insurance ID #:	444-55-4444A	SSN:	444-55-4444		

Insurance Name:	Medicare/ Ball Insurance Carriers
Insurance Group #:	62958
Employer Name:	XYZ Corporation

Authorization

☒ Authorization to Release Information
☒ Authorization for Assignment of Benefits
☐ Authorization for Consent for Treatment
☐ My insurance will be billed but there may be a balance due.

Signature: _Chris Conners_   Date: _11/19/CCYY_

Clinical Information

Principal Diagnosis:	Chronic Renal Failure	
Other Diagnosis:		
Surgical Procedure:	Hemodialysis	11/20/CCYY
Other Procedures:		
Remarks:	ESRD diagnosed 8/21 three years prior	

Previous Balance:	$3050.00	Payment:		Copay:		Adjustment:	
Total Fee:	$2706.00	Cash ☐ Check ☐ Credit ☐	Cash ☐ Check ☐ Credit ☐	Remarks:	New Balance:	$5756.00

Castle Memorial Medical Center
P.O. Box 79364
Collins, CO 81234

Patient Name	Patient No.	Sex	Date of Birth	Admission Date	Discharge Date	Page No.
CHRIS CONNERS	10092	M	06/24/CCYY-75	11/19/CCYY	11/19/CCYY	1

Guarantor Name and Address
CHRIS CONNERS
9009 CAMELIA COURT
COLLINS, CO 81221

Insurance Company: MEDICARE/ BALL INS CARRIERS
Claim Number: DOCUMENT 185
Attending Physician: CAROL CANCER, M.D.

Date of Service	Description of Hospital Services	Service Code	Qty.	Charges	Total Charges
	SUMMARY OF CHARGES				
	ROOM & BOARD – SEMI		2	$700.00	
	PHARMACY		10	$184.00	
	LABORATORY		17	$247.00	
	MED-SURG SUPPLIES		28	$489.00	
	DIALYSIS TREATMENT		1	$1086.00	
	SUBTOTAL OF CHARGES				$2706.00
	PAYMENTS AND ADJUSTMENTS			NONE	
	SUBTOTAL PAYMENTS/ADJ				NONE
	BALANCE DUE				$2706.00

Medicare and Medicaid Claims Beginning Financials
HANAKA FAMILY

Insurance Plan	Rover Insurers, Inc.—Ninja Enterprises			
Patient:	**HIRO**	**HOLLY**		
C/O DEDUCTIBLE	0.00	0.00		
DEDUCTIBLE	100.00	25.00		
COINSURANCE	0.00	0.00		
ACCIDENT BENEFIT	0.00	0.00		
LIFETIME MAXIMUM	52,772.00	41,263.42		
M/N OFFICE VISITS				
OFFICE VISITS				
HOSPITAL VISITS				
DXL				
SURGERY				
ASSISTANT SURGERY				
ANESTHESIA				

Encounter Form

Provider Information

Name:	Harold Hamada, M.D.					
Address:	89347 Hialia Street					
City:	Hilo	State:	HI	Zip Code:	96825	
Telephone #:		Fax #:				
Medicare ID#:		UPIN #:	C32145			
Tax ID #:	69-2159735	Accepts Medicare Assignment:	☒			
Provider's Signature:	*Harold Hamada, MD*		Date: 3/14/CCYY			

Appointment Information

Appointment Date:		Time:	
Next Appt. Date:		Time:	
Date of First Visit:	03/14/CCYY	Date of Injury:	
Referring Physician:			

Patient Information

Name:	Hiro Hanaka				
Address:	293 Huronea Street				
City:	Hilo	State:	HI	Zip Code:	96823
Telephone #:	(808) 555-9682	Account #:	10094		
Date of Birth:	01/15/CCYY-75	Gender:	Male		
Marital Status:	Married	Relationship to Guarantor:	Self		
Student Status:	☐ Full-time	☐ Part-time			
Insurance Type:	☒ Pvt ☒ M/care ☐ M/caid ☐ WC ☐ Other ____ COB ____				
Hospitalization Date:					
Hospital Information:					

Guarantor Information

Name:	Hiro Hanaka
Address:	293 Huronea Street
City: Hilo State: HI Zip Code: 96823	
Insurance ID #:	666-77-8901A/ 77-8901 NIN
Insurance Name:	Medicare/ Rover Insurers, Inc.
Insurance Group #:	21088
Employer Name:	Ninja Enterprises

Authorization

☒ Authorization to Release Information
☒ Authorization for Assignment of Benefits
☐ Authorization for Consent for Treatment
☐ My insurance will be billed but there may be a balance due.
Signature: *Hiro Hanaka*   Date: 3/14/CCYY

Clinical Information

	DOS	POS	CPT® /HCPCS Description	ICD-9-CM (*Indicates diagnosis for all lines)	Amount
1	03/14/CCYY	Office	Est pt, comprehensive exam, moderate complexity	Chronic Sinusitis	$ 75.00
2					
3					
4					
5					
6					
Remarks:					

Previous Balance:		Payment:		Copay:		Adjustment:		
Total Fee:	$75.00	Cash ☐ Check ☐ Credit ☐		Cash ☐ Check ☐ Credit ☐		Remarks:	New Balance:	$75.00

Encounter Form

Provider Information

Name:	Hillary Holt, M.D.
Address:	8348 Hamilton Drive

City:	Hilo	State:	HI	Zip Code:	96827

Telephone #:		Fax #:	
Medicare ID#:		UPIN #:	D54306
Tax ID #:	69-2486224	Accepts Medicare Assignment:	☒

Provider's Signature:	*Hillary Holt, MD*	Date: *5/14/CCYY*

Appointment Information

Appointment Date:		Time:	
Next Appt. Date:		Time:	
Date of First Visit:	05/14/CCYY	Date of Injury:	
Referring Physician:			

Guarantor Information

Name:	Hiro Hanaka
Address:	293 Huronea Street

City:	Hilo	State:	HI	Zip Code:	96823

Patient Information

Name:	Hiro Hanaka
Address:	293 Huronea Street

City:	Hilo	State:	HI	Zip Code:	96823

Telephone #:	(808) 555-9682	Account #:	10094
Date of Birth:	01/15/CCYY-75	Gender:	Male
Marital Status:	Married	Relationship to Guarantor:	Self

Insurance ID #:	666-77-8901A/ 77-8901 NIN
Insurance Name:	Medicare/ Rover Insurers, Inc.
Insurance Group #:	21088
Employer Name:	Ninja Enterprises

Student Status: ☐ Full-time ☐ Part-time

Insurance Type: ☒ Pvt ☒ M/care ☐ M/caid ☐ WC ☐ Other _____ COB

Hospitalization Date:

Hospital Information:

Authorization

☒ Authorization to Release Information
☒ Authorization for Assignment of Benefits
☐ Authorization for Consent for Treatment
☐ My insurance will be billed but there may be a balance due.

Signature: *Hiro Hanaka*   Date: *5/14/CCYY*

Clinical Information

	DOS	POS	CPT® /HCPCS Description	ICD-9-CM (*Indicates diagnosis for all lines)	Amount
1	05/14/CCYY	Office	Excision, malignant lesion, face, 1.0 cm	Removal of Malignant Facial Moles	$260.00
2					
3					
4					
5					
6					

Remarks:						
Previous Balance:	$75.00	Payment:		Copay:		Adjustment:	
Total Fee:	$260.00	Cash ☐ Check ☐ Credit ☐	Cash ☐ Check ☐ Credit ☐	Remarks:	New Balance:	$335.00

Encounter Form

Provider Information

Name:	Harry Henson, M.D.
Address:	P.O. Box 8459

City:	Hilo	State:	HI	Zip Code:	96821

Telephone #:		Fax #:	
Medicare ID#:		UPIN #:	E52203
Tax ID #:	69-7896214	Accepts Medicare Assignment:	☒

Provider's Signature:	*Harry Henson, MD*	Date: *11/04/CCYY*

Appointment Information

Appointment Date:		Time:	
Next Appt. Date:		Time:	
Date of First Visit:	11/04/CCYY	Date of Injury:	
Referring Physician:			

Guarantor Information

Name:	Holly Hanaka
Address:	293 Huronea Street

City:	Hilo	State:	HI	Zip Code:	96823

Patient Information

Name:	Holly Hanaka
Address:	293 Huronea Street

City:	Hilo	State:	HI	Zip Code:	96823

Telephone #:	(808) 555-9682	Account #:	10095
Date of Birth:	12/18/CCYY-73	Gender:	Female
Marital Status:	Married	Relationship to Guarantor:	Self

Insurance ID #:	666-77-8901B/ 77-8901 NIN
Insurance Name:	Medicare/ Rover Insurers, Inc.
Insurance Group #:	21088
Employer Name:	Ninja Enterprises

Student Status: ☐ Full-time ☐ Part-time

Insurance Type: ☒ Pvt ☒ M/care ☐ M/caid ☐ WC ☐ Other _____ COB

Hospitalization Date:

Hospital Information:

Authorization

☒ Authorization to Release Information
☒ Authorization for Assignment of Benefits
☐ Authorization for Consent for Treatment
☐ My insurance will be billed but there may be a balance due.

Signature: *Holly Hanaka*   Date: *11/04/CCYY*

Clinical Information

	DOS	POS	CPT® /HCPCS Description	ICD-9-CM (*Indicates diagnosis for all lines)	Amount
1	11/04/CCYY	Office	Routine ECG; 12 leade w/ interp and report	*Chest Pain; *1Cardiac Arrhythmia	$ 38.88
2	11/04/CCYY	Office	Cardiovascular stress test using treadmill	*; *1	$169.63
3	11/04/CCYY	Office	Handling of specimen for transfer	*; *1; *2Ulcer Duodenal	$ 3.00
4	11/04/CCYY	Office	Complete (CBC), automated	*; *1; *2	$ 34.00
5	11/04/CCYY	Office	Thyroid hormone uptake	*2	$ 35.00
6	11/04/CCYY	Office	Hepatic function panel	*2	$ 63.00

Remarks:						
Previous Balance:		Payment:		Copay:		Adjustment:	
Total Fee:	$343.51	Cash ☐ Check ☐ Credit ☐	Cash ☐ Check ☐ Credit ☐	Remarks:	New Balance:	$343.51

Hospital Admission Form

Provider Information

Name:	Hilo General Hospital
Address:	P.O. Box 192

City:	Hilo	State:	HI	Zip Code:	96829

Telephone#:		Fax#:	
Medicare ID#:	120034	UPIN#:	

Tax ID #:	69-7593048	Accepts Medicare Assignment: ☒
Provider's Signature:	*Betty Biller*	Date: _11/15/CCYY_

Patient Information

Name:	Holly Hanaka
Address:	293 Huronea Street

City:	Hilo	State:	HI	Zip Code:	96823
Telephone#:	(808) 555-9682	Control #:	10095		
Date of Birth:	12/18/CCYY-73	Gender:	Female		

Marital Status:	Married	Relationship to Guarantor:	Self
Student Status:	☐ Full-time	☐ Part-time	
Insurance Type:	☒ Pvt ☒ M/care ☐ M/caid ☐ WC ☐ Other _____		

Admission Information

Admission Date:	11/14/CCYY	Time:	9:00 AM
Discharge Date:	11/15/CCYY	Time:	10:00 AM
Attending Phy's ID#:	F40005	Date of Injury:	
Attending Physician:	Hashedi Hada, M.D.		

Guarantor Information

Name:	Holly Hanaka
Address:	293 Huronea Street

City:	Hilo	State:	HI	Zip Code:	96823
Insurance ID #:	666-77-8901B	SSN:	666-77-8901		
Insurance Name:	Medicare/ Rover Insurers, Inc.				
Insurance Group #:	21088				
Employer Name:	Ninja Enterprises				

Authorization

☒ Authorization to Release Information
☒ Authorization for Assignment of Benefits
☐ Authorization for Consent for Treatment
☐ My insurance will be billed but there may be a balance due.

Signature: _Holly Hanaka_ Date: _11/14/CCYY_

Clinical Information

Principal Diagnosis:	Coronary Arthrosclerosis	
Other Diagnosis:		
Surgical Procedure:	Right/Left Heart Cardiac Catheterization	11/14/CCYY
Other Procedures:		
Remarks:		

Previous Balance:	$343.51	Payment:		Copay:		Adjustment:		
Total Fee:	$6049.00	Cash ☐ Check ☐ Credit ☐		Cash ☐ Check ☐ Credit ☐		Remarks:	New Balance:	$6392.51

Hilo General Hospital
P.O. Box 192
Hilo, HI 96829

Patient Name	Patient No.	Sex	Date of Birth	Admission Date	Discharge Date	Page No.
HOLLY HANAKA	10095	F	12/18/CCYY-73	11/14/CCYY	11/15/CCYY	1

Guarantor Name and Address
HOLLY HANAKA
293 HURONEA STREET
HILO, HI 96823

Insurance Company: MEDICARE/ ROVER INS INC.
Claim Number: DOCUMENT 190
Attending Physician: HASHEDI HADA, M.D.

Date of Service	Description of Hospital Services	Service Code	Qty.	Charges	Total Charges
	SUMMARY OF CHARGES				
	ROOM & BOARD/SEMI		1	$620.00	
	PHARMACY		2	$82.00	
	MED-SURG SUPPLIES		5	$175.00	
	CARDIAC CATH LAB		31	$5172.00	
	SUBTOTAL OF CHARGES				$6049.00
	PAYMENTS AND ADJUSTMENTS			NONE	
	SUBTOTAL PAYMENTS/ADJ				NONE
	BALANCE DUE				$6049.00

Encounter Form

Provider Information

Name:	Herbert Harnsen, M.D.
Address:	P.O. Box 2598

City:	Hilo	State:	HI	Zip Code:	96828

Telephone #:		Fax #:	
Medicare ID#:		UPIN #:	G32150

Tax ID #:	69-2589436	Accepts Medicare Assignment:	☒
Provider's Signature:	_Herbert Harnsen, MD_	Date:	11/15/CCYY

Appointment Information

Appointment Date:		Time:	
Next Appt. Date:		Time:	
Date of First Visit:		Date of Injury:	
Referring Physician:			

Guarantor Information

Name:	Holly Hanaka
Address:	293 Huronea Street

City:	Hilo	State:	HI	Zip Code:	96823

Insurance ID #:	666-77-8901B/ 77-8901 NIN
Insurance Name:	Medicare/ Rover Insurers, Inc.
Insurance Group #:	21088
Employer Name:	Ninja Enterprises

Patient Information

Name:	Holly Hanaka
Address:	293 Huronea Street

City:	Hilo	State:	HI	Zip Code:	96823

Telephone #:	(808) 555-9682	Account #:	10095
Date of Birth:	12/18/CCYY-73	Gender:	Female
Marital Status:	Married	Relationship to Guarantor:	Self
Student Status:	☐ Full-time	☐ Part-time	
Insurance Type:	☒ Pvt ☒ M/care ☐ M/caid ☐ WC ☐ Other	COB	
Hospitalization Date:	From: 11/14/CCYY	To: 11/15/CCYY	
Hospital Information:	Hilo Memorial Center, P.O. Box 171821, Hilo, HI 96828		

Authorization

☒ Authorization to Release Information
☒ Authorization for Assignment of Benefits
☐ Authorization for Consent for Treatment
☐ My insurance will be billed but there may be a balance due.

Signature: _Holly Hanaka_ Date: 11/15/CCYY

Clinical Information

	DOS	POS	CPT® /HCPCS Description	ICD-9-CM (*Indicates diagnosis for all lines)	Amount
1	11/14/CCYY	Office	Blood typing Rh (D)	*Coronary Arthrosclerosis; *1	$ 25.00
2	11/14/CCYY	Office	Blood, gases, pH only	*; *1 Aortocoronary Bypass Status	$ 63.00
3	11/14/CCYY	Office	Hepatic function panel	*; *1	$ 70.00
4	11/14/CCYY	Inpt Hosp	Hosp care, comp hist & exam, high complexity	*; *1	$ 202.21
5	11/14/CCYY	Inpt Hosp	Rt heart cath; transseptal left heart cath, intact septum	*; *1	$1508.88
6	11/15/CCYY	Inpt Hosp	Sub hosp care, expand prob foc exam, moderate comp	*; *1	$ 176.42

Remarks:

Previous Balance:	$6392.51	Payment:		Copay:		Adjustment:	
Total Fee:	$2045.51	Cash ☐ Check ☐ Credit ☐	Cash ☐ Check ☐ Credit ☐	Remarks:	New Balance: $8438.02

Health Claims Examining Exercises

(**Instructor's Note**: Medical Billing exercises in the entire text should be completed prior to students starting Health Claims Examining Exercise 10–A. New files should be set up for the Health Claims Examining exercises.)

Exercise **10-A**

Directions: Complete an Insurance Coverage Form (located in the **Forms** chapter) and set up Family Files for all families in this chapter. Refer to the Family Data Tables (**Documents 171–173**) located in the beginning of this chapter, and the Contracts located in the **Contracts, UCR Conversion Factor Report, and Relative Value Study** chapter.

Exercise **10-B**

Directions: Complete a Payment Worksheet (located in the **Forms** chapter) for CMS-1500 (**Documents 175–179, 181–185, and 187–191**) and UB-92 (**Documents 184–185 and 190**) claims using the guidelines contained in the **Introduction** chapter and using the UCR Conversion Factor Report, Relative Value Study, and Contracts located in the **Contracts, UCR Conversion Factor Report, and Relative Value Study** chapter. Also, complete a Coordination of Benefits Calculation Worksheet (located in the **Forms** chapter) for applicable claims. The following Medicare Remittance Notices (**Document 192**) should be referred to for claims payment and coordination of benefit information.

When processing claims, the Beginning Financials (**Documents 174, 180, and 186**) should be incorporated as payment history and claim calculations should be adjusted accordingly. Any carryover deductible listed should be included in the current year deductible for that individual. Therefore, in figuring current year deductible, students should be instructed to subtract the carryover deductible from the current year's amount.

Upon completion of each claim complete or update the Family Benefits Tracking Sheet (located in the **Forms** chapter) by compiling all of the claims payment data for the family.

MEDICARE REMITTANCE NOTICE

DATE: DECEMBER 21, CCYY
CHECK SEQUENCE NO.: 1203-09782-003
PAGE 1 OF 2

BENEFICIARY NAME	SVC FR MO-DY	TO DY-YR	PLACE TYPE	PROCEDURE DESCRIPTION	AMOUNT BILLED	AMOUNT APPROVED	SEE NOTE	DEDUCTIBLE	COINSURANCE	PAYMENT	INTEREST
VERNON VAUGHN	06-26	26-CCYY	1	90782	35.00	3.00	56				
	06-26	26-CCYY	1	J3260	25.00	3.00	56				
	06-26	26-CCYY	1	A4550-ZP	35.00	20.00	56				
	06-26	26-CCYY	1	53620	100.00	70.13	56				
	06-26	26-CCYY	1	81000-XL	20.00	4.72	56				
	06-26	26-CCYY	1	87205	20.00	6.38	56				
*777-77-0000A				TOTALS	235.00	107.23	442	0.00	19.23	88.00	0.00
CHRIS CONNERS	06-26	26-CCYY	1	99214	50.00	37.70	56				
*444-55-4444A				TOTALS	50.00	37.70	442	0.00	7.54	30.16	0.00
HOLLY HANAKA	11-14	13-CCYY	1	86901	25.00	0.00	61				
	11-14	13-CCYY	1	82800	63.00	0.00	61				
	11-14	13-CCYY	1	80058	70.00	0.00	61				
	11-14	14-CCYY	1	99223	202.21	164.40	56				
	11-14	14-CCYY	1	93527	1508.88	1225.60	56				
	11-15	15-CCYY	1	99232	176.42	153.40	56				
*666-77-8901B				TOTALS	2045.51	1543.40	442	0.00	308.68	1234.72	0.00
VICKI VAUGHN	06-01	01-CCYY	1	99214	50.00	37.70	56				
*777-77-0000B				TOTALS	50.00	37.70	442	0.00	7.54	30.16	0.00
VICKI VAUGHN	06-10	10-CCYY	1	99213	50.00	35.00	56				
	06-10	10-CCYY	1	11100-LT	75.00	53.95	56				
	06-10	10-CCYY	1	88305	45.00	40.00	56				
	06-10	10-CCYY	1	A4550-ZP	20.00	20.00	56				
*777-77-0000B				TOTALS	190.00	148.95	442	0.00	29.79	119.16	0.00
CLARA CONNERS	09-04	04-CCYY	3	99255	175.00	115.40	56				
	09-05	05-CCYY	3	27365-51	2860.00	1999.40	56				
	09-05	05-CCYY	3	27506-22	3750.00	862.82	236				
	09-05	05-CCYY	3	27506-80	937.50	138.05	238				
	09-05	05-CCYY	3	27365-80	715.00	319.91	238				
*444-55-4444B				TOTALS	8437.50	3435.58	442	0.00	687.12	2748.46	0.00
VERNON VAUGHN	07-10	10-CCYY	1	90782	35.00	3.00	56				
	07-10	10-CCYY	1	J3260	25.00	3.00	56				
	07-10	10-CCYY	1	A4550-ZP	35.00	20.00	56				
	07-10	10-CCYY	1	52281	375.00	323.60	56				
	07-10	10-CCYY	1	81000-XL	20.00	4.72	56				
	07-10	10-CCYY	1	87205-XL	20.00	6.38	56				
	07-10	10-CCYY	1	99214	75.00	50.30	56				
*777-77-0000A				TOTALS	585.00	411.00	442	0.00	79.98	331.02	0.00

56 - Medicare limits payment to this amount.
61 - Medicare can only pay for laboratory tests when assignment is accepted.
236 - Indicated amount has been adjusted for unusual procedural services.
238 - Indicated amount has been adjusted for assistant surgeon.
442 - Total for these charges.

MEDICARE REMITTANCE NOTICE

DATE: DECEMBER 21, CCYY
CHECK SEQUENCE NO.: 1203-09782-003
PAGE 2 OF 2

BENEFICIARY NAME	SVC FR MO-DY	TO DY-YR	PLACE TYPE	PROCEDURE DESCRIPTION	AMOUNT BILLED	AMOUNT APPROVED	SEE NOTE	DEDUCTIBLE	COINSURANCE	PAYMENT	INTEREST
CLARA CONNERS	07-07	TO									
	08-06	CCYY	2	E0450-RR	1000.00	637.43	56				
*444-44-4444B				TOTALS	1000.00	637.43	442	0.00	127.49	509.94	0.00
CLARA CONNERS	08-07	TO									
	09-06	CCYY	2	E0450-RR	1000.00	637.43	56				
*444-44-4444B				TOTALS	1000.00	637.43	442	0.00	127.49	509.94	0.00
HOLLY HANAKA	11-04	04-CCYY	1	93000	38.88	0.00	58				
	11-04	04-CCYY	1	93015	169.63	135.70	56				
	11-04	04-CCYY	1	99000	3.00	0.00	61				
	11-04	04-CCYY	1	85027	34.00	0.00	61				
	11-04	04-CCYY	1	80091	35.00	0.00	61				
	11-04	04-CCYY	1	80058	63.00	0.00	61				
*666-77-8901B				TOTALS	343.51	135.70	442	0.00	27.14	108.56	0.00
HIRO HANAKA	03-14	14-CCYY	1	99214	75.00	50.30	56				
*666-77-8901A				TOTALS	75.00	50.30	442	0.00	10.06	40.24	0.00
VERNON VAUGHN	07-29	29-CCYY	1	90782	35.00	3.00	56				
	07-29	29-CCYY	1	A4550-ZP	35.00	20.00	56				
	07-29	29-CCYY	1	53600	55.00	36.65	56				
*777-77-0000A				TOTALS	125.00	59.65	442	0.00	11.93	47.72	0.00
CHRIS CONNERS	05-28	28-CCYY	3		3000.00	1251.25	56				
*444-44-4444A				TOTALS	3000.00	1251.25	442	0.00	250.25	1001.00	0.00
CHRIS CONNERS	11-19	21-CCYY	3		2706.00	2358.99	56				
*444-44-4444A				TOTALS	2706.00	2358.99	442	952.00	0.00	1406.99	0.00
HIRO HANAKA	05-14	14-CCYY	1	11641	260.00	250.00	56				
*666-77-8901A				TOTALS	260.00	250.00	442	0.00	50.00	200.00	0.00
VICKI VAUGHN	08-13	13-CCYY	1	92083-YB	175.00	74.80	56				
	08-14	14-CCYY	1	92014-AP	95.00	86.86	56				
*777-77-0000B				TOTALS	270.00	161.66	442	0.00	32.33	129.33	0.00
HOLLY HANAKA	11-14	15-CCYY	1		6049.00	3648.65	56				
*666-77-8901B				TOTALS	6049.00	3648.65	442	952.00	0.00	2696.65	0.00

56 - Medicare limits payment to this amount.
58 - Medicare does not pay for this.
61 - Medicare can only pay for laboratory tests when assignment is accepted.
236 - Indicated amount has been adjusted for unusual procedural services.
238 - Indicated amount has been adjusted for assistant surgeon.
442 - Total for these charges.

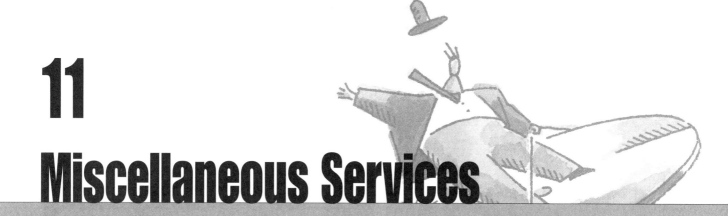

11
Miscellaneous Services

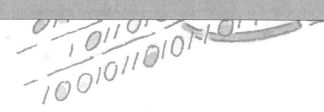

Medical Billing Exercises

Exercise 11-1

Directions: Complete Patient Information Sheets (leave **Assigned Provider** field blank), Ledger Cards, and Insurance Coverage Forms and set up patient charts for the following families using copies of the forms in the **Forms** chapter. Refer to the Family Data Tables **(Documents 193–195)** for information.

Individual folders with dividers may be used to store information for each family. One Patient Information Sheet and Insurance Coverage Form should be filled out for the entire family.

FAMILY DATA TABLE

RUBBLE FAMILY	INSURED'S INFORMATION	SPOUSE'S INFORMATION	CHILD #1	CHILD #2	CHILD #3
Name	Ronny Rubble	Raisa Rubble	Royal Rubble	Renee Rubble	
Address	1234 Rufus Blvd. Rockwell, RI 02845	1234 Rufus Blvd. Rockwell, RI 02845	1234 Rufus Blvd. Rockwell, RI 02845	1234 Rufus Blvd. Rockwell, RI 02845	
Email Address	ronnyr@rubble.com				
TELEPHONE #					
Home:	(401) 555-0284	(401) 555-0284	(401) 555-0284	(401) 555-0284	
Work:	(401) 555-0285				
Cell:	(401) 555-0286				
Date of Birth	06/15/CCYY-45	06/07/CCYY-43	06/02/CCYY-18	07/01/CCYY-16	
Social Security #	001-00-0001	001-00-0002	001-00-0003	001-00-0004	
Marital Status/Gender	Married/Male	Married/Female	Single/Male	Single/Female	
Student Status			Full-time	Full-time	
Patient Account #	10055	10096	10098	10097	
Allergies/Medical Conditions	None	None	None	None	
PRIMARY INSURANCE CARRIER					
Name Address	Winter Insurance Company 9763 Western Way Whittier, CO 82963	Winter Insurance Company 9763 Western Way Whittier, CO 82963	Winter Insurance Company 9763 Western Way Whittier, CO 82963	Winter Insurance Company 9763 Western Way Whittier, CO 82963	
Effective Date	01/01/CCPY	01/01/CCPY	01/01/CCPY	01/01/CCPY	
Member's ID #	00-0001 ABC	00-0001 ABC	00-0001 ABC	00-0001 ABC	
Group Policy #	36928	36928	36928	36928	
Policy/Employer	ABC Corporation 1234 Whitaker Lane Colter, CO 81222				
OTHER INSURANCE CARRIER					
Name Address					
Effective Date					
Member's ID #					
Group Policy #					
Policy/Employer					
Responsible Party	Self	Self	Insured	Insured	
EMERGENCY CONTACT					
Name Telephone # Address	Roy Ronter (410) 555-0287 4321 Rufus Blvd. Rockwell, RI 02845	Roy Ronter (410) 555-0287 4321 Rufus Blvd. Rockwell, RI 02845	Roy Ronter (410) 555-0287 4321 Rufus Blvd. Rockwell, RI 02845	Roy Ronter (410) 555-0287 4321 Rufus Blvd. Rockwell, RI 02845	

DOCUMENT 194

FAMILY DATA FORM

MINNETOMA FAMILY	INSURED'S INFORMATION	SPOUSE'S INFORMATION	CHILD #1	CHILD #2	CHILD #3
Name	Miles Minnetoma	Mindy Minnetoma	Monty Minnetoma	Morey Minnetoma	Melanie Minnetoma
Address	1800 Moonriver Drive Monte Mort, MN 55621	1800 Moonriver Drive Monte Mort, MN 55621	1800 Moonriver Drive Monte Mort, MN 55621	1800 Moonriver Drive Monte Mort, MN 55621	1800 Moonriver Drive Monte Mort, MN 55621
Email Address	milesm@minnetoma.com				
TELEPHONE #					
Home:	(507) 555-5562	(507) 555-5562	(507) 555-5562	(507) 555-5562	(507) 555-5562
Work:	(507) 555-5563				
Cell:	(507) 555-5564				
Date of Birth	02/17/CCYY-43	04/19/CCYY-41	11/04/CCYY-16	07/01/CCYY-17	04/01/CCYY-18
Social Security #	002-00-0002	002-00-0006	002-00-0003	002-00-0004	002-00-0005
Marital Status/Gender	Married/Male	Married/Female	Single/Male	Single/Male	Single/Female
Student Status			Full-time	Full-time	Full-time
Patient Account #	10052	10107	10099	10101	10100
Allergies/Medical Conditions	None	None	None	None	None
PRIMARY INSURANCE CARRIER					
Name Address	Ball Insurance Carriers 3895 Bubble Blvd. Ste. 283 Boxwood, CO 85926		Ball Insurance Carriers 3895 Bubble Blvd. Ste. 283 Boxwood, CO 85926	Ball Insurance Carriers 3895 Bubble Blvd. Ste. 283 Boxwood, CO 85926	Ball Insurance Carriers 3895 Bubble Blvd. Ste. 283 Boxwood, CO 85926
Effective Date	01/01/CCPY	01/01/CCPY	01/01/CCPY	01/01/CCPY	01/01/CCPY
Member's ID #	00-0002 XYZ	00-0002 XYZ	00-0002 XYZ	00-0002 XYZ	00-0002 XYZ
Group Policy #	62958	62958	62958	62958	62958
Policy/Employer	XYZ Corporation 9817 Bobcat Blvd. Bastion, CO 81319				
OTHER INSURANCE CARRIER					
Name Address					
Effective Date					
Member's ID #					
Group Policy #					
Policy/Employer					
Responsible Party	Self	Self	Insured	Insured	Insured
EMERGENCY CONTACT					
Name Telephone # Address	Mario Milwaukee (507) 555-5565 81 Moonriver Drive Monte Mort, MN 55621	Mario Milwaukee (507) 555-5565 81 Moonriver Drive Monte Mort, MN 55621	Mario Milwaukee (507) 555-5565 81 Moonriver Drive Monte Mort, MN 55621	Mario Milwaukee (507) 555-5565 81 Moonriver Drive Monte Mort, MN 55621	Mario Milwaukee (507) 555-5565 81 Moonriver Drive Monte Mort, MN 55621

FAMILY DATA TABLE

TALAWAN FAMILY	INSURED'S INFORMATION	SPOUSE'S INFORMATION	CHILD #1	CHILD #2	CHILD #3
Name	Tiron Talawan	Tara Talawan	Taura Talawan	Tabari Talawan	Tanya Talawan
Address	426 Tata Street Turnville, TN 37062	426 Tata Street Turnville, TN 37062	426 Tata Street Turnville, TN 37062	426 Tata Street Turnville, TN 37062	426 Tata Street Turnville, TN 37062
Email Address	tiront@talawan.com				
TELEPHONE #					
Home:	(423) 555-3706	(423) 555-3706	(423) 555-3706	(423) 555-3706	(423) 555-3706
Work:	(423) 555-3707				
Cell:	(423) 555-3708				
Date of Birth	07/25/CCYY-45	09/27/CCYY-43	06/04/CCYY-13	03/10/CCYY-18	05/12/CCYY-16
Social Security #	003-00-0003	003-00-0006	003-00-0004	003-00-0005	003-00-0007
Marital Status/Gender	Married/Male	Married/Female	Single/Female	Single/Male	Single/Female
Student Status			Full-time	Full-time	Full-time
Patient Account #	10104	10105	10102	10103	10106
Allergies/Medical Conditions	None	None	None	None	None
PRIMARY INSURANCE CARRIER					
Name Address	Rover Insurers, Inc. 5931 Rolling Road Ronson, CO 81369	Rover Insurers, Inc. 5931 Rolling Road Ronson, CO 81369	Rover Insurers, Inc. 5931 Rolling Road Ronson, CO 81369	Rover Insurers, Inc. 5931 Rolling Road Ronson, CO 81369	Rover Insurers, Inc. 5931 Rolling Road Ronson, CO 81369
Effective Date	01/01/CCPY	01/01/CCPY	01/01/CCPY	01/01/CCPY	01/01/CCPY
Member's ID #	00-0003 NIN	00-0003 NIN	00-0003 NIN	00-0003 NIN	00-0003 NIN
Group Policy #	21088	21088	21088	21088	21088
Policy/Employer	Ninja Enterprises 1234 Nockout Road Newton, NM 88012				
OTHER INSURANCE CARRIER					
Name Address					
Effective Date					
Member's ID #					
Group Policy #					
Policy/Employer					
Responsible Party	Self	Self	Insured	Insured	Insured
EMERGENCY CONTACT					
Name	Trishaw Tyrone	Trishaw Tyrone	Trishaw Tyrone	Trishaw Tyrone	Trishaw Tyrone
Telephone #	(423) 555-3709	(423) 555-3709	(423) 555-3709	(423) 555-3709	(423) 555-3709
Address	624 Tata Street Turnville, TN 37062	624 Tata Street Turnville, TN 37062	624 Tata Street Turnville, TN 37062	624 Tata Street Turnville, TN 37062	624 Tata Street Turnville, TN 37062

Exercise **11-2**

Directions: Complete a CMS-1500 for each of the Encounter Forms (**Documents 197–201, 203–207, and 209–213**) in this chapter. CMS-1500 forms may be provided by your instructor or purchased from a stationery store.

   After completion of each CMS-1500 form complete a Patient Receipt (if a payment was made), and post the transaction(s) to the patient Ledger Card/Statement of Account previously created.

Exercise **11-3**

Directions: Upon completion of all of the activities in Exercise 11–2 complete a Bank Deposit Slip/Ticket (located in the **Forms** chapter) for all payments made on the patient's account in this chapter.

Exercise **11-4**

Directions: Using an Insurance Claims Register (located in the **Forms** Chapter) list all claims that have been fully prepared and are ready for submission to the insurance carrier for payment. Enter the date that you created the CMS-1500 in the **Date Claim Filed** column.

Exercise **11-5**

Directions: Using the stationery or Request for Additional Information Form (located in the **Forms** chapter), write a letter or request information for the following scenario. In each case, you are the medical biller working for Any Billing Services. Addresses and personal information are contained in the patient files that were previously set up. Also, refer to the Family Data Table (**Document 195**) for required information.

1. Create a correspondence for TiRon Talawan advising him that his doctor, Tessa Tamsen, M.D. is retiring from the practice of medicine at the end of the year. Dr. Tessa Tamsen's practice is being taken over by Dr. Tamara Tehachipi.

Miscellaneous Claims Beginning Financials

RUBBLE FAMILY

Insurance Plan	Winter Insurance Company—ABC Corporation				
Patient:	**RONNY**	**RAISA**	**ROYAL**	**RENEE***	**ROLF**
C/O DEDUCTIBLE	0.00	0.00	0.00	0.00	0.00
DEDUCTIBLE	27.50	100.00	0.00	100.00	0.00
COINSURANCE	0.00	427.50	0.00	500.00	0.00
ACCIDENT BENEFIT	0.00	0.00	0.00	0.00	0.00
LIFETIME MAXIMUM	3,752.19	31,377.11	272.16	7,777.27	0.00
M/N OFFICE VISITS					
OFFICE VISITS					
HOSPITAL VISITS					
DXL					
SURGERY					
ASSISTANT SURGERY					
ANESTHESIA					

*Renee - Total rental payments for apnea monitor = $1,125.00.

Encounter Form

Provider Information

Name:	Rockwell Emergency Medical Services
Address:	P.O. Box 221
City:	Rockwell State: RI Zip Code: 02831
Telephone #:	Fax #:
Medicare ID#:	UPIN #:
Tax ID #:	55-5555555 Accepts Medicare Assignment: ☒
Provider's Signature:	Betty Biller Date: 3/2/CCYY

Appointment Information

Appointment Date:	Time:
Next Appt. Date:	Time:
Date of First Visit:	Date of Injury:
Referring Physician:	

Guarantor Information

Name:	Ronny Rubble
Address:	1234 Rufus Road
City: Rockwell	State: RI Zip Code: 02845
Insurance ID #:	00-0001 ABC
Insurance Name:	Winter Insurance Company
Insurance Group #:	36928
Employer Name:	ABC Corporation

Patient Information

Name:	Raisa Rubble
Address:	1234 Rufus Road
City:	Rockwell State: RI Zip Code: 02845
Telephone #:	(401) 555-0284 Account #: 10096
Date of Birth:	06/07/CCYY-43 Gender: Female
Marital Status:	Married Relationship to Guarantor: Spouse
Student Status:	☐ Full-time ☐ Part-time
Insurance Type:	☒ Pvt ☐ M/care ☐ M/caid ☐ WC ☐ Other _____
Hospitalization Date:	
Hospital Information:	Rockwell community Hospital, P.O. Box 900, Rockwell, RI 02831

Authorization

☒ Authorization to Release Information
☐ Authorization for Assignment of Benefits
☐ Authorization for Consent for Treatment
☐ My insurance will be billed but there may be a balance due.

Signature: Raisa Rubble Date: 3/3/CCYY

Clinical Information

	DOS	POS	CPT® /HCPCS Description	ICD-9-CM (*Indicates diagnosis for all lines)	Amount
1	03/03/CCYY	Ambulance	ALS-1, emergency	Diabetic Coma	$527.00
2					
3					
4					
5					
6					

Remarks:	Patient was transported from 627 River Street to Rockwell Hospital in an ambulance with advance life support.				
Previous Balance:		Payment:	Copay:	Adjustment:	
Total Fee:	$527.00	Cash ☐ Check ☐ Credit ☐	Cash ☐ Check ☐ Credit ☐	Remarks:	New Balance: $527.00

Encounter Form

DOCUMENT 198

Provider Information

Name:	Round Health Care Services
Address:	4444 West Road

City:	Rockwell	State:	RI	Zip Code:	02831
Telephone #:		Fax #:			
Medicare ID#:		UPIN #:			
Tax ID #:	55-5555666	Accepts Medicare Assignment:	☒		
Provider's Signature:	*Betty Biller*		Date: *4/7/CCYY*		

Patient Information

Name:	Raisa Rubble
Address:	1234 Rufus Road

City:	Rockwell	State:	RI	Zip Code:	02845
Telephone #:	(401) 555-0284	Account #:	10096		
Date of Birth:	06/07/CCYY-43	Gender:	Female		
Marital Status:	Married	Relationship to Guarantor:		Spouse	
Student Status:	☐ Full-time	☐ Part-time			
Insurance Type:	☒ Pvt ☐ M/care ☐ M/caid ☐ WC ☐ Other _____				
Hospitalization Date:					
Hospital Information:					

Appointment Information

Appointment Date:		Time:	
Next Appt. Date:		Time:	
Date of First Visit:		Date of Injury:	
Referring Physician:			

Guarantor Information

Name:	Ronny Rubble
Address:	1234 Rufus Road

City:	Rockwell	State:	RI	Zip Code:	02845
Insurance ID #:	00-0001 ABC				
Insurance Name:	Winter Insurance Company				
Insurance Group #:	36928				
Employer Name:	ABC Corporation				

Authorization

☒ Authorization to Release Information
☐ Authorization for Assignment of Benefits
☐ Authorization for Consent for Treatment
☐ My insurance will be billed but there may be a balance due.

Signature: *Raisa Rubble*   Date: *4/7/CCYY*

Clinical Information

	DOS	POS	CPT® /HCPCS Description	ICD-9-CM (*Indicates diagnosis for all lines)	Amount
1	04/07/CCYY	Inpt Hosp	Home blood glucose monitor	Diabetic Coma	$273.00
2					
3					
4					
5					
6					
Remarks:	Ronald Reed, M.D. UPIN #: I12287 prescribed a glucometer for patient.				
Previous Balance:	$527.00	Payment:		Copay:		Adjustment:			
Total Fee:	$273.00	Cash ☐ Check ☐ Credit ☐	Cash ☐ Check ☐ Credit ☐	Remarks:		New Balance:	$800.00

Encounter Form

DOCUMENT 199

Provider Information

Name:	Rockwell Emergency Medical Services
Address:	P.O. Box 221

City:	Rockwell	State:	RI	Zip Code:	02831
Telephone #:		Fax #:			
Medicare ID#:		UPIN #:			
Tax ID #:	55-5555555	Accepts Medicare Assignment:	☐		
Provider's Signature:	*Betty Biller*		Date: *7/21/CCYY*		

Patient Information

Name:	Renee Rubble
Address:	1234 Rufus Road

City:	Rockwell	State:	RI	Zip Code:	02845
Telephone #:	(401) 555-0284	Account #:	10097		
Date of Birth:	07/01/CCYY-16	Gender:	Female		
Marital Status:	Single	Relationship to Guarantor:		Child	
Student Status:	☒ Full-time	☐ Part-time			
Insurance Type:	☒ Pvt ☐ M/care ☐ M/caid ☐ WC ☐ Other _____				
Hospitalization Date:					
Hospital Information:	Rockwell Community Hospital, P.O. Box 900, Rockwell, RI 02831				

Appointment Information

Appointment Date:		Time:	
Next Appt. Date:		Time:	
Date of First Visit:		Date of Injury:	
Referring Physician:			

Guarantor Information

Name:	Ronny Rubble
Address:	1234 Rufus Road

City:	Rockwell	State:	RI	Zip Code:	02845
Insurance ID #:	00-0001 ABC				
Insurance Name:	Winter Insurance Company				
Insurance Group #:	36928				
Employer Name:	ABC Corporation				

Authorization

☒ Authorization to Release Information
☐ Authorization for Assignment of Benefits
☐ Authorization for Consent for Treatment
☐ My insurance will be billed but there may be a balance due.

Signature: *Ronny Rubble*   Date: *7/21/CCYY*

Clinical Information

	DOS	POS	CPT® /HCPCS Description	ICD-9-CM (*Indicates diagnosis for all lines)	Amount
1	07/21/CCYY	Ambulance	ALS-1, emergency	Respiratory Distress	$387.00
2					
3					
4					
5					
6					
Remarks:	Patient was transported from 1234 Rufus Road to Rockwell Hospital in an ambulance with advance life support.				
Previous Balance:		Payment:		Copay:		Adjustment:			
Total Fee:	$387.00	Cash ☐ Check ☐ Credit ☐	Cash ☐ Check ☐ Credit ☐	Remarks:		New Balance:	$387.00

Encounter Form

Provider Information

Name:	Robert Rotweiler, D.P.M.
Address:	622 E. Rivergrove

City:	Rockwell	State:	RI	Zip Code:	02831

Telephone #:		Fax #:	
Medicare ID#:		UPIN #:	T64003

Tax ID #:	55-5555777	Accepts Medicare Assignment:	☐

Provider's Signature:	*Robert Rotweiler, DPM*	Date: *7/2/CCYY*

Appointment Information

Appointment Date:		Time:	
Next Appt. Date:		Time:	
Date of First Visit:		Date of Injury:	
Referring Physician:			

Guarantor Information

Name:	Ronny Rubble
Address:	1234 Rufus Road

City:	Rockwell	State:	RI	Zip Code:	02845

Patient Information

Name:	Royal Rubble
Address:	1234 Rufus Road

City:	Rockwell	State:	RI	Zip Code:	02845

Telephone #:	(401) 555-0284	Account #:	10093

Date of Birth:	06/02/CCYY-18	Gender:	Male

Marital Status:	Single	Relationship to Guarantor:	Child

Student Status:	☒ Full-time	☐ Part-time	

Insurance Type:	☒ Pvt ☐ M/care ☐ M/caid ☐ WC ☐ Other _____

Hospitalization Date:	
Hospital Information:	Rockwell Community Hospital, P.O. Box 900, Rockwell, RI 02831

Insurance Information

Insurance ID #:	00-0001 ABC
Insurance Name:	Winter Insurance Company
Insurance Group #:	36928
Employer Name:	ABC Corporation

Authorization

☒ Authorization to Release Information
☒ Authorization for Assignment of Benefits
☐ Authorization for Consent for Treatment
☐ My insurance will be billed but there may be a balance due.

Signature: *Ronny Rubble*　　Date: *7/2/CCYY*

Clinical Information

	DOS	POS	CPT® /HCPCS Description	ICD-9-CM (*Indicates diagnosis for all lines)	Amount
1	07/02/CCYY	Otpt Hosp	Radial keratotomy	Degenerative Myopia	$1800.00
2					
3					
4					
5					
6					
Remarks:					

Previous Balance:		Payment:		Copay:		Adjustment:		
Total Fee:	$1800.00	Cash ☐ Check ☐ Credit ☐	Cash ☐ Check ☐ Credit ☐	Remarks:			New Balance:	$1800.00

Encounter Form

Provider Information

Name:	Rossman Medical Supply
Address:	2121 Rosemont Avenue

City:	Rockwell	State:	RI	Zip Code:	02831

Telephone #:		Fax #:	
Medicare ID#:		UPIN #:	

Tax ID #:	55-5555333	Accepts Medicare Assignment:	☒

Provider's Signature:	*Betty Biller*	Date: *8/1/CCYY*

Appointment Information

Appointment Date:		Time:	
Next Appt. Date:		Time:	
Date of First Visit:		Date of Injury:	
Referring Physician:			

Guarantor Information

Name:	Ronny Rubble
Address:	1234 Rufus Road

City:	Rockwell	State:	RI	Zip Code:	02845

Patient Information

Name:	Renee Rubble
Address:	1234 Rufus Road

City:	Rockwell	State:	RI	Zip Code:	02845

Telephone #:	(401) 555-0284	Account #:	10097

Date of Birth:	07/01/CCYY-16	Gender:	Female

Marital Status:	Single	Relationship to Guarantor:	Child

Student Status:	☒ Full-time	☐ Part-time	

Insurance Type:	☒ Pvt ☐ M/care ☐ M/caid ☐ WC ☐ Other _____

Hospitalization Date:	
Hospital Information:	

Insurance Information

Insurance ID #:	00-0001 ABC
Insurance Name:	Winter Insurance Company
Insurance Group #:	36928
Employer Name:	ABC Corporation

Authorization

☒ Authorization to Release Information
☒ Authorization for Assignment of Benefits
☐ Authorization for Consent for Treatment
☐ My insurance will be billed but there may be a balance due.

Signature: *Ronny Rubble*　　Date: *8/1/CCYY*

Clinical Information

	DOS	POS	CPT® /HCPCS Description	ICD-9-CM (*Indicates diagnosis for all lines)	Amount
1	8/1-8/31/CCYY	Home	Apnea monitor, without recording feature	Sleep Apnea	$175.00
2					
3					
4					
5					
6					
Remarks:	Ronald Rosales, M.D. UPIN #: L54478 prescribed an apnea monitor for patient.				

Previous Balance:	$387.00	Payment:		Copay:		Adjustment:		
Total Fee:	$175.00	Cash ☐ Check ☐ Credit ☐	Cash ☐ Check ☐ Credit ☐	Remarks:			New Balance:	$562.00

Miscellaneous Claims Beginning Financials

MINNETOMA FAMILY

Insurance Plan	Ball Insurance Carriers—XYZ Corporation				
Patient:	MILES*	MINDY	MONTY	MOREY	MELANIE
C/O DEDUCTIBLE	0.00	0.00	0.00	0.00	0.00
DEDUCTIBLE	0.00	0.00	25.00	0.00	115.00
COINSURANCE	0.00	0.00	0.00	0.00	0.00
ACCIDENT BENEFIT	0.00	0.00	0.00	0.00	0.00
LIFETIME MAXIMUM	0.00	0.00	29,621.70	0.00	3,721.62
M/N OFFICE VISITS					
OFFICE VISITS					
HOSPITAL VISITS					
DXL					
SURGERY					
ASSISTANT SURGERY					
ANESTHESIA					

Encounter Form

Provider Information

Name:	Michael Miller, D.P.M.
Address:	1750 South Mole
City:	Monte Mort　State: MN　Zip Code: 55634
Telephone #:	Fax #:
Medicare ID#:	UPIN #: T42301
Tax ID #:	31-3335777　Accepts Medicare Assignment: ☐
Provider's Signature:	*Michael Miller, DPM*　Date: 3/7/CCYY

Appointment Information

Appointment Date:	Time:
Next Appt. Date:	Time:
Date of First Visit:	Date of Injury:
Referring Physician:	

Guarantor Information

Name:	Miles Minnetoma
Address:	1800 Moonriver Drive
City:	Monte Mort　State: MN　Zip Code: 55621
Insurance ID #:	00-0002 XYZ
Insurance Name:	Ball Insurance Carriers
Insurance Group #:	62958
Employer Name:	XYZ Corporation

Patient Information

Name:	Monty Minnetoma
Address:	1800 Moonriver Drive
City:	Monte Mort　State: MN　Zip Code: 55621
Telephone #:	(507) 555-5562　Account #: 10099
Date of Birth:	11/04/CCYY-16　Gender: Male
Marital Status:	Single　Relationship to Guarantor: Child
Student Status:	☒ Full-time　☐ Part-time
Insurance Type:	☒ Pvt ☐ M/care ☐ M/caid ☐ WC ☐ Other _____
Hospitalization Date:	From: 03/06/CCYY　To: 03/09/CCYY
Hospital Information:	Monte Mort Hospital, P.O. Box 3000, Monte Mort, MN 55634

Authorization

☒ Authorization to Release Information
☐ Authorization for Assignment of Benefits
☐ Authorization for Consent for Treatment
☐ My insurance will be billed but there may be a balance due.

Signature: _Miles Minnetoma_　Date: 3/7/CCYY

Clinical Information

	DOS	POS	CPT® /HCPCS Description	ICD-9-CM (*Indicates diagnosis for all lines)	Amount
1	03/07/CCYY	Inpt Hosp	Capsulotomy; midfoot, extensive, tendon lengthening	Clubfoot	$2851.00
2					
3					
4					
5					
6					
Remarks:					
Previous Balance:		Payment:	Copay:	Adjustment:	
Total Fee:	$2851.00	Cash ☐ Check ☐ Credit ☐	Cash ☐ Check ☐ Credit ☐	Remarks:	New Balance: $2851.00

Encounter Form   DOCUMENT 204

Provider Information

Name:	Monte Mort Medical Supply
Address:	1289 Montrose Avenue
City:	Monte Mort State: MN Zip Code: 55662
Telephone #:	Fax #:
Medicare ID#:	UPIN #:
Tax ID #:	31-3335333 Accepts Medicare Assignment: ☐
Provider's Signature:	*Betty Biller* Date: 3/10/CCYY

Appointment Information

Appointment Date:	Time:
Next Appt. Date:	Time:
Date of First Visit:	Date of Injury:
Referring Physician:	

Guarantor Information

Name:	Miles Minnetoma
Address:	1800 Moonriver Drive
City: Monte Mort	State: MN Zip Code: 55621
Insurance ID #:	00-0002 XYZ
Insurance Name:	Ball Insurance Carriers
Insurance Group #:	62958
Employer Name:	XYZ Corporation

Patient Information

Name:	Monty Minnetoma
Address:	1800 Moonriver Drive
City:	Monte Mort State: MN Zip Code: 55621
Telephone #:	(507) 555-5562 Account #: 10099
Date of Birth:	11/04/CCYY-16 Gender: Male
Marital Status:	Single Relationship to Guarantor: Child
Student Status:	☒ Full-time ☐ Part-time
Insurance Type:	☒ Pvt ☐ M/care ☐ M/caid ☐ WC ☐ Other ____
Hospitalization Date:	
Hospital Information:	

Authorization

☒ Authorization to Release Information
☐ Authorization for Assignment of Benefits
☐ Authorization for Consent for Treatment
☐ My insurance will be billed but there may be a balance due.

Signature: *Miles Minnetoma*   Date: 3/10/CCYY

Clinical Information

	DOS	POS	CPT® /HCPCS Description	ICD-9-CM (*Indicates diagnosis for all lines)	Amount
1	03/10/CCYY	Office	AFO; single, upright w/ static stop; custom	Clubfoot	$397.00
2					
3					
4					
5					
6					

Remarks:	Marvin Moody, M.D. UPIN#: C33445 prescribed services for patient.
Previous Balance:	$2851.00 Payment: Copay: Adjustment:
Total Fee:	$397.00 Cash ☐ Check ☐ Credit ☐ Cash ☐ Check ☐ Credit ☐ Remarks: New Balance: $3248.00

Encounter Form   DOCUMENT 205

Provider Information

Name:	Monte Mort Medical Supply
Address:	1289 Montrose Avenue
City:	Monte Mort State: MN Zip Code: 55634
Telephone #:	Fax #:
Medicare ID#:	UPIN #:
Tax ID #:	31-3335333 Accepts Medicare Assignment: ☐
Provider's Signature:	*Betty biller* Date: 11/2/CCYY

Appointment Information

Appointment Date:	Time:
Next Appt. Date:	Time:
Date of First Visit:	Date of Injury:
Referring Physician:	

Guarantor Information

Name:	Miles Minnetoma
Address:	1800 Moonriver Drive
City: Monte Mort	State: MN Zip Code: 55621
Insurance ID #:	00-0002 XYZ
Insurance Name:	Ball Insurance Carriers
Insurance Group #:	62958
Employer Name:	XYZ Corporation

Patient Information

Name:	Melanie Minnetoma
Address:	1800 Moonriver Drive
City:	Monte Mort State: MN Zip Code: 55621
Telephone #:	(507) 555-5562 Account #: 10100
Date of Birth:	04/01/CCYY-18 Gender: Female
Marital Status:	Single Relationship to Guarantor: Child
Student Status:	☒ Full-time ☐ Part-time
Insurance Type:	☒ Pvt ☐ M/care ☐ M/caid ☐ WC ☐ Other ____
Hospitalization Date:	
Hospital Information:	

Authorization

☒ Authorization to Release Information
☐ Authorization for Assignment of Benefits
☐ Authorization for Consent for Treatment
☐ My insurance will be billed but there may be a balance due.

Signature: *Miles Minnetoma*   Date: 11/2/CCYY

Clinical Information

	DOS	POS	CPT® /HCPCS Description	ICD-9-CM (*Indicates diagnosis for all lines)	Amount
1	11/2-12/1/CCYY	Home	Nebulizer Rental, with compressor	Chronic Bronchitis	$127.50
2					
3					
4					
5					
6					

Remarks:	Marlene Moore, M.D. UPIN #: D44556 prescribed nebulizer.
Previous Balance:	Payment: Copay: Adjustment:
Total Fee:	$127.50 Cash ☐ Check ☐ Credit ☐ Cash ☐ Check ☐ Credit ☐ Remarks: New Balance: $127.50

Encounter Form

Provider Information

Name:	Molly Moline, M.D.				
Address:	2127 Moreno Avenue				
City:	Monte Mort	State:	MN	Zip Code:	55602
Telephone #:		Fax #:			
Medicare ID#:		UPIN #:	C40650		
Tax ID #:	31-3335999	Accepts Medicare Assignment:	☐		
Provider's Signature:	*Molly Moline, MD*		Date: *6/30/CCYY*		

Appointment Information

Appointment Date:		Time:	
Next Appt. Date:		Time:	
Date of First Visit:		Date of Injury:	
Referring Physician:			

Guarantor Information

Name:	Miles Minnetoma				
Address:	1800 Moonriver Drive				
City:	Monte Mort	State:	MN	Zip Code:	55621
Insurance ID #:	00-0002 XYZ				
Insurance Name:	Ball Insurance Carriers				
Insurance Group #:	62958				
Employer Name:	XYZ Corporation				

Patient Information

Name:	Morey Minnetoma				
Address:	1800 Moonriver Drive				
City:	Monte Mort	State:	MN	Zip Code:	55621
Telephone #:	(507) 555-5562	Account #:	10101		
Date of Birth:	07/01/CCYY-17	Gender:	Male		
Marital Status:	Single	Relationship to Guarantor:	Child		
Student Status:	☒ Full-time	☐ Part-time			
Insurance Type:	☒ Pvt ☐ M/care ☐ M/caid ☐ WC ☐ Other _____				
Hospitalization Date:					
Hospital Information:					

Authorization

☒ Authorization to Release Information
☒ Authorization for Assignment of Benefits
☐ Authorization for Consent for Treatment
☐ My insurance will be billed but there may be a balance due.

Signature: *Miles Minnetoma*   Date: *6/30/CCYY*

Clinical Information

	DOS	POS	CPT® /HCPCS Description	ICD-9-CM (*Indicates diagnosis for all lines)	Amount
1	06/30/CCYY	Office	Office visit, established patient, minimal	Bronchitis	$50.00
2					
3					
4					
5					
6					
Remarks:					
Previous Balance:		Payment:		Copay:		Adjustment:		
Total Fee:	$50.00	Cash ☐ Check ☐ Credit ☐	Cash ☐ Check ☐ Credit ☐	Remarks:	New Balance:	$50.00

Encounter Form

Provider Information

Name:	Monte Mort Ambulance				
Address:	212 Moffat Avenue				
City:	Monte Mort	State:	MN	Zip Code:	55602
Telephone #:		Fax #:			
Medicare ID#:		UPIN #:			
Tax ID #:	31-3335111	Accepts Medicare Assignment:	☐		
Provider's Signature:	*Betty Biller*		Date: *12/10/CCYY*		

Appointment Information

Appointment Date:		Time:	
Next Appt. Date:		Time:	
Date of First Visit:		Date of Injury:	
Referring Physician:			

Guarantor Information

Name:	Miles Minnetoma				
Address:	1800 Moonriver Drive				
City:	Monte Mort	State:	MN	Zip Code:	55621
Insurance ID #:	00-0002 XYZ				
Insurance Name:	Ball Insurance Carriers				
Insurance Group #:	62958				
Employer Name:	XYZ Corporation				

Patient Information

Name:	Melanie Minnetoma				
Address:	1800 Moonriver Drive				
City:	Monte Mort	State:	MN	Zip Code:	55621
Telephone #:	(507) 555-5562	Account #:	10100		
Date of Birth:	04/01/CCYY-18	Gender:	Female		
Marital Status:	Single	Relationship to Guarantor:	Child		
Student Status:	☒ Full-time	☐ Part-time			
Insurance Type:	☒ Pvt ☐ M/care ☐ M/caid ☐ WC ☐ Other _____				
Hospitalization Date:					
Hospital Information:	Monte Mort Hospital, P.O. Box 3000, Monte Mort, MN 55634				

Authorization

☒ Authorization to Release Information
☐ Authorization for Assignment of Benefits
☐ Authorization for Consent for Treatment
☐ My insurance will be billed but there may be a balance due.

Signature: *Miles Minnetoma*   Date: *12/10/CCYY*

Clinical Information

	DOS	POS	CPT® /HCPCS Description	ICD-9-CM (*Indicates diagnosis for all lines)	Amount
1	12/10/CCYY	Ambulance	BLS-emergency	Chronic Bronchitis	$242.50
2					
3					
4					
5					
6					
Remarks:	Patient was transported from 1800 Moonriver Drive to Monte Mort Hospital.				
Previous Balance:	$127.50	Payment:		Copay:		Adjustment:		
Total Fee:	$242.50	Cash ☐ Check ☐ Credit ☐	Cash ☐ Check ☐ Credit ☐	Remarks:	New Balance:	$370.00

Miscellaneous Claims Beginning Financials
TALAWAN FAMILY

Insurance Plan	Rover Insurers, Inc.—Ninja Enterprises				
Patient:	TIRON	TARA	TANYA	TABARI	TAURA
C/O DEDUCTIBLE	0.00	0.00	0.00	0.00	0.00
DEDUCTIBLE	0.00	0.00	10.50	15.00	150.00
COINSURANCE	875.00	0.00	0.00	0.00	962.17
ACCIDENT BENEFIT	0.00	0.00	0.00	0.00	0.00
LIFETIME MAXIMUM	12,027.62	1,276.47	625.16	2,291.19	9,472.13
M/N OFFICE VISITS					
OFFICE VISITS					
HOSPITAL VISITS					
DXL					
SURGERY					
ASSISTANT SURGERY					
ANESTHESIA					

Encounter Form

Provider Information

Name:	Tessa Tamsen, D.P.M.
Address:	404 Tadeo Street
City:	Turnville State: TN Zip Code: 37041
Telephone #:	Fax #:
Medicare ID#:	UPIN #: T34591
Tax ID #:	27-3219519 Accepts Medicare Assignment: ☐
Provider's Signature:	Tessa Tamsen, DPM Date: 2/14/CCYY

Appointment Information

Appointment Date:	Time:
Next Appt. Date:	Time:
Date of First Visit:	Date of Injury: 2/14/CCYY
Referring Physician:	

Guarantor Information

Name:	TiRon Talawan
Address:	426 Tata Street
City: Turnvillle	State: TN Zip Code: 37062
Insurance ID #:	00-0003 NIN
Insurance Name:	Rover Insurers, Inc.
Insurance Group #:	21088
Employer Name:	Ninja Enterprises

Patient Information

Name:	Taura Talawan
Address:	426 Tata Street
City:	Turnville State: TN Zip Code: 37062
Telephone #:	(423) 555-3706 Account #: 10102
Date of Birth:	06/04/CCYY-13 Gender: Female
Marital Status:	Single Relationship to Guarantor: Child
Student Status:	☒ Full-time ☐ Part-time
Insurance Type:	☒ Pvt ☐ M/care ☐ M/caid ☐ WC ☐ Other _____
Hospitalization Date:	From: 02/14/CCYY To:02/15/CCYY
Hospital Information:	Turnville Medical Center, P.O. Box 1700, Turnville, TN 37041

Authorization

☒ Authorization to Release Information
☒ Authorization for Assignment of Benefits
☐ Authorization for Consent for Treatment
☐ My insurance will be billed but there may be a balance due.

Signature: _TiRon Talawan_   Date: 2/14/CCYY

Clinical Information

	DOS	POS	CPT® /HCPCS Description	ICD-9-CM (*Indicates diagnosis for all lines)	Amount
1	02/14/CCYY	Inpt Hosp	Open treatment of talus fracture, w/ internal fixation	Fracture Foot, Open	$662.00
2					
3					
4					
5					
6					

Remarks:	Patient fell from jungle gym on the playground.				
Previous Balance:		Payment:	Copay:	Adjustment:	
Total Fee:	$662.00	Cash ☐ Check ☐ Credit ☐	Cash ☐ Check ☐ Credit ☐	Remarks:	New Balance: $662.00

Encounter Form · DOCUMENT 210

Provider Information

Name:	Turnville Ambulance Service
Address:	424 Taft Street
City:	Turnville	State: TN	Zip Code: 37021
Telephone #:		Fax #:
Medicare ID#:		UPIN #:
Tax ID #:	27-3211119	Accepts Medicare Assignment: ☐
Provider's Signature:	*Betty Biller*	Date: 4/11/CCYY

Appointment Information

Appointment Date:		Time:
Next Appt. Date:		Time:
Date of First Visit:		Date of Injury: 04/11/CCYY
Referring Physician:		

Guarantor Information

Name:	TiRon Talawan
Address:	426 Tata Street
City: Turnville	State: TN	Zip Code: 37062
Insurance ID #:	00-0003 NIN
Insurance Name:	Rover Insurers, Inc.
Insurance Group #:	21088
Employer Name:	Ninja Enterprises

Patient Information

Name:	Tabari Talawan
Address:	426 Tata Street
City:	Turnville	State: TN	Zip Code: 37062
Telephone #:	(423) 555-3706	Account #: 10103
Date of Birth:	03/10/CCYY-18	Gender: Male
Marital Status:	Single	Relationship to Guarantor: Child
Student Status:	☒ Full-time	☐ Part-time
Insurance Type:	☒ Pvt ☐ M/care ☐ M/caid ☐ WC ☐ Other
Hospitalization Date:	
Hospital Information:	Turnville Medical Center, P.O. Box 1700, Turnville, TN 37041

Authorization

☒ Authorization to Release Information
☐ Authorization for Assignment of Benefits
☐ Authorization for Consent for Treatment
☐ My insurance will be billed but there may be a balance due.
Signature: *TiRon Talawan*   Date: 4/11/CCYY

Clinical Information

	DOS	POS	CPT® /HCPCS Description	ICD-9-CM (*Indicates diagnosis for all lines)	Amount
1	04/11/CCYY	Ambulance	Ambulance service, basic life support, emergency	Unconsciousness	$497.00
2					
3					
4					
5					
6					

Remarks:	Patient was transported from 426 Tata Street to Turnville Medical Center.				
Previous Balance:		Payment:		Copay:	Adjustment:
Total Fee:	$497.00	Cash ☐ Check ☐ Credit ☐	Cash ☐ Check ☐ Credit ☐	Remarks:	New Balance: $497.00

Encounter Form · DOCUMENT 211

Provider Information

Name:	Turnville Medical Supply
Address:	6721 Taggert Street
City:	Turnville	State: TN	Zip Code: 37020
Telephone #:		Fax #:
Medicare ID#:		UPIN #:
Tax ID #:	27-3222229	Accepts Medicare Assignment: ☒
Provider's Signature:	*Betty Biller*	Date: 6/2/CCYY

Appointment Information

Appointment Date:		Time:
Next Appt. Date:		Time:
Date of First Visit:		Date of Injury:
Referring Physician:		

Guarantor Information

Name:	TiRon Talawan
Address:	426 Tata Street
City: Turnville	State: TN	Zip Code: 37062
Insurance ID #:	00-0003 NIN
Insurance Name:	Rover Insurers, Inc.
Insurance Group #:	21088
Employer Name:	Ninja Enterprises

Patient Information

Name:	Tabari Talawan
Address:	426 Tata Street
City:	Turnville	State: TN	Zip Code: 37062
Telephone #:	(423) 555-3706	Account #: 10103
Date of Birth:	03/10/CCYY-18	Gender: Male
Marital Status:	Single	Relationship to Guarantor: Child
Student Status:	☒ Full-time	☐ Part-time
Insurance Type:	☒ Pvt ☐ M/care ☐ M/caid ☐ WC ☐ Other
Hospitalization Date:	
Hospital Information:	

Authorization

☒ Authorization to Release Information
☐ Authorization for Assignment of Benefits
☐ Authorization for Consent for Treatment
☐ My insurance will be billed but there may be a balance due.
Signature: *TiRon Talawan*   Date: 6/2/CCYY

Clinical Information

	DOS	POS	CPT® /HCPCS Description	ICD-9-CM (*Indicates diagnosis for all lines)	Amount
1	06/02/CCYY	Home	Fully-reclining wheelchair, fixed full length arm,	Cerebral Palsy	$1324.00
2			Swing away, detachable, elevating leg rests		
3					
4					
5					
6					

Remarks:	Tiron Twang, M.D. UPIN #: G42112 prescribed a purchase of a juvenile wheelchair for patient.				
Previous Balance:	$497.00	Payment:		Copay:	Adjustment:
Total Fee:	$1324.00	Cash ☐ Check ☐ Credit ☐	Cash ☐ Check ☐ Credit ☐	Remarks:	New Balance: $1821.00

Encounter Form

Provider Information

Name:	Turnville Ambulance Service
Address:	424 Taft Street
City:	Turnville	State:	TN	Zip Code:	37201
Telephone #:		Fax #:	
Medicare ID#:		UPIN #:	
Tax ID #:	27-3211119	Accepts Medicare Assignment: ☐
Provider's Signature:	*Betty Biller*	Date: *2/14/CCYY*

Appointment Information

Appointment Date:		Time:	
Next Appt. Date:		Time:	
Date of First Visit:		Date of Injury: 02/14/CCYY
Referring Physician:	

Patient Information

Name:	Taura Talawan
Address:	426 Tata Street
City:	Turnville	State:	TN	Zip Code:	37062
Telephone #:	(423) 555-3706	Account #:	10102
Date of Birth:	06/04/CCYY-13	Gender:	Female
Marital Status:	Single	Relationship to Guarantor:	Child
Student Status:	☒ Full-time	☐ Part-time
Insurance Type:	☒ Pvt ☐ M/care ☐ M/caid ☐ WC ☐ Other _____
Hospitalization Date:	
Hospital Information:	Turnville Medical Center, P.O. Box 1700, Turnville, TN 37041

Guarantor Information

Name:	TiRon Talawan
Address:	426 Tata Street
City:	Turnville	State:	TN	Zip Code:	37062
Insurance ID #:	00-0003 NIN
Insurance Name:	Rover Insurers, Inc.
Insurance Group #:	21088
Employer Name:	Ninja Enterprises

Authorization

☒ Authorization to Release Information
☐ Authorization for Assignment of Benefits
☐ Authorization for Consent for Treatment
☐ My insurance will be billed but there may be a balance due.

Signature: *TiRon Talawan* Date: *2/14/CCYY*

Clinical Information

	DOS	POS	CPT® /HCPCS Description	ICD-9-CM (*Indicates diagnosis for all lines)	Amount
1	02/14/CCYY	Ambulance	Ambulance services, basic life support, non-emergency	Fracture Foot, Open	$376.00
2					
3					
4					
5					
6					

Remarks:	Patient fell from jungle gym on the playground.				
Previous Balance:	$662.00	Payment:		Copay:		Adjustment:		
Total Fee:	$376.00	Cash ☐ Check ☐ Credit ☐	Cash ☐ Check ☐ Credit ☐	Remarks:	New Balance:	$1038.00

Encounter Form

Provider Information

Name:	Ted Tagliari, D.P.M.
Address:	P.O. Box 8927
City:	Turnville	State:	TN	Zip Code:	37062
Telephone #:		Fax #:	
Medicare ID#:		UPIN #:	T58056
Tax ID #:	27-3333339	Accepts Medicare Assignment: ☒
Provider's Signature:	*Ted Tagliari, DPM*	Date: *10/7/CCYY*

Appointment Information

Appointment Date:		Time:	
Next Appt. Date:		Time:	
Date of First Visit:		Date of Injury:	
Referring Physician:	

Patient Information

Name:	TiRon Talawan
Address:	426 Tata Street
City:	Turnville	State:	TN	Zip Code:	37062
Telephone #:	(423) 555-3706	Account #:	10104
Date of Birth:	07/25/CCYY-45	Gender:	Male
Marital Status:	Married	Relationship to Guarantor:	Self
Student Status:	☐ Full-time	☐ Part-time
Insurance Type:	☒ Pvt ☐ M/care ☐ M/caid ☐ WC ☐ Other _____
Hospitalization Date:	From: 10/06/CCYY To: 10/08/CCYY
Hospital Information:	Turnville Medical Center, P.O. Box 1700, Turnville, TN 37041

Guarantor Information

Name:	TiRon Talawan
Address:	426 Tata Street
City:	Turnvillle	State:	TN	Zip Code:	37062
Insurance ID #:	00-0003 NIN
Insurance Name:	Rover Insurers, Inc.
Insurance Group #:	21088
Employer Name:	Ninja Enterprises

Authorization

☒ Authorization to Release Information
☒ Authorization for Assignment of Benefits
☐ Authorization for Consent for Treatment
☐ My insurance will be billed but there may be a balance due.

Signature: *TiRon Talawan* Date: *10/7/CCYY*

Clinical Information

	DOS	POS	CPT® /HCPCS Description	ICD-9-CM (*Indicates diagnosis for all lines)	Amount
1	10/07/CCYY	Inpt Hosp	Correction, hallux valgus, w/ sesamoidectomy;	Hallux Valgus	$850.00
2			simple exostectomy		
3					
4					
5					
6					

Remarks:	Second surgical procedure was performed by Terry Thomas, M.D. UPIN #: J33392				
Previous Balance:		Payment:		Copay:		Adjustment:		
Total Fee:	$850.00	Cash ☐ Check ☐ Credit ☐	Cash ☐ Check ☐ Credit ☐	Remarks:	New Balance:	$850.00

Health Claims Examining Exercises

(**Instructor's Note:** Medical Billing exercises in the entire text should be completed prior to students starting Health Claims Examining Exercise 11–A. New files should be set up for the Health Claims Examining exercises.)

Exercise **11-A**

Directions: Complete an Insurance Coverage Form (located in the **Forms** chapter) and set up Family Files for all families in this chapter. Refer to the Family Data Table **(Documents 193–195)**, located in the beginning of this chapter, and the Contracts located in the **Contracts, UCR Conversion Factor Report, and Relative Value Study** chapter.

Exercise **11-B**

Directions: Complete a Payment Worksheet (located in the **Forms** chapter) for CMS-1500 claims **(Documents 197–201, 203–207, and 209–213)** using the guidelines contained in the **Introduction** chapter and using the UCR Conversion Factor Report, Relative Value Study, and Contracts located in the **Contracts, UCR Conversion Factor Report, and Relative Value Study** chapter.

When processing claims, the Beginning Financials **(Documents 196, 202, and 208)** should be incorporated as payment history and claim calculations should be adjusted accordingly. Any carryover deductible listed should be included in the current year deductible for that individual. Therefore, in figuring current year deductible, students should be instructed to subtract the carryover deductible from the current year's amount.

Upon completion of each claim complete or update the Family Benefits Tracking Sheet (located in the **Forms** chapter) by compiling all of the claims payment data for the family.

12
Forms

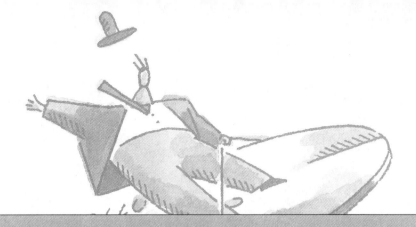

F ollowing are the forms you will need to complete the exercises in this text. Two copies of each of the forms have been included. While these forms are copyrighted by ICDC Publishing, Inc., purchase of this text allows you the right to copy these forms as needed to complete the exercises.

Patient Information Sheet

Ledger Card/Statement of Account

Insurance Coverage Form

Patient Receipt

Deposit Slip/Ticket

Insurance Claims Register

Insurance Tracer

Charge Slip

Treatment Authorization Request

Stationery (Any Billing Services)

Request for Additional Information Form

Payment Worksheet

Family Benefits Tracking Sheet

Coordination of Benefits Calculation Worksheet

Stationery (Any Insurance Carrier, Inc.)

Request for Additional Information Forms

ANY BILLING SERVICES
123 Any Way
Anytown, USA 12345
(123) 456-7890

PATIENT INFORMATION SHEET

INSURED'S INFORMATION

Patient Account #: _____ Assigned Provider: _____ Birth Date: _____

Name: (Last, First, Middle) _____ Gender: _____

Address: (include City, State, Zip) _____

Home Phone: _____ Marital Status: _____ Social Security #: _____

Employer Name: _____ Work Phone: _____

Employer Address: _____ Cell Phone: _____

Employment Status: _____ Referred by: _____

Allergies/Medical Conditions: _____ Email Address: _____

Primary Ins Policy: _____ Address: _____

Member's ID #: _____ Group Policy #: _____ Insured's Name: _____

Secondary Ins Policy: _____ Address: _____

Member's ID #: _____ Group Policy #: _____ Insured's Name: _____

SPOUSE'S INFORMATION

Patient Account #: _____ Assigned Provider: _____ Birth Date: _____

Name: (Last, First, Middle) _____ Gender: _____

Social Security #: _____ Employment Status: _____

Employer Name: _____ Work Phone: _____

Employer Address: _____

Allergies/Medical Conditions: _____

Primary Ins Policy: _____ Address: _____

Member's ID #: _____ Group Policy #: _____ Insured's Name: _____

Secondary Ins Policy: _____ Address: _____

Member's ID #: _____ Group Policy #: _____ Insured's Name: _____

CHILD #1

Patient Account #: _____ Assigned Provider: _____ Birth Date: _____

Name of Minor Child: _____ Social Security #: _____

Gender: _____ Marital Status: _____ Relationship to Insured: _____

Allergies/Medical Conditions: _____ Student Status: _____

Primary Ins Policy: _____ Insured's Name: _____

Secondary Ins Policy: _____ Insured's Name: _____

CHILD #2

Patient Account #: _____ Assigned Provider:_____ Birth Date:_____

Name of Minor Child: _____ Social Security #: _____

Gender: _____ Marital Status:_____ Relationship to Insured: _____

Allergies/Medical Conditions:_____ Student Status:_____

Primary Ins Policy: _____ Insured's Name: _____

Secondary Ins Policy: _____ Insured's Name: _____

CHILD #3

Patient Account #: _____ Assigned Provider: _____ Birth Date:_____

Name of Minor Child: _____ Social Security #: _____

Gender:_____ Marital Status:_____ Relationship to Insured: _____

Allergies/Medical Conditions:_____ Student Status:_____

Primary Ins Policy: _____ Insured's Name: _____

Secondary Ins Policy:_____ Insured's Name: _____

EMERGENCY CONTACT

Name:_____ Home Phone: _____Other Phone: _____

Address: (include City, State, Zip) _____

_____

(This Patient Information Sheet has been modified for usage with this text.)

ANY BILLING SERVICES
123 Any Way
Anytown, USA 12345
(123) 456-7890

PATIENT INFORMATION SHEET

INSURED'S INFORMATION

Patient Account #: _____ Assigned Provider: _____ Birth Date:_____

Name: (Last, First, Middle) _____ Gender: _____

Address: (include City, State, Zip)_____

Home Phone: _____ Marital Status:_____ Social Security #: _____

Employer Name: _____ Work Phone: _____

Employer Address: _____ Cell Phone: _____

Employment Status:_____ Referred by: _____

Allergies/Medical Conditions:_____ Email Address: _____

Primary Ins Policy: _____ Address: _____

Member's ID #:_____ Group Policy #: _____ Insured's Name:_____

Secondary Ins Policy:_____ Address: _____

Member's ID #:_____ Group Policy #:_____ Insured's Name: _____

SPOUSE'S INFORMATION

Patient Account #: _____ Assigned Provider: _____ Birth Date: _____

Name: (Last, First, Middle) _____ Gender: _____

Social Security #: _____ Employment Status:_____

Employer Name: _____ Work Phone: _____

Employer Address: _____

Allergies/Medical Conditions: _____

Primary Ins Policy: _____ Address: _____

Member's ID #: _____ Group Policy #: _____ Insured's Name: _____

Secondary Ins Policy: _____ Address: _____

Member's ID #: _____ Group Policy #:_____ Insured's Name: _____

CHILD #1

Patient Account #: _____ Assigned Provider: _____ Birth Date: _____

Name of Minor Child: _____ Social Security #: _____

Gender: _____ Marital Status: _____ Relationship to Insured: _____

Allergies/Medical Conditions: _____ Student Status: _____

Primary Ins Policy: _____ Insured's Name: _____

Secondary Ins Policy: _____ Insured's Name: _____

CHILD #2

Patient Account #: _____ Assigned Provider: _____ Birth Date: _____

Name of Minor Child: _____ Social Security #: _____

Gender: _____ Marital Status: _____ Relationship to Insured: _____

Allergies/Medical Conditions: _____ Student Status: _____

Primary Ins Policy: _____ Insured's Name: _____

Secondary Ins Policy: _____ Insured's Name: _____

CHILD #3

Patient Account #: _____ Assigned Provider: _____ Birth Date: _____

Name of Minor Child: _____ Social Security #: _____

Gender: _____ Marital Status: _____ Relationship to Insured: _____

Allergies/Medical Conditions: _____ Student Status: _____

Primary Ins Policy: _____ Insured's Name: _____

Secondary Ins Policy: _____ Insured's Name: _____

EMERGENCY CONTACT

Name: _____ Home Phone: _____Other Phone: _____

Address: (include City, State, Zip) _____

_____

(This Patient Information Sheet has been modified for usage with this text.)

ANY BILLING SERVICES
123 Any Way
Anytown, USA 12345
(123) 456-7890

Ledger Card/Statement of Account

RESPONSIBLE PARTY: _____

ADDRESS: _____

TELEPHONE #: _____

PATIENT NAME: _____ PATIENT ACCOUNT #: _____

SPECIAL NOTES: _____

_____

Date	Description of Service	Charge	Payments	Adjustments	Remaining Balance

ANY BILLING SERVICES
123 Any Way
Anytown, USA 12345
(123) 456-7890

Ledger Card/Statement of Account

RESPONSIBLE PARTY: _____

ADDRESS: _____

TELEPHONE #: _____

PATIENT NAME: _____ PATIENT ACCOUNT #: _____

SPECIAL NOTES: _____

_____

Date	Description of Service	Charge	Payments	Adjustments	Remaining Balance

ANY BILLING SERVICES
123 Any Way
Anytown, USA 12345
(123) 456-7890

Insurance Coverage Form

INSURED: _____ BIRTH DATE: _____

SSN: _____ EFFECTIVE DATE: _____

INSURANCE NAME: _____

ADDRESS: _____

ID/MEMBER #: _____ GROUP #: _____

DEPENDENT AGE LIMIT: _____

_____

INDIV. DEDUCTIBLE AMOUNT: _____ 3 MO CARRYOVER: _____

FAMILY DEDUCTIBLE: _____ AGGREGATE/NONAGGREGATE

STANDARD COINSURANCE: _____ LIFETIME MAXIMUM: _____

COINSURANCE LIMIT: _____

_____

BENEFITS PAID AT OTHER THAN THE STANDARD COINSURANCE % (Including benefit, coinsurance

amount and special circumstances, [SSO allowed at 100%, required for hysterectomy, coronary bypass, etc.]):

_____

_____

_____

PREAUTHORIZATION REQUIRED FOR: _____

_____

_____

ACCIDENT BENEFIT AMOUNT: _____ TREATMENT TO BE RECEIVED WITHIN _____ DAYS

OTHER NOTES/COMMENTS: _____

_____

Total Payments (CCYY)

Indicate below the name of the insured and his/her dependents. When any of the following information is received, write it in pencil followed by the date. This will help you to realize when a patient's deductible has been met and if he/she is nearing any maximum benefit.

	INSURED	DEPENDENT	DEPENDENT	DEPENDENT	DEPENDENT
NAME:	_____	_____	_____	_____	_____
DEDUCTIBLE:	_____	_____	_____	_____	_____
COINS PD:	_____	_____	_____	_____	_____
LIFETIME:	_____	_____	_____	_____	_____

ANY BILLING SERVICES
123 Any Way
Anytown, USA 12345
(123) 456-7890

Insurance Coverage Form

INSURED: _____ BIRTH DATE: _____

SSN: _____ EFFECTIVE DATE: _____

INSURANCE NAME: _____

ADDRESS: _____

ID/MEMBER #: _____ GROUP #: _____

DEPENDENT AGE LIMIT: _____

_____

INDIV. DEDUCTIBLE AMOUNT: _____ 3 MO CARRYOVER: _____

FAMILY DEDUCTIBLE: _____ AGGREGATE/NONAGGREGATE

STANDARD COINSURANCE: _____ LIFETIME MAXIMUM: _____

COINSURANCE LIMIT: _____

_____

BENEFITS PAID AT OTHER THAN THE STANDARD COINSURANCE % (Including benefit, coinsurance

amount and special circumstances, [SSO allowed at 100%, required for hysterectomy, coronary bypass, etc.]):

_____

_____

_____

PREAUTHORIZATION REQUIRED FOR: _____

_____

_____

ACCIDENT BENEFIT AMOUNT: _____ TREATMENT TO BE RECEIVED WITHIN _____ DAYS

OTHER NOTES/COMMENTS: _____

_____

Total Payments (CCYY)

Indicate below the name of the insured and his/her dependents. When any of the following information is received, write it in pencil followed by the date. This will help you to realize when a patient's deductible has been met and if he/she is nearing any maximum benefit.

	INSURED	DEPENDENT	DEPENDENT	DEPENDENT	DEPENDENT
NAME:	_____	_____	_____	_____	_____
DEDUCTIBLE:	_____	_____	_____	_____	_____
COINS PD:	_____	_____	_____	_____	_____
LIFETIME:	_____	_____	_____	_____	_____

PATIENT RECEIPTS

ANY BILLING SERVICE
123 Any Way
Anytown, USA 12345
(123) 456-7890

RECEIPT   Date _____ CC _____ No.

Received From _____

Address _____

_____ Dollars $ _____

For _____

ACCOUNT			HOW PAID			
AMT OF ACCOUNT			CASH			
AMT PAID			CHECK			
BALANCE DUE			MONEY ORDER			By _____

ANY BILLING SERVICE
123 Any Way
Anytown, USA 12345
(123) 456-7890

RECEIPT   Date _____ CC _____ No.

Received From _____

Address _____

_____ Dollars $ _____

For _____

ACCOUNT			HOW PAID			
AMT OF ACCOUNT			CASH			
AMT PAID			CHECK			
BALANCE DUE			MONEY ORDER			By _____

ANY BILLING SERVICE
123 Any Way
Anytown, USA 12345
(123) 456-7890

RECEIPT   Date _____ CC _____ No.

Received From _____

Address _____

_____ Dollars $ _____

For _____

ACCOUNT			HOW PAID			
AMT OF ACCOUNT			CASH			
AMT PAID			CHECK			
BALANCE DUE			MONEY ORDER			By _____

ANY BILLING SERVICE
123 Any Way
Anytown, USA 12345
(123) 456-7890

RECEIPT   Date _____ CC _____ No.

Received From _____

Address _____

_____ Dollars $ _____

For _____

ACCOUNT			HOW PAID			
AMT OF ACCOUNT			CASH			
AMT PAID			CHECK			
BALANCE DUE			MONEY ORDER			By _____

PATIENT RECEIPTS

Receipt 1

ANY BILLING SERVICE
123 Any Way
Anytown, USA 12345
(123) 456-7890

RECEIPT Date _____ CC _____ No.

Received From _____

Address _____

Dollars $ _____

For _____

ACCOUNT			HOW PAID		
AMT OF ACCOUNT			CASH		
AMT PAID			CHECK		
BALANCE DUE			MONEY ORDER		

By _____

Receipt 2

ANY BILLING SERVICE
123 Any Way
Anytown, USA 12345
(123) 456-7890

RECEIPT Date _____ CC _____ No.

Received From _____

Address _____

Dollars $ _____

For _____

ACCOUNT			HOW PAID		
AMT OF ACCOUNT			CASH		
AMT PAID			CHECK		
BALANCE DUE			MONEY ORDER		

By _____

Receipt 3

ANY BILLING SERVICE
123 Any Way
Anytown, USA 12345
(123) 456-7890

RECEIPT Date _____ CC _____ No.

Received From _____

Address _____

Dollars $ _____

For _____

ACCOUNT			HOW PAID		
AMT OF ACCOUNT			CASH		
AMT PAID			CHECK		
BALANCE DUE			MONEY ORDER		

By _____

Receipt 4

ANY BILLING SERVICE
123 Any Way
Anytown, USA 12345
(123) 456-7890

RECEIPT Date _____ CC _____ No.

Received From _____

Address _____

Dollars $ _____

For _____

ACCOUNT			HOW PAID		
AMT OF ACCOUNT			CASH		
AMT PAID			CHECK		
BALANCE DUE			MONEY ORDER		

By _____

DEPOSIT SLIP/TICKET

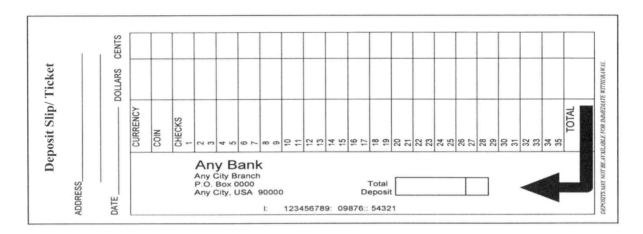

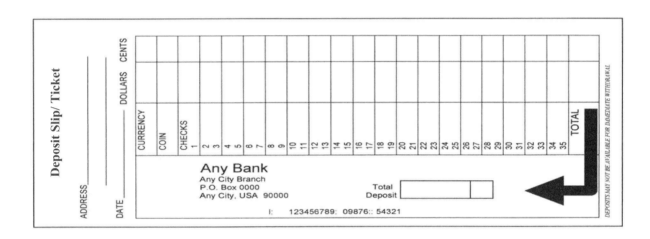

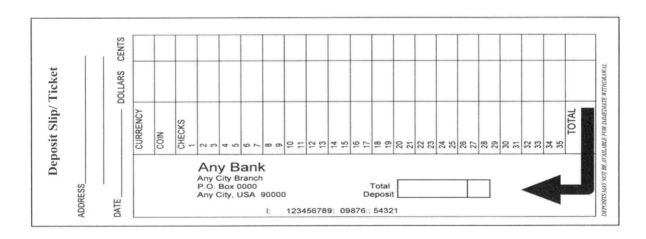

DEPOSIT SLIP/TICKET

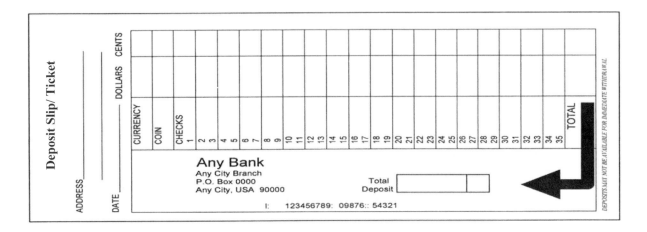

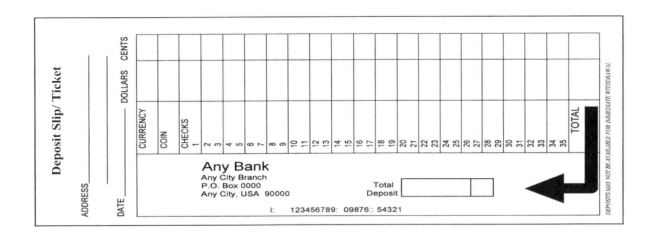

ANY BILLING SERVICES
123 Any Way
Anytown, USA 12345
(123) 456-7890

Insurance Claims Register

Page No. _____

Date Claims Filed	Patient Name	Name of Insurance Policy	Place Claim Sent	Claim Amount	Follow-Up Date	Paid Amount	Remaining Balance

ANY BILLING SERVICES
123 Any Way
Anytown, USA 12345
(123) 456-7890

Insurance Claims Register

Page No. _____

Date Claims Filed	Patient Name	Name of Insurance Policy	Place Claim Sent	Claim Amount	Follow-Up Date	Paid Amount	Remaining Balance

ANY BILLING SERVICES
123 Any Way
Anytown, USA 12345
(123) 456-7890

INSURANCE TRACER

Date: _____

Dear Insurance Carrier:

    We sent a claim to you over six weeks ago and have not heard back from you.
Patient:
Insured:
Address:
SSN/Birth Date:
Group Number:
Claim Amount:
Date Billed:
Date of Services:
Date of Illness or Injury:
Diagnosis:
Employer:
Address:

    Please supply the following information on the above named claim within ten days. Payment on this claim is overdue, and we would like to avoid involving the patient and the state insurance commissioner in a reimbursement complaint.

Claim pending because:_____

Payment in progress. Check will be mailed on:_____

Payment previously made. Date: _____

To whom: _____

Check #: _____ Payment Amount: _____

Claim denied. Reason: _____

Patient notified: Yes   No

Remarks: _____

Thank you for your assistance.

Completed by: _____

ANY BILLING SERVICES
123 Any Way
Anytown, USA 12345
(123) 456-7890

INSURANCE TRACER

Date: _____

Dear Insurance Carrier:

    We sent a claim to you over six weeks ago and have not heard back from you.
Patient:
Insured:
Address:
SSN/Birth Date:
Group Number:
Claim Amount:
Date Billed:
Date of Services:
Date of Illness or Injury:
Diagnosis:
Employer:
Address:

    Please supply the following information on the above named claim within ten days. Payment on this claim is overdue, and we would like to avoid involving the patient and the state insurance commissioner in a reimbursement complaint.

Claim pending because:_____

Payment in progress. Check will be mailed on:_____

Payment previously made. Date: _____

To whom: _____

Check #: _____ Payment Amount: _____

Claim denied. Reason: _____

Patient notified: Yes   No

Remarks: _____

Thank you for your assistance.

Completed by: _____

ANY BILLING SERVICES
123 Any Way
Anytown, USA 12345
(123) 456-7890

Charge Slip

Patient's Name: _____ Account/ID Number: _____

Patient's Address: _____

Phone Number: _____ Date of Service: _____

Provider's Name: _____ Provider's TIN: _____

Provider's Address: _____

X	Code	Description	Fee	X	Code	Description	Fee	X	Code	Description	Fee
Initial				**Established**				**Special Procedures**			
	99202	Expanded Exam	60.00		99211	Minimal Exam	35.00				
	99203	Detailed Low Complexity	100.00		99212	Brief Straightforward Exam	40.00				
	99204	Comp Moderate Complexity Exam	140.00		99213	Expanded Low Complexity Exam	45.00				
	99205	Comp High Complexity Exam	160.00		99214	Detailed Moderate Complexity Exam	60.00				
					99215	Comp High Complexity Exam	90.00				
Consultations				**Laboratory**				**Prescriptions**			
	99244	Comprehensive	150.00		36415	Venipuncture	20.00				
	99221	Straightforward Detailed Exam Inpatient Hospital	175.00		81000	Urinalysis	30.00				
	99301	Straightforward Detailed History & Exam Nursing Home	150.00		82948	Glucose Fingerstick	18.00				
					93000	EKG	55.00				

X	Code	Diagnosis	X	Code	Diagnosis	X	Code	Diagnosis
	466	Bronchitis, Acute		401	Hypertension		460	Upper Resp Tract Infection
	428	Congestive Heart Failure		414	Ischemic Heart Disease		599.0	Urinary Tract Infection
	431	CVA		724.2	Low Back Syndrome		616	Vaginitis
	250.0	Diabetes Mellitus		278.0	Obesity		490	Bronchitis
	625.3	Dysmenorrhea		715	Osteoarthritis		244	Acquired Hypothyroidism
	345	Epilepsy		462	Pharyngitis. Acute		**ICD-9**	**Other Diagnosis**
	0009.0	Gastroenteritis		714	Rheumatoid Arthritis			

Remarks/Special Instructions	New Appointment	Statement of Account	
		Old Balance	
		Today's Fee	
Referring Physician	Recall	Payment	
		New Balance	

CPT® codes, descriptions, and two digit numeric modifiers only are copyright American Medical Association. All Rights Reserved.

ANY BILLING SERVICES
123 Any Way
Anytown, USA 12345
(123) 456-7890

Charge Slip

Patient's Name: _____ Account/ID Number: _____

Patient's Address: _____

Phone Number: _____ Date of Service: _____

Provider's Name: _____ Provider's TIN: _____

Provider's Address: _____

X	Code	Description	Fee	X	Code	Description	Fee	X	Code	Description	Fee
Initial				**Established**				**Special Procedures**			
	99202	Expanded Exam	60.00		99211	Minimal Exam	35.00				
	99203	Detailed Low Complexity	100.00		99212	Brief Straightforward Exam	40.00				
	99204	Comp Moderate Complexity Exam	140.00		99213	Expanded Low Complexity Exam	45.00				
	99205	Comp High Complexity Exam	160.00		99214	Detailed Moderate Complexity Exam	60.00				
					99215	Comp High Complexity Exam	90.00				
Consultations				**Laboratory**				**Prescriptions**			
	99244	Comprehensive	150.00		36415	Venipuncture	20.00				
	99221	Straightforward Detailed Exam Inpatient Hospital	175.00		81000	Urinalysis	30.00				
	99301	Straightforward Detailed History & Exam Nursing Home	150.00		82948	Glucose Fingerstick	18.00				
					93000	EKG	55.00				

X	Code	Diagnosis	X	Code	Diagnosis	X	Code	Diagnosis
	466	Bronchitis, Acute		401	Hypertension		460	Upper Resp Tract Infection
	428	Congestive Heart Failure		414	Ischemic Heart Disease		599.0	Urinary Tract Infection
	431	CVA		724.2	Low Back Syndrome		616	Vaginitis
	250.0	Diabetes Mellitus		278.0	Obesity		490	Bronchitis
	625.3	Dysmenorrhea		715	Osteoarthritis		244	Acquired Hypothyroidism
	345	Epilepsy		462	Pharyngitis. Acute		**ICD-9**	**Other Diagnosis**
	0009.0	Gastroenteritis		714	Rheumatoid Arthritis			

Remarks/Special Instructions	**New Appointment**	**Statement of Account**	
		Old Balance	
		Today's Fee	
Referring Physician	Recall	Payment	
		New Balance	

ANY BILLING SERVICES
123 Any Way, Anytown, USA 12345
(123) 456-7890

TREATMENT AUTHORIZATION REQUEST

Verbal Control No.	Type of Service Requested ☐ ☐ Drug Other	Is Request Retroactive? ☐ ☐ YES NO	Is Patient Medicare Eligible? ☐ ☐ YES NO	Provider Phone No.	Patient's Authorized Representative (IF ANY) Enter name and address:

Provider Name and Address　　　　**Provider Number**

FOR STATE USE
Provider your request is:
☐ Approved as Requested
☐ Approved as Modified (items marked below as authorized may be claimed)
☐ Denied
☐ Deferred

By: _____
　　Medi-Cal Consultant

Name and Address of Patient
Patient Name (Last, First, MI)　　**Medicaid Identification Number**

Street Address　　**Gender**　**Age**　**Date of Birth** | |

City, State, Zip Code　　**Patient Status**
☐ Home　☐ Board & Care

Comments/Explanation
_____
_____
_____
_____
_____

Phone Number
☐ SNF/ICF　☐ Acute

Diagnosis Description　　**ICD-9-CM Diagnosis Code**

Medical Justification

Line No.	Authorized Yes	No	Approved Units	Specific Services Requested	Units of Service	NDC/UPC or Procedure Code	Quantity	Charges
1	☐	☐						
2	☐	☐						
3	☐	☐						
4	☐	☐						
5	☐	☐						
6	☐	☐						

To the best of my knowledge, the above information is true, accurate and complete, and the requested services are medically indicated and necessary to the health of the patient.

Authorization is valid for services provided

From　Date　　**To　Date**
| |　　| |

_____　_____　_____
Signature of Physician or Provider　Title　Date

Sequence Number

ANY BILLING SERVICES
123 Any Way, Anytown, USA 12345
(123) 456-7890

TREATMENT AUTHORIZATION REQUEST

Verbal Control No.	Type of Service Requested ☐ ☐ Drug Other	Is Request Retroactive? ☐ ☐ YES NO	Is Patient Medicare Eligible? ☐ ☐ YES NO	Provider Phone No.	Patient's Authorized Representative (IF ANY) Enter name and address:

Provider Name and Address	Provider Number	**FOR STATE USE** Provider your request is: ☐ Approved as Requested ☐ Approved as Modified (items marked below as authorized may be claimed) ☐ Denied ☐ Deferred
Name and Address of Patient Patient Name (Last, First, MI)	**Medicaid Identification Number**	
Street Address	**Gender Age Date of Birth**	By: _____ Medi-Cal Consultant
City, State, Zip Code	**Patient Status** ☐ Home ☐ Board & Care	**Comments/Explanation**
Phone Number	☐ SNF/ICF ☐ Acute	_____
Diagnosis Description	**ICD-9-CM Diagnosis Code**	_____
Medical Justification		_____
		_____

Line No.	Authorized Yes	No	Approved Units	Specific Services Requested	Units of Service	NDC/UPC or Procedure Code	Quantity	Charges
1	☐	☐						
2	☐	☐						
3	☐	☐						
4	☐	☐						
5	☐	☐						
6	☐	☐						

To the best of my knowledge, the above information is true, accurate and complete, and the requested services are medically indicated and necessary to the health of the patient.

_____ _____ _____
Signature of Physician or Provider   Title   Date

Authorization is valid for services provided

From Date	To Date
| |	| |

Sequence Number

ANY BILLING SERVICES
123 Any Way
Anytown, USA 12345
(123) 456-7890

Serving all your medical needs for 17 years

ANY BILLING SERVICES
123 Any Way
Anytown, USA 12345
(123) 456-7890

Serving all your medical needs for 17 years

ANY BILLING SERVICES
123 Any Way
Anytown, USA 12345
(123) 456-7890

Date: _____

Re: Policyholder: _____

Patient Account #: _____

Employee: _____

Dependent: _____

Dear _____ :

We need additional information from you.

We are writing to _____

_____

_____

_____

_____

_____

Please respond on the reverse of this letter or attach additional information or documentation. Thank you.

Sincerely yours,

ANY BILLING SERVICES
123 Any Way
Anytown, USA 12345
(123) 456-7890

Date: _____

Re: Policyholder: _____

Patient Account #: _____

Employee: _____

Dependent: _____

Dear _____ :

We need additional information from you.

We are writing to _____

_____

_____

_____

_____

_____

Please respond on the reverse of this letter or attach additional information or documentation. Thank you.

Sincerely yours,

ANY INSURANCE CARRIER, INC.
P.O. Box 1111, Anywhere, USA 12345 (123) 456-7890

Payment Worksheet

Eligible Employee:		**Accident Benefit:**	$	(CCYY)
Company:		**Lifetime Max:**	$	
Insured's ID Number:		**Deductible:**	$	(CCYY)
Patient:		**Carryover Ded:**	$	(CCNY)
Relationship:		**Coinsurance:**	$	(CCYY)
Provider's Zip Code:		**Date of Injury:**		

Procedure Type of Service	Dates of Service	Billed Amount	Excluded Amounts*	Allowed	Basic/ Accident 100%	Maj. Med. ___ %	___ %	UCR Calculations
1.		$	$	$	$			
2.								
3.								
4.								
5.								
6.								
⇩Remarks:	Totals:	$	$	$	$			
	Deductible:				$			
	Amount Subject to Coinsurance:				$			
	Coinsurance:				$			
	Amount Subject to Adjustment:				$			
	Adjustment (See Remarks):				$			
	Payment Amount:	$			$			

*Denial Reasons
1.
2.
3.
4.
5.
6.

Payees
1.
2.
3.
4.
5.
6.

If you disagree with our decision on your claim, you have the right by law to request that your claim be reviewed by your plan administrator. This request must be made in writing within 60 days of receipt of this notice. If you wish, you may submit your written comments and views. Please consult your plan's claim review procedures. See your employer regarding any other ERISA questions.

ANY INSURANCE CARRIER, INC.
P.O. Box 1111, Anywhere, USA 12345 (123) 456-7890

Payment Worksheet

Eligible Employee:		Accident Benefit:	$	(CCYY)
Company:		Lifetime Max:	$	
Insured's ID Number:		Deductible:	$	(CCYY)
Patient:		Carryover Ded:	$	(CCNY)
Relationship:		Coinsurance:	$	(CCYY)
Provider's Zip Code:		Date of Injury:		

Procedure Type of Service	Dates of Service	Billed Amount	Excluded Amounts*	Allowed	Basic/ Accident 100%	Maj. Med. ___%	___%	UCR Calculations
1.		$	$	$	$			
2.								
3.								
4.								
5.								
6.								
⇩Remarks:	Totals:	$	$	$	$			

Deductible:	$	
Amount Subject to Coinsurance:	$	
Coinsurance:	$	
Amount Subject to Adjustment:	$	
Adjustment (See Remarks):	$	
Payment Amount:	$	$

*Denial Reasons
1.
2.
3.
4.
5.
6.

Payees
1.
2.
3.
4.
5.
6.

If you disagree with our decision on your claim, you have the right by law to request that your claim be reviewed by your plan administrator. This request must be made in writing within 60 days of receipt of this notice. If you wish, you may submit your written comments and views. Please consult your plan's claim review procedures. See your employer regarding any other ERISA questions.

FAMILY BENEFITS TRACKING SHEET

FAMILY DEDUCTIBLE

Patient Name	Document #	Amount	Total

Contract: _____

Ind. Ded.: _____

Family Ded.: _____

Aggregate   Nonaggregate

Coins. Limit: _____

Family Coins. Limit: _____

Aggregate   Nonaggregate

	Individual Deductible		Coinsurance		Lifetime Maximum	
Document #	Amount	Total	Amount	Total	Amount	Total

Patient Name:

Prior C/O	------		-------		-------	

Patient Name:

Prior C/O	------		-------		-------	

Patient Name:

Prior C/O	------		-------		-------	

Patient Name:

Prior C/O	------		-------		-------	

FAMILY BENEFITS TRACKING SHEET

FAMILY DEDUCTIBLE

Patient Name	Document #	Amount	Total

Contract: _____

Ind. Ded.: _____

Family Ded.: _____

Aggregate   Nonaggregate

Coins. Limit: _____

Family Coins. Limit: _____

Aggregate   Nonaggregate

Document #	Individual Deductible		Coinsurance		Lifetime Maximum	
	Amount	Total	Amount	Total	Amount	Total

Patient Name:

Prior C/O	------		-------		-------	

Patient Name:

Prior C/O	------		-------		-------	

Patient Name:

Prior C/O	------		-------		-------	

Patient Name:

Prior C/O	------		-------		-------	

ANY INSURANCE CARRIER, INC.
P.O. Box 1111, Anywhere, USA 12345 (123) 456-7890

Coordination of Benefits Calculation Worksheet

Patient's Name: _____   Year: _____

Payment Calculation:

1. Total allowable amount for this claim is the higher of either the primary plan's
   allowable amount or the secondary plan's allowable amount.   _____

2. Total primary insurance carrier payment for this claim.   _____

3. Difference between Line 1 and Line 2.   _____

4. Secondary insurance carrier's normal liability for this claim.   _____

5. The lesser of Line 3 or Line 4.   _____
   This is the amount of the secondary insurance carrier actual payment on this claim.

Credit Reserve:

6. Normal liability for this claim (Line 4 above).   _____

7. Actual payment for this claim (line 5 above).   _____

8. Subtract Line 7 from Line 6.   _____

9. Credit reserve on all previous claims for this patient.   _____

10. Total credit reserve (add Line 8 and Line 9).   _____

Instructions:
Place the patient's name and the year that services were rendered in the box on the top of the COB calculation sheet.
1. Enter the total allowable amount on this claim. The total allowable amount is the greater of either the primary plan's allowable amount or the secondary plan's allowable amount.
2. Enter the total amount that other insurance companies have paid on this claim.
3. Subtract line 2 from line 1.
4. Enter the normal liability amount for this insurance company for this claim.
5. Enter the lesser of either Line 3 or Line 4. This is the actual amount of the secondary insurance payer on this claim.

To Calculate Credit Reserve:
6. Enter the normal liability amount for the secondary insurance carrier for this claim.
7. Enter the actual payment for the secondary insurance carrier for this claim.
8. Subtract Line 7 from Line 6. This is the amount of money the secondary carrier has saved by paying secondary on this claim. This amount becomes part of the credit reserve.
9. Enter the credit reserve amount for all previous claims for this patient.
10. Add Line 8 and Line 9. This is the total credit reserve for this patient.

ANY INSURANCE CARRIER, INC.
P.O. Box 1111, Anywhere, USA 12345 (123) 456-7890

Coordination of Benefits Calculation Worksheet

Patient's Name: _____   Year: _____

Payment Calculation:

1. Total allowable amount for this claim is the higher of either the primary plan's
   allowable amount or the secondary plan's allowable amount.   _____

2. Total primary insurance carrier payment for this claim.   _____

3. Difference between Line 1 and Line 2.   _____

4. Secondary insurance carrier's normal liability for this claim.   _____

5. The lesser of Line 3 or Line 4.
   This is the amount of the secondary insurance carrier actual payment on this claim.   _____

Credit Reserve:

6. Normal liability for this claim (Line 4 above).   _____

7. Actual payment for this claim (line 5 above).   _____

8. Subtract Line 7 from Line 6.   _____

9. Credit reserve on all previous claims for this patient.   _____

10. Total credit reserve (add Line 8 and Line 9).   _____

Instructions:
Place the patient's name and the year that services were rendered in the box on the top of the COB calculation sheet.
1. Enter the total allowable amount on this claim. The total allowable amount is the greater of either the primary plan's allowable amount or the secondary plan's allowable amount.
2. Enter the total amount that other insurance companies have paid on this claim.
3. Subtract line 2 from line 1.
4. Enter the normal liability amount for this insurance company for this claim.
5. Enter the lesser of either Line 3 or Line 4. This is the actual amount of the secondary insurance payer on this claim.

To Calculate Credit Reserve:
6. Enter the normal liability amount for the secondary insurance carrier for this claim.
7. Enter the actual payment for the secondary insurance carrier for this claim.
8. Subtract Line 7 from Line 6. This is the amount of money the secondary carrier has saved by paying secondary on this claim. This amount becomes part of the credit reserve.
9. Enter the credit reserve amount for all previous claims for this patient.
10. Add Line 8 and Line 9. This is the total credit reserve for this patient.

ANY INSURANCE CARRIER, INC.
P.O. Box 1111, Anywhere, USA 12345
(123) 456-7890

Serving all your medical needs for 17 years

ANY INSURANCE CARRIER, INC.
P.O. Box 1111, Anywhere, USA 12345
(123) 456-7890

Serving all your medical needs for 17 years

ANY INSURANCE CARRIER, INC.
P.O. Box 1111, Anywhere, USA 12345
(123) 456-7890

Claim No.: _____

Name: _____

Please refer to the paragraph checked below.

☐ Careful attention is being given to this claim. We will write you further about it in a short time.

☐ As you requested, we are returning the _____

☐ Please let us know whether this claimant has returned to work and, if so, when _____
  If not, does total disability still exist? _____ Will proofs of claim be submitted? _____
  Information as to the claimant's present condition will be appreciated.

☐ Please have the _____ statement completed and return the attached form to us.

☐ Consideration of further benefits can be given only after we receive the _____

_____

_____

☐ The attached furnished our first knowledge of this claim. Please arrange for
  submission of the required proofs of claim if this is properly covered under our insurance.

ANY INSURANCE CARRIER, INC.
P.O. Box 1111, Anywhere, USA 12345
(123) 456-7890

Claim No.: _____

Name: _____

Please refer to the paragraph checked below.

□ Careful attention is being given to this claim. We will write you further about it in a short time.

□ As you requested, we are returning the _____

□ Please let us know whether this claimant has returned to work and, if so, when _____
  If not, does total disability still exist? _____ Will proofs of claim be submitted? _____
  Information as to the claimant's present condition will be appreciated.

□ Please have the _____ statement completed and return the attached form to us.

□ Consideration of further benefits can be given only after we receive the _____

_____
_____

□ The attached furnished our first knowledge of this claim. Please arrange for
  submission of the required proofs of claim if this is properly covered under our insurance.

ANY INSURANCE CARRIER, INC.
P.O. Box 1111, Anywhere, USA 12345
(123) 456-7890

REQUEST FORM
☐ Medical   ☐ Dental

Please return requested information to: _____

☐ **First Request**   ☐ **Second Request**   ☐ **Third and Final Request**

Insured:_____   Date: _____

Patient: _____   Claim #:_____

BEFORE WE CAN PROCESS YOUR CLAIM, WE NEED THE ADDITIONAL INFORMATION CHECKED BELOW:

☐ Please complete in full the member portion of the claim form. Dental (employee section).

☐ Itemized Statements from: _____
_____

☐ Copies of other Insurance Payments from: _____
_____

☐ Full-time Student Eligibility Form Request: Please have the Registrar of the College or University that
_____ attends complete the attached Student Eligibility Form for the _____
Semester/Quarter.

☐ Other: _____

☐ THE FOLLOWING EXPENSES WILL BE HELD UNTIL THE ABOVE REQUESTED ITEMS ARE
RECEIVED IN THIS OFFICE _____

☐ We attempted on _____ to obtain the above necessary information to properly
process your claim. As of this date, it has not been received. The file will **now** be considered **closed**
until the information is received and proper evaluation can be given to your claim.

Thank you,

ANY INSURANCE CARRIER, INC.
P.O. Box 1111, Anywhere, USA 12345
(123) 456-7890

REQUEST FORM
☐ Medical ☐ Dental

Please return requested information to: _____

☐ **First Request**   ☐ **Second Request**   ☐ **Third and Final Request**

Insured: _____   Date: _____

Patient: _____   Claim #: _____

BEFORE WE CAN PROCESS YOUR CLAIM, WE NEED THE ADDITIONAL INFORMATION CHECKED BELOW:

☐ Please complete in full the member portion of the claim form. Dental (employee section).

☐ Itemized Statements from: _____
_____

☐ Copies of other Insurance Payments from: _____
_____

☐ Full-time Student Eligibility Form Request: Please have the Registrar of the College or University that
_____ attends complete the attached Student Eligibility Form for the _____
Semester/Quarter.

☐ Other: _____

☐ THE FOLLOWING EXPENSES WILL BE HELD UNTIL THE ABOVE REQUESTED ITEMS ARE
RECEIVED IN THIS OFFICE _____

☐ We attempted on _____ to obtain the above necessary information to properly
process your claim. As of this date, it has not been received. The file will **now** be considered **closed**
until the information is received and proper evaluation can be given to your claim.

Thank you,

13
Contracts, UCR & RVS

Following are the Contracts and other information you will need to complete the exercises in this text.

Contract 1—ABC Corporation/ Winter Insurance Company

Contract 2—Ninja Enterprises/ Rover Insurers, Inc.

Contract 3—XYZ Corporation/ Ball Insurance Carriers

UCR Conversion Factor Report

Relative Value Study

Assistant Surgeon Procedures Listing

Network Provider Listing

Contract 1 – ABC Corporation

WINTER INSURANCE CO, 9763 WESTERN WAY, WHITTIER, CO 82963, (970) 555-2963
POLICY: ABC Corporation, 1234 Whitaker Lane, Colter, CO 81222   EFFECTIVE DATE: 06/01/PY
INSURANCE GROUP # and SUFFIX: 54321/WHI
INSURANCE CONTACT:_____Wilma Williams_____   PHONE NUMBER:_____(970) 555-1234_____

ELIGIBILITY
EMPLOYEE: Must work a minimum of 35 hours per week. Is eligible for coverage the first of the month following 60 consecutive days of continuous employment.
DEPENDENTS: Are eligible for coverage from birth to age 19, or to age 24 if a full-time student or handicapped prior to age 19/24 (proof of disability must be furnished within 31 days after dependent reaches limiting age). Dependent is not eligible as a dependent if eligible as an employee. Unmarried natural children, legally adopted and foster children are included (also includes legal guardianship). If both parents are covered by the plan, children may be covered by one employee only.

EFFECTIVE DATE
EMPLOYEE: If written application is made prior to the eligibility date, coverage becomes effective the first of the month following 60 days of employment.
DEPENDENTS: The date acquired by the covered employee becomes the effective date if written application is made within 31 days of the eligibility date. Newborns are automatically covered for the first seven days following birth; well-baby charges excluded. Coverage will terminate after seven days unless written application for coverage is submitted by the employee within 31 days of birth.

TERMINATION OF COVERAGE
EMPLOYEE: Coverage terminates the last day of the month following termination of employment or when the employee ceases to qualify as an eligible employee, or following request for termination of coverage.
DEPENDENTS: Coverage terminates the date the employee's coverage terminates, or the last day of the month during which the dependent no longer qualifies as an eligible dependent.

EXTENSION OF BENEFITS - If covered under the plan when disabled, employee may continue coverage for 12 months following the date of termination or until no longer disabled, whichever is less.

COMPREHENSIVE MEDICAL BENEFITS

SUPPLEMENTAL ACCIDENT EXPENSE - 100% of first $300 for services incurred within 120 days of date of accident. Not subject to deductible.

PLAN BENEFITS
INDIVIDUAL CALENDAR YEAR DEDUCTIBLE: $100; three month carry-over provision.
FAMILY MAXIMUM DEDUCTIBLE: $200, aggregate.
STANDARD COINSURANCE: 90% except 100% of hospital room and board expenses for 365 days per lifetime.
COINSURANCE LIMIT: $750 out-of-pocket per individual; $1,500 out-of-pocket per family. Two separate members must satisfy the individual limit, not to include deductible. Applies only in the calendar year in which the limit is met.
LIFETIME MAXIMUM: $300,000 per person.
PRE-EXISTING LIMITATION: On 6/1/PY no restriction. After 6/1/PY, if treatment received within 90 days prior to effective date, no coverage for that condition for 12 months from the effective date (continuously covered for 12 months) unless treatment free for three consecutive months ending after the effective date of coverage.

X-RAY AND LABORATORY
REMARKS: Professional component charges covered at 40% of UCR allowance for procedure. Routine procedures are not covered.

INPATIENT HOSPITAL EXPENSE
Room and board payable at 100% of semi-private room rate. Miscellaneous expenses covered at 90%. Nonmedically necessary, well baby care and cosmetic services excluded. Personal comfort items not covered.

MENTAL/NERVOUS/PSYCHONEUROTIC
INCLUDES SUBSTANCE ABUSE AND ALCOHOLISM.
   OUTPATIENT MENTAL/NERVOUS TREAT-MENT
COINSURANCE: 50% while not hospital confined.
CALENDAR YEAR MAXIMUM: None.
   INPATIENT MENTAL/NERVOUS TREATMENT
PHYSICIAN SERVICES: Covered at 90%.
HOSPITAL SERVICES: Covered at 90%.
ALLOWED PROVIDERS: Psychiatrists and clinical psychologists. Marriage and Family Child Counselor and Licensed Clinical Social Worker allowed with referral from M.D.

EXTENDED CARE FACILITY
LIFETIME MAXIMUM: 60 days.
HOSPITAL SERVICES: 80% of billed room and board charge.
REQUIREMENTS: Stay must begin within 14 days of acute hospital stay of at least three days. Extended

care must be due to same disability that caused hospitalization and continued hospital care would otherwise be required.

DURABLE MEDICAL EQUIPMENT
COINSURANCE: Covered at 90%.
REQUIREMENTS: Must be prescribed by M.D. Must not be primarily necessary for exercise, environmental control, convenience, comfort, or hygiene. Must only be useful for the prescribed patient. Covered up to purchase price only.

ANESTHESIA
Computed using block time.

REMARKS: Covered expenses include charges for the initial set of contact lenses which are necessary due to cataract surgery. Handicapped children are limited to a $15,000 lifetime maximum after attainment of age 19. Coordination of Benefits according to National Association of Insurance Carriers (NAIC) guidelines. Subject to Third Party Liability and subrogation.

MEDICARE INTEGRATION
TYPE: Nonduplication of benefits applies.
REMARKS: Assume all Medicare benefits whether or not individual actually enrolled.

EXCLUSIONS
1. Expenses resulting from self-inflicted injuries, work related injuries, or illnesses.
2. Charges or services: in excess of UCR, not medically necessary, for completion of claim forms, for failure to keep appointments; for routine, preventative or experimental services.
3. Eye refractions; contacts or glasses; orthotics (eye exercises); radial keratotomy or other procedures for surgical correction of refractive errors.
4. Custodial care and/or convalescent facility coverage.
5. Cosmetic surgery unless for repair of an injury or surgery incurred while covered or result of mastectomy.
6. Diagnosis or treatment of infertility including artificial insemination, in vitro fertilization, etc., contraceptive materials or devices, non-therapeutic abortions except where the life of the mother is endangered, reversal of voluntary sterilization.
7. Pregnancy-related expenses for dependent children.
8. Expenses for obesity, weight reduction, or diet control unless at least 100 lbs. overweight.
9. Vitamins, food supplements, and/or protein supplements.
10. Sex altering treatments or surgeries or related studies.
11. Orthopedic shoes or other devices for support or treatment of feet except as medically necessary following foot surgery.
12. Bio-feedback related services or treatment, EDTA chelation therapy.

COMPREHENSIVE DENTAL BENEFITS

INTEGRATED: Deductible provisions, lifetime maximum and coinsurance limit combined with comprehensive Major Medical.
CALENDAR YEAR DEDUCTIBLE: $100.
DEDUCTIBLE CARRYOVER: No carryover.
FAMILY DEDUCTIBLE LIMIT: $200, aggregate.
COINSURANCE: 90%.
COINSURANCE LIMIT: $500 (Patient responsibility, not to include disallowed amounts or the deductible.)
APPLICATION OF COINSURANCE LIMIT: Applies only in the calendar year in which the limit is met.
FAMILY COINSURANCE LIMIT: $1,000.
MAXIMUM: $300,000 lifetime.
MAXIMUM PER CALENDAR YEAR: $1,500.
ORTHODONTIA ELIGIBILITY: Dependents only.
SPACE MAINTAINER ELIGIBILITY: Dependents only.
FLUORIDE ELIGIBILITY: Employees and dependents.
ORTHODONTIC: 90% coinsurance.
ORTHODONTIC MAXIMUM: $800 lifetime; not subject to the $1,500 calendar year maximum.
CLAIM COST CONTROL OPTIONS: Predetermination of benefits required on claims over $500; alternate course of treatment based on customarily employed method. Benefits cut to 50% if no pre-determination done.
PROSTHETIC REPLACEMENTS: Five-year rule applies to replacement of any previously installed prosthetics.
ORDERED AND UNDELIVERED: Excludes expenses for any devices installed or delivered after 30 days following termination date of insurance.
MISSING AND UNREPLACED EXCLUSION: Applies.
REMARKS: Orthodontic benefits are payable as incurred, rather than amortized over the period of time during which work is performed.

Contract 2 – Ninja Enterprises

ROVER INSURERS, INC.
5931 ROLLING ROAD
RONSON, CO 81369
(970) 555-1369

INSURANCE CONTACT: _____**Ravyn Ranger**_____   PHONE NUMBER: _____**(970) 555-0863**_____
POLICY: **NINJA ENTERPRISES, 1234 Nockout Road, Newton, NM 88012**   EFFECTIVE DATE: 01/01/PY
INSURANCE GROUP # AND SUFFIX: **21088/NIN**

ELIGIBILITY EMPLOYEES must work a minimum of 30 hours per week. They are eligible for coverage the first of the month following one consecutive month of continuous employment. DEPENDENTS are eligible for coverage from birth to age 19, or to age 25 if a full-time student or handicapped prior to age 19/25. Is not eligible as a dependent if eligible as an employee. Unmarried natural children, legally adopted children, foster children, and legal guardianship children are included. If both parents are covered by the plan, children may be covered by one parent only.

EFFECTIVE DATE - EMPLOYEE becomes effective, if written application is made prior to eligibility date, on the first of the month following 30 days of continuous employment. If employee is absent from work due to disability on the date of eligibility, coverage will not start until the first of the month following the date of return to active work.

DEPENDENTS become effective on the date the covered employee becomes effective, if written application is made within 31 days of eligibility date. If confined in a hospital on the date of eligibility, coverage will not start until the first of the month following the date the confinement ends. Newborns are automatically covered for the first 14 days following birth. Coverage terminates after 14 days unless written application for coverage is submitted by the employee within 31 days of birth.

TERMINATION OF COVERAGE - EMPLOYEE'S coverage terminates the last day of the month following termination of employment or when the employee ceases to qualify as an eligible employee, or following request for termination of coverage.

DEPENDENTS' coverage terminates the date the employee's coverage terminates, or the last day of the month during which the dependent no longer qualifies as an eligible dependent.

EXTENSION OF BENEFITS - If covered under the plan when disabled, may continue coverage in accordance with COBRA. No other extension available.

COMPREHENSIVE MEDICAL BENEFITS

PREADMISSION TESTING - Outpatient diagnostic tests performed prior to inpatient admissions are paid at 100% whether through a network provider or not.

PRECERTIFICATION - Voluntary, nonemergency inpatient admissions must be approved at least five days prior to admission. Emergency admissions must be precertified within 48 hrs. of admission. Benefits are reduced to 50% if not performed as required.

SECOND SURGICAL OPINION - The SSO is paid at 100% of UCR. It is required for the following: bunionectomy, cataract extraction, chemonucleolysis, cholecystectomy, coronary bypass, hemorrhoidectomy, hysterectomy, inguinal herniorrhaphy, laparotomy, laminectomy, mastectomy, meniscectomy, oophorectomy, prostatectomy, salpingectomy, submucous resection, total joint replacement (hip or knee), tenotomy, varicose veins (all procedures).
                              IF SSO NOT PERFORMED, ALL RELATED EXPENSES PAYABLE AT 50%.

SUPPLEMENTAL ACCIDENT EXPENSE - 100% is paid on the first $500 for services incurred within 90 days of the date of accident. Subject to $20 copayment. After $500, payments are subject to calendar year deductible. Provider does not have to be a network member to receive 100% benefit. Common accident provision applies.

OUTPATIENT FACILITY CHARGES PAYABLE AT 100% - Network outpatient facility expenses for following procedures paid 100%. Does not include professional charges: arthroscopy, breast biopsy, cataract removal, bronchoscopy, deviated nasal septum, pilonidal cyst, myringotomy w/tubes, esophagoscopy, colonoscopy, herniorrhaphy (umbilical, to five years old), skin and subsequent lesions, benign and malignant (2cms+).

INDIVIDUAL CALENDAR YEAR DEDUCTIBLE - $150; three month carryover provision. All plan services subject to deductible unless otherwise indicated.

FAMILY MAXIMUM DEDUCTIBLE - $300, nonaggregate. Two family members must meet individual deductible limit.

STANDARD COINSURANCE - 80% for Network providers; 60% for Non-network providers.

COINSURANCE LIMIT - $1,250 out-of-pocket per individual; $2,500 out-of-pocket per family. Two individuals must meet their individual out-of-pocket limit to satisfy the family limit. Limits not to include deductible, surgery expenses reduced because SSO not performed, or hospital benefits reduced because precertification not performed. 100% of allowed amount paid thereafter for network providers; 80% for non-network providers.

<u>LIFETIME MAXIMUM</u> - $1,000,000 per person.

<u>PRE-EXISTING LIMITATION</u> - If treatment is received within 90 days prior to effective date, no coverage on that condition for six months from the effective date (continuously covered for six consecutive months) unless treatment free for three consecutive months which ends after the effective date of coverage.

<u>INPATIENT HOSPITAL EXPENSE</u>   **IF NO PRECERTIFICATION, ADMISSION PAID AT 50%**

<u>DEDUCTIBLE</u> **- $200,** waived for network facilities, applies to non-network. Inpatient hospital expenses not subject to regular Major Medical deductible.

ROOM AND BOARD - Network providers: 80% of semi-private/ICU; Non-network providers: 60% of semi-private/ICU.

MISCELLANEOUS FEES - Network: 80%; Non-network: 60%.

EXCLUSIONS - Well baby care. Automatic coverage for first seven days if baby is ill. Otherwise, no coverage.

<u>MENTAL/NERVOUS/PSYCHONEUROTIC</u> - Includes substance abuse and alcoholism.

> <u>OUTPATIENT MENTAL AND NERVOUS TREATMENT</u>
>
> PAYABLE - $60 per visit for first 5 visits; $30 per visit for next 21 visits.
>
> COINSURANCE - 80% for first five visits (maximum payable: $60 per visit), 50% per visit for next 21 visits (maximum payable: $30 per visit).
>
> CALENDAR YEAR MAXIMUM - 26 visits.
>
> <u>INPATIENT MENTAL AND NERVOUS TREATMENT</u>
>
> PHYSICIAN SERVICES - 70% applies to network and non-network providers.
>
> HOSPITAL SERVICES - 70% network and non-network providers.

<u>MAMMOGRAMS</u>

COINSURANCE - 80% Network providers; 60% Non-network providers.

REQUIREMENTS - Baseline mammogram for women age 35–39; for ages 40–49, one allowed every two years; for ages 50+, one allowed every year.

<u>X-RAY AND LABORATORY</u> - PROFESSIONAL COMPONENTS - Professional charges paid at 25% of UCR.

<u>DURABLE MEDICAL EQUIPMENT</u>

COINSURANCE - 50%.

REQUIREMENTS - Prescribed by M.D.; must not be primarily necessary for exercise, environmental control, convenience, comfort or hygiene. Must be an article only useful for the prescribed patient. Covered up to purchase price only.

<u>ANESTHESIA:</u> Use actual time.

<u>MEDICARE</u>

TYPE - Maintenance of benefits.

REMARKS - Assume all Medicare benefits whether or not individual actually enrolled. Subject to all other plan provisions.

<u>EXCLUSIONS</u>

1. Expenses resulting from self-inflicted injuries.
2. Work-related injuries or illnesses.
3. Services for which there is no charge in the absence of insurance.
4. Charges or services in excess of UCR or not medically necessary.
5. Pre-existing conditions.
6. Charges for completion of claim forms and failure to keep appointments.
7. Routine or preventative or experimental services.
8. Eye refractions; contacts or glasses; orthotics (eye exercises); radial keratotomy or other procedures for surgical correction of refractive errors.
9. Custodial care.
10. Cosmetic surgery unless for repair of an injury or surgery incurred while covered or result of mastectomy.
11. Biofeedback related services or treatment.
12. Dental care of teeth, gums or alveolar process (TMJ) except: a) reduction of fractures of the jaw or facial bones; b) surgical correction of harelip, cleft palate or prognathism; c) removal of salivary duct stones; d) removal of bony cysts of jaw, torus palatinus, leukoplakia, or malignant tissues.
13. Reversal of voluntary sterilization.
14. Diagnosis or treatment of infertility including artificial insemination, in vitro fertilization, etc.
15. Contraceptive materials or devices.
16. Pregnancy; pregnancy-related expenses of dependent children for the delivery including Caesarian section. Related illnesses may be covered such as pre-eclampsia, vaginal bleeding, etc.
17. Non-therapeutic abortions except where the life of the mother is endangered.
18. Vitamins.

Contract 3 – XYZ Corporation

BALL INSURANCE CARRIERS　　　*(800) 555-5432*

3895 Bubble Blvd. Ste. 283, Boxwood, CO 85926　　　(970) 555-5432

INSURANCE CONTACT:　Betty Bell　　　PHONE NUMBER:　(970) 555-9876

Policy: **XYZ Corporation, 9817 Bobcat Blvd., Bastion, CO 81319**　　Insurance Group # and Suffix:　**62958/XYZ**

Basic/Major Medical Plan　　　Effective Date: 09/01/PY

ELIGIBILITY

EMPLOYEE: Must work a minimum of 30 hours per week. Is eligible for coverage the first of the month following three consecutive months of continuous employment.

DEPENDENTS: Are eligible for coverage from birth to age 19 or to age 23 if a full-time student or handicapped prior to age 19/23 (proof of disability must be furnished within 31 days after dependent reaches limiting age). Not eligible as a dependent if eligible as an employee. Unmarried natural children, legally adopted and foster children are included (includes legal guardianship). If both parents are covered by the plan, children may be covered by one employee only.

EFFECTIVE DATE

EMPLOYEE: If written application is made prior to eligibility date, coverage becomes effective the first of the month following three months of continuous employment.

DEPENDENTS: The date acquired by the covered employee becomes the effective date if written application is made within 31 days of eligibility date. If confined in a hospital on date of eligibility, coverage will not start until the first of the month following the date the confinement ends. Newborns are automatically covered for the first 30 days following birth. Coverage will be terminated after 30 days unless written application for coverage is submitted by the employee within 31 days of birth.

TERMINATION OF COVERAGE

EMPLOYEE: Coverage terminates the last day of the month following termination of employment, or when the employee ceases to qualify as an eligible employee, or following request for termination of coverage.

DEPENDENTS: Coverage terminates the date the employee's coverage terminates or the last day of the month during which the dependent no longer qualifies as an eligible dependent.

BASIC BENEFITS

PREADMISSION TESTING

Outpatient diagnostic tests performed prior to inpatient admissions; paid at 100% of UCR.

SUPPLEMENTAL ACCIDENT EXPENSE

100% of the first $300 for services incurred within 90 days of accident.

INPATIENT HOSPITAL EXPENSE

DEDUCTIBLE: $50.

ROOM AND BOARD: 100% Up to semi-private room charge. ICU up to $600 per day.

MISCELLANEOUS FEES: 100% Unlimited.

MAXIMUM PERIOD: Ten days per period of disability.

SURGERY

CONVERSION FACTOR: $8.50.

CALENDAR YEAR MAXIMUM: $1,600 per person.

REMARKS: Voluntary sterilizations covered.

ASSISTANT SURGERY

CONVERSION FACTOR: $8.50.

CALENDAR YEAR MAXIMUM ALLOWANCE: $320 per person. Maximum of 20% of surgeon's allowance or billed charge, whichever is less.

REMARKS: Voluntary sterilizations covered for women only.

IN-HOSPITAL PHYSICIANS

DAILY MAXIMUM: $21 for the first day; $8 per day thereafter.

MAXIMUM PERIOD: Ten days per period of disability.

REMARKS: Only one doctor can be paid per day.

ANESTHESIA

CONVERSION FACTOR: $7.50.

CALENDAR YEAR MAXIMUM: $300 per person.

REMARKS: Voluntary sterilizations covered.

OUTPATIENT PHYSICIANS VISITS

CONVERSION FACTOR: $7.50.

CALENDAR YEAR MAXIMUM: $300 per person.

REMARKS: Chiropractors, M.D.s, D.O.s and acupuncturists allowed.

X-RAY AND LABORATORY

CONVERSION FACTOR: $7.

CALENDAR YEAR MAXIMUM: $200 per person.

REMARKS: Professional component charges covered at 40% of UCR allowance for procedure. Routine procedures are not covered.

MAJOR MEDICAL EXPENSES

INDIVIDUAL CALENDAR YEAR DEDUCTIBLE: $125; three month carryover provision.

FAMILY MAXIMUM DEDUCTIBLE: Two family members must satisfy their individual calendar year deductible in order to satisfy the family deductible.

STANDARD COINSURANCE: 80%.

COINSURANCE LIMIT: $400 out-of-pocket per individual; $800 out-of-pocket per family (not to include deductible); aggregate.

APPLICATION OF COINSURANCE LIMIT: Coinsurance limit applies in the calendar year in which the limit is met and the following calendar year.

OUTPATIENT MENTAL/NERVOUS EXPENSE: 50% coinsurance while not a hospital inpatient.

LIFETIME MAXIMUM: $1,000,000 per person.

ROOM LIMIT: Semi-private room rate.

HOSPITAL DEDUCTIBLE: Not covered.

HOME HEALTH CARE: 120 visits per calendar year. Prior hospital confinement required.

PRE-EXISTING LIMITATION: If treatment received within six months prior to effective date, $2,000 maximum payment until patient has been covered continuously under the plan for 12 months.

ANESTHESIA: Calculated using actual time.

MEDICARE

TYPE: Coordination of Benefits.

REMARKS: Assume all Medicare benefits whether or not individual actually enrolled. Subject to all other plan provisions.

EXCLUSIONS

1. Expenses resulting from self-inflicted injuries.
2. Work-related injuries or illnesses.
3. Services for which there is no charge in the absence of insurance.
4. Charges or services in excess of UCR or not medically necessary.
5. Charges for completion of claim forms and failure to keep appointments.
6. Routine or preventative or experimental services.
7. Eye refractions; contacts or glasses; orthotics (eye exercises); radial keratotomy or other procedures for surgical correction of refractive errors.
8. Custodial care.
9. Cosmetic surgery unless for repair of an injury or surgery incurred while covered or result of mastectomy.
10. Dental care of teeth, gums or alveolar process (TMJ) except: a) reduction of fractures of the jaw or facial bones; b) surgical correction of harelip, cleft palate or prognathism; c) removal of salivary duct stones; d) removal of bony cysts of jaw, torus palatinus, leukoplakia, or malignant tissues.
11. Reversal of voluntary sterilization.
12. Diagnosis or treatment of infertility including artificial insemination, in vitro fertilization, etc.
13. Contraceptive materials or devices.
14. Non-therapeutic abortions except where the life of the mother is endangered.
15. Expenses for obesity, weight reduction, or diet control unless at least 100 lbs. overweight.
16. Vitamins, food supplements and/or protein supplements.
17. Sex-altering treatments or surgeries or related studies.
18. Orthopedic shoes or other devices for support or treatment of feet except as medically necessary following foot surgery.
19. Bio-feedback related services or treatment.
20. Experimental transplants.
21. EDTA Chelation therapy.

COMPREHENSIVE DENTAL BENEFITS

DEDUCTIBLE: $50.

FAMILY DEDUCTIBLE LIMIT: $150; nonaggregate. COINSURANCE: 80%.

MAXIMUM: No lifetime maximum. $1,000 per calendar year maximum.

SPACE MAINTAINER ELIGIBILITY: Employees and dependents.

FLUORIDE ELIGIBILITY: Dependents up to age 18 only.

ORTHODONTIA: No coverage.

CLAIM COST CONTROL: Predetermination of benefits and alternate course of treatment based on customarily employed methods.

PROSTHETIC REPLACEMENTS: Five-year replacement rule applies to replacements of any previously installed prosthetics.

ORDERED AND UNDELIVERED: Excludes expenses for any devices installed or delivered after 30 days following termination of insurance.

ORAL SURGERY: Covered at regular coinsurance rate, subject to calendar year maximum.

EXTENSION OF BENEFITS: 12 months.

MISSING AND UNREPLACED: Applies.

UCR Conversion Factor Report

The following list of UCR Conversion Factors is intended to be used for training and reference purposes only.

Zip	Area	Including Zip Codes	Surgery	Medicine	X-Ray & Lab	Anesthesia
006	Puerto Rico	006-009	35.58	31.13	26.68	22.14
010	Western & Southern Mass	010, 012-018, 025-027	40.40	35.35	30.30	27.10
011	Eastern Mass	011, 018, 020, 023, 024	40.68	35.59	30.51	29.37
021	Boston	021, 023	42.18	36.91	31.63	43.99
028	Rhode Island	028, 029	37.57	32.87	28.18	25.94
030	New Hampshire	030-038	32.16	28.14	24.12	34.57
039	Maine	039-049	31.01	27.13	23.26	31.34
050	Vermont	050-054, 056-059	29.49	25.80	22.11	20.17
060	No. CT incl. Hartford	060-062, 067	37.29	32.63	27.96	23.35
063	New Haven-New London Area	063, 064	38.26	33.48	28.70	31.24
065	Bridgeport & New Haven	065, 066	42.92	37.55	32.19	33.18
068	Stamford Norwalk Area incl. Darien & Greenwich	068, 069	47.70	41.73	25.77	26.21
070	Newark Suburbs incl. The Oranges, Montclair & Plainfield	070, 078, 079	46.92	41.06	35.19	41.06
071	Newark, Paterson & Trenton Suburbs	071, 075, 085	46.46	40.65	34.85	29.89
072	Elizabeth & Paterson Area	072, 074	45.24	39.59	33.93	31.89
073	Northeastern & Southern New Jersey	073, 076, 077, 083, 087	45.71	40.00	34.28	39.44
080	Southern NJ incl. Atlantic City	080-082, 084	41.70	36.49	31.27	35.63
086	Central NJ incl. Trenton	086, 088, 089	42.90	37.54	32.17	41.73
100	New York City	100-102	72.49	63.41	54.35	56.39
103	Staten Island & Brooklyn	103, 112	66.02	57.77	49.51	30.30

Zip	Area	Including Zip Codes	Surgery	Medicine	X-Ray & Lab	Anesthesia
104	Bronx, White Plains, Yonkers, New Rochelle	104, 106-108	62.50	54.69	46.87	37.84
105	Westchester County	105	57.68	50.47	43.26	37.76
109	Orange County, incl. Suffern	109, 126	57.06	49.92	42.79	51.42
110	Queens	110	63.60	55.65	47.70	41.49
111	Long Island	111, 113-119	64.62	56.54	48.46	47.27
120	Albany Area	120, 121	38.22	33.44	28.66	32.85
122	Kingston, Schenectady & Albany	122-124	39.47	34.54	28.60	27.74
125	Poughkeepsie, Monticello & N.E. NY	125, 127-129, 136	40.71	35.62	30.53	32.71
130	Syracuse, Utica Area	130-131, 133-134	34.17	29.90	25.63	30.86
132	Syracuse & Birmingham	132, 139	37.55	32.86	28.16	42.65
135	Northwestern NY incl. Niagara Falls & Elmira	135, 140-141, 143, 145, 149	33.91	29.67	25.43	26.08
137	Southwestern NY incl. Rochester	137-138, 144, 146-148	32.38	28.33	24.28	34.26
142	Buffalo	142	31.96	27.96	23.97	19.84
150	Pittsburgh Area	150, 151	39.09	34.21	29.32	25.25
152	Pittsburgh	152	38.69	33.85	29.01	38.24
153	Southwestern PA	153-158	36.76	32.16	27.57	25.25
159	Johnstown, Harrisburg, Allentown & Wilkes-Barre	159, 171, 181, 185, 187	39.97	34.97	29.98	39.50
160	Pennsylvania–Miscellaneous	160, 163-166, 169, 172, 177-179, 182-184, 188-189	37.95	33.21	28.46	33.77
162	Bradford, Wilsboro, York, Lancaster, Lehigh Valley	162, 167-168, 174-176, 180, 186	34.21	29.93	25.65	33.22

Zip	Area	Including Zip Codes	Surgery	Medicine	X-Ray & Lab	Anesthesia
170	Lancaster & Harrisburg	170, 173	33.90	29.66	25.42	35.03
190	Philadelphia Area	190	41.61	36.40	31.20	39.96
191	Philadelphia	191	46.24	40.46	34.68	44.80
193	Reading-Norristown	193-196	39.07	34.18	29.30	30.79
197	Delaware excl. Wilmington	197, 199	35.59	31.14	26.69	27.26
198	Wilmington	198	37.40	32.70	28.05	30.63
200	Washington DC	200, 207, 223	48.67	42.59	36.50	48.45
206	MD excl. Baltimore Area	206, 216-219	40.36	35.32	30.27	39.70
208	MD & VA Suburbs of Wash. DC	208, 209, 220-222	44.88	39.27	33.66	42.25
210	Baltimore Area	210, 211, 214	48.00	42.00	36.00	35.35
212	Baltimore	212	47.10	41.21	35.33	41.29
224	Virginia–Miscellaneous	224-229, 239, 242-246	30.46	26.65	22.84	33.18
230	Richmond Area	230-232	31.56	27.62	23.67	30.41
233	Norfolk, Newport News & Pt Smith	233-238	34.19	29.92	25.64	33.28
240	Roanoke & Area	240, 241	28.85	25.24	21.63	26.64
247	West Virginia–Miscellaneous	247-250, 252, 258-259, 262-264, 266-268, 215	33.95	29.70	25.46	32.88
251	Charleston Area	251, 253, 254, 256	35.27	30.86	26.45	31.56
255	Huntington, Wheeling, Parkesburg, Morgantown	255, 257, 260, 261, 265	32.94	28.82	24.70	31.14
270	Eastern North Carolina	270, 272-273, 280-281	28.35	24.81	21.26	29.79
271	Winston-Salem, Durham	271, 277	32.90	28.79	24.68	31.49

Zip	Area	Including Zip Codes	Surgery	Medicine	X-Ray & Lab	Anesthesia
274	Greensboro & Raleigh Area	274, 275	29.93	26.19	22.45	25.63
276	Raleigh	276	30.49	26.68	22.87	31.11
278	North Carolina	278-279, 285, 287-288	30.01	26.26	22.51	30.05
282	Charlotte	282	32.02	28.02	24.01	31.45
283	Fayetteville-Wilmington	283-284	29.35	25.68	22.01	21.30
286	Western North Carolina	286, 289	27.46	24.03	20.60	24.53
290	South Carolina–Miscellaneous	290-291, 293, 295-299	28.20	24.68	21.15	34.63
292	Columbia-Charleston Area	292, 294	29.80	26.07	22.35	28.40
300	Atlanta Area	300, 301	36.99	32.37	27.74	46.64
302	Atlanta	302, 303	38.86	34.00	29.14	47.43
304	Gainesville, Augusta, Savannah, Columbus Suburbs	304-305, 308, 313 315, 314, 316, 319	34.02	29.76	25.51	32.74
306	Augusta, Macon, Savannah, Columbus Cities	306-307, 309-310, 312, 314, 316, 319	36.86	32.25	27.64	38.73
320	Northern & West Central FL incl. Jacksonville & Ft. Myers	320, 323, 325, 338 339	35.95	31.46	26.96	43.69
322	Jacksonville & Gainesville Area	322, 326	37.72	33.01	28.29	41.83
327	St. Petersburg & Orlando Area	327, 337	37.04	32.41	27.78	45.31
328	Tampa & Orlando Cities	328, 329, 336	39.00	34.12	29.25	46.99
330	Miami Area	330-332	53.94	47.19	40.45	54.17
333	Ft. Lauderdale Area incl. West Palm Beach	333, 334, 349	44.63	39.05	33.47	51.72
335	Tampa Area	335, 342, 346	35.56	31.11	26.67	44.16

Zip	Area	Including Zip Codes	Surgery	Medicine	X-Ray & Lab	Anesthesia
350	Birmingham-Huntsville, Montgomery, Mobile	350-351, 358, 361-362, 366-367, 369	31.80	27.83	23.85	36.47
352	Birmingham	352	31.93	27.94	23.94	33.50
354	Alabama–Miscellaneous	354-357, 359-360, 363,-365, 368, 324	30.90	27.04	23.18	32.06
370	Nashville Area	370-371, 384-385	28.31	24.77	21.23	29.18
372	Nashville	372	29.75	26.03	22.31	30.93
373	Tennessee–Miscellaneous	373, 377, 378	26.18	22.91	19.63	30.83
374	Chattanooga	374, 376	29.08	25.45	21.18	35.21
379	Knoxville-Memphis Area	379-380, 382-383	27.43	24.00	20.57	51.34
381	Memphis	381	31.33	27.41	23.50	36.92
386	Mississippi–Miscellaneous	386-387, 389-390, 394-397	29.05	25.42	21.79	35.58
388	Jackson Area	388, 391-393	29.76	26.04	22.32	32.66
400	Kentucky–Miscellaneous	400-401, 403-404, 406-409, 413-418, 420-427	29.46	25.77	22.09	33.62
402	Louisville	402	31.39	27.47	23.54	39.18
405	Lexington Area	405, 410-412	31.44	27.51	23.58	33.90
430	Columbus-Marion Areas	430-431, 433, 457	30.35	26.56	22.76	28.89
432	Columbus Areas	432	34.11	29.85	25.58	34.72
434	Ohio–Miscellaneous	434-435, 437-438, 446, 448, 456	31.67	27.71	23.75	29.21
436	Toledo	436	32.63	28.55	24.47	30.12
439	Central Northeast Ohio Incl. Akron & Canton	439, 442-443, 447, 449, 458	32.89	28.78	24.67	39.83

Zip	Area	Including Zip Codes	Surgery	Medicine	X-Ray & Lab	Anesthesia
440	Cleveland Area, Youngstown	440, 445	33.89	29.65	25.42	37.46
441	Cleveland, Youngstown Area	441, 444	37.10	32.46	27.83	38.69
450	Cincinnati, Dayton, Springfield Area	450, 451, 453, 455	30.63	26.80	22.97	39.55
452	Cincinnati	452	33.34	29.17	25.00	34.56
454	Dayton	454	32.41	28.36	24.31	32.74
460	Northeast Indiana Area	460, 465-467, 469, 473	28.37	24.82	21.28	30.38
461	Indianapolis Area	461, 462	32.88	28.77	24.66	31.17
463	Gary-South Bend Area	463	32.75	28.77	24.56	30.29
468	Southwest IN excl. Washington, Incl. Ft. Wayne	468, 474, 477, 478	28.87	25.26	21.65	28.56
470	Southern Indiana incl. Lafayette	470-472, 475, 476, 479	27.87	24.39	20.90	30.13
480	Detroit	480-482, 485	36.63	32.05	27.47	31.41
483	Suburb Detroit, Flint & Grand Rapids incl. Iron Mount	483, 484, 491, 494, 499	28.77	25.17	21.57	26.22
486	Central & Northeast MI	486-489, 497	31.41	27.48	23.56	28.87
490	Western & Southern MI Incl. Grand Rapids	490, 492, 493, 495, 496, 498	30.72	26.88	23.04	28.41
500	Des Moines Area	500-502	26.82	23.47	20.11	23.18
503	Des Moines	503	29.27	25.61	21.95	34.22
504	Western Iowa & Cedar Rapids, Decorah	504, 505, 510-513, 521, 523	26.99	23.62	20.24	29.59
506	Southern Iowa excl. Des Moines	506-508, 520, 522, 524-528	28.89	25.28	21.66	36.70
530	Milwaukee Area	531, 531, 534	29.72	26.01	22.29	23.25

Zip	Area	Including Zip Codes	Surgery	Medicine	X-Ray & Lab	Anesthesia
532	Milwaukee	532	32.11	28.10	24.08	26.46
535	Madison-La Crosse-Oshkosh Area	535, 546, 549	29.22	25.57	21.92	25.56
537	North-South Central Wisconsin	537, 539, 544, 545	29.44	25.76	22.08	25.91
538	Wisconsin–Miscellaneous, Incl. Green Bay	538, 540-543, 547, 548	26.99	23.62	20.24	25.61
550	Minneapolis-St. Paul Area	550, 551, 553	26.42	23.12	19.81	29.46
554	Minneapolis-St. Paul	554	29.01	25.39	21.76	28.08
556	Minnesota–Miscellaneous	556, 560-567	26.93	23.48	20.12	25.53
557	Rochester Area	557-559	27.72	24.25	20.79	34.16
570	South Dakota	570-577	27.42	24.00	20.57	27.56
580	North Dakota	580-588	28.00	24.50	21.00	23.12
590	Montana	590-599	28.54	24.97	21.40	35.46
600	Chicago N & S Suburban Area	600, 605	42.66	37.32	31.99	46.09
601	Chicago Area	601-604, 464	41.84	36.61	31.38	45.27
606	Chicago	606	45.64	39.94	34.23	49.57
609	Northern Illinois	609, 611-613	30.13	26.36	22.60	37.41
610	Illinois–Miscellaneous	610, 614, 624, 626	28.86	25.25	21.65	30.73
615	Central & Southern Illinois	615-619, 623, 625, 627-629	31.64	27.69	23.73	33.16
630	St. Louis incl. East St. Louis	630, 620	32.80	28.70	24.60	36.89
631	St Louis incl. East St. Louis Area	631, 633, 622	34.91	30.55	26.18	41.98
634	Missouri – Miscellaneous, incl. Hannibal, Jefferson	634-635, 638, 644, 646-648, 650-651, 653-658	28.69	25.10	21.52	32.26

Zip	Area	Including Zip Codes	Surgery	Medicine	X-Ray & Lab	Anesthesia
636	Southern & Mid MO & St. Joseph	636-637, 639, 645, 652	28.33	24.79	21.25	32.99
640	Kansas City Area	640-641, 661-661	33.48	29.29	25.11	40.30
660	Kansa–Miscellaneous, incl. Topeka Area	660, 664-665, 667-671, 673-677, 679	28.15	24.63	21.11	32.93
666	Topeka-Wichita	666, 672, 678	28.64	25.06	21.48	38.34
680	Nebraska–Miscellaneous	680, 683-693	23.56	20.61	17.67	29.93
681	Omaha	681	26.22	22.95	19.67	34.40
700	New Orleans	700, 701	37.46	32.78	28.09	53.50
703	Louisiana–Miscellaneous	703, 710, 712-714	30.58	26.76	22.94	42.98
704	Baton Rouge Area	704-707	31.98	27.98	23.99	35.12
708	Baton Rouge, Shreveport	708, 711	31.67	27.71	23.75	42.25
716	Arkansas–Miscellaneous	716-720, 723-725, 727	27.62	24.17	20.71	24.73
721	Little Rock Area	721-722, 726, 728, 729	29.69	25.98	22.27	31.11
730	Oklahoma–Miscellaneous	730, 734-735, 737-740, 743-744, 747-748	29.30	25.64	21.98	34.05
731	Oklahoma City	731, 736	31.89	27.90	23.92	36.25
741	Tulsa and Area	741, 745, 746, 749	31.56	27.62	23.67	35.11
750	Dallas Area	750	36.92	32.31	27.69	47.77
751	Dallas-Ft. Worth Area	751, 760, 767	34.34	30.05	25.75	45.20
752	Dallas	752	38.93	34.07	29.20	52.54
753	Northeast Texas, Abilene & Midland Areas	753, 755, 757, 759, 769, 778, 796, 797	32.03	28.02	24.02	43.06

Zip	Area	Including Zip Codes	Surgery	Medicine	X-Ray & Lab	Anesthesia
754	Texas–Miscellaneous	754, 756, 758, 762, 764-766, 768, 771, 780-781, 789, 790, 792-793, 795	30.96	27.09	23.22	41.63
761	Ft. Worth, Houston & Corpus Christi Suburbs	761, 774, 776, 783	35.53	31.09	26.65	43.28
763	Amarillo, Wichita Falls & Conroe	763, 773, 791	33.61	29.41	25.20	41.62
770	Houston	770, 772, 775	40.60	35.52	30.45	42.66
777	Austin & Beaumont	777, 779, 787, 788	33.10	28.96	24.82	50.31
782	San Antonio, Corpus Christi	782, 784, 785	34.15	29.88	25.61	42.62
794	Lubbock-El Paso	794, 798, 799	32.18	28.16	24.14	60.46
800	Colorado–Miscellaneous	800, 804, 805, 807, 809, 810, 812-815	30.87	27.01	23.15	37.39
801	Denver, Colorado Springs, Alamosa, Glenwood Spring Areas	801-803, 806, 808, 811, 816	32.32	28.28	24.24	41.69
820	Wyoming	820, 822-831	28.30	24.77	21.23	28.45
832	Idaho	832-838	29.04	25.41	21.78	33.03
840	Utah excl. Ogden	840-843, 845-847	26.20	22.92	19.65	29.88
844	Ogden	844	24.46	21.41	18.35	29.10
850	Phoenix & Area	850, 852, 853, 864	35.55	31.10	26.66	41.73
855	Arizona–Miscellaneous	855-857, 859-860, 863, 865	33.14	28.99	24.85	40.94
870	New Mexico	870-875, 877-884	31.86	27.88	23.89	43.10
890	Reno & Area	890, 895, 897	34.38	30.08	25.78	49.11
891	Las Vegas & Area, Nathan	891	39.67	34.71	29.75	60.65
893	Nevada–Miscellaneous	893, 894, 898	30.46	26.65	22.85	41.55

Zip	Area	Including Zip Codes	Surgery	Medicine	X-Ray & Lab	Anesthesia
900	Downtown Los Angeles, Princeton, Sorlete, Backdoor, Brighton	900, 901	50.64	44.31	37.98	47.55
902	Inglewood, Pansy, Espana, Bell Gardens, Beverly Hills, Western Los Angeles, Huntington Beach, South Gate	902, 903	49.16	43.02	36.87	52.84
904	Santa Monica, Long Beach, Glendale, Eldorado, Shereville	904, 908, 912	45.18	39.53	33.89	47.94
905	Torrance & Long Beach Suburbs, Southern Los Angeles, Seattle, Santa View, S. Whittier, Montebello	905-907	42.83	37.48	32.12	46.02
910	Pasadena, Altadena, Glendora, Gardena, San Fernando, Bayport	910, 911	41.03	35.90	30.77	43.33
913	Northern Los Angeles Area, Canoga, Huntington Park	913-916	44.92	39.30	33.69	48.45
917	West Covina, Pomona, Ontario Area, Hacienda Heights	917	41.85	36.62	31.39	47.11
918	Alhambra, San Bernardino, Riverside	918, 923-925	37.55	32.85	28.16	47.14
920	San Diego & Area	920, 921	39.37	34.45	29.53	40.38
922	Palm Springs, Anaheim, Santa Ana, Bridle	922, 926-928	43.37	37.95	32.52	48.90
930	Ventura & Area	930, 933, 935	38.43	33.63	28.82	42.55
931	Santa Barbara, Fresno & Bakersfield	931-932, 934, 936-937	36.62	32.04	27.46	43.94
939	Salinas, San Rafael, Stockton, Santa Rosa	393, 949, 952, 954	36.39	31.84	27.29	43.41
940	San Francisco	940	39.54	34.59	29.65	46.71
941	San Francisco Bay Area	941, 944	40.86	35.75	30.65	46.29
943	Palo Alto, Berkeley, San Jose, & Sacramento Suburbs	943, 947, 951, 957	40.74	35.65	30.56	44.43
945	Oakland, Richmond & Suburbs of San Jose & Stockton	955, 956, 948, 950, 953	39.00	34.12	29.25	41.95
955	Sacramento & Northern California	955, 956, 958-961	33.87	29.64	25.40	39.97
967	Hawaii	967, 968	39.30	34.39	29.47	30.21
970	Portland & Western Oregon	970, 971, 974, 975	30.87	27.01	23.15	34.20

Zip	Area	Including Zip Codes	Surgery	Medicine	X-Ray & Lab	Anesthesia
972	Portland	972	31.74	27.77	23.80	35.54
973	Oregon–Miscellaneous	973, 976-979	28.94	25.32	21.70	34.45
980	Seattle, Tacoma & Area, Western	980-984	34.45	30.14	25.83	36.48
985	Washington excl. Seattle & Tacoma, Walla Walla	985, 986, 988-994	29.24	25.58	21.93	34.96
995	Alaska	995-999	36.72	32.13	27.54	49.12

Relative Value Study

The following list of Relative Value Study Units is to be used with the Health Claims Examining program. This listing is intended to be used for training and reference purposes only.

Relative Value Units

CPT®/HCPCS*	Description	Total RVUs	Follow-Up Days
00100	ANESTHESIA FOR INTEG SUSTEM – HEAD	5.00	–
00162	ANES FOR RADICAL SURGERY OF NOSE OR SINUSES	7.00	–
00170	ANESTHESIA FOR INTRAORAL PROCEDURE	5.00	–
00300	ANESTHESIA, INTEGUMENTARY SYSTEM	5.00	–
00600	ANESTHESIA FOR PROCEDURE ON CERVICAL	7.00	–
00740	ANESTHESIA FOR UPPER G.I. PROCEDURES	4.00	–
00790	ANESTHESIA FOR LAPAROSCOPIC PROCEDURE	6.00	–
00900	ANES FOR PROCEDURE ON PERINEAL INTEGUMENTARY	3.00	–
00902	PERINEUM, ANORECTAL PROCOEDURE	4.00	–
00910	ANESTHESIA FOR TRANSURETHRAL PROCEDURE	3.00	–
00955	VAGINAL DELIVERY CONT EPIDURAL ANALGESIC	5.00	–
01758	ANES EXCISION OF CYST – UPPER ARM	5.00	–
11044	CLEANSING TISSUE/MUSCLE/BONE	6.10	10
11050	TRIM SKIN LESION	0.86	–
11051	TRIM 2 TO 4 SKIN LESIONS	1.28	–
11052	TRIM OVER 4 SKIN LESIONS	1.38	–
11100	BIOPSY OF SKIN LESION	1.24	–
11101	BIOPSY, EACH ADDED LESION	0.65	–
11421	EXCISION BIOPSY VULVA	2.38	10
11641	EXCISION OF LESION	4.74	10
11740	DRAIN BLOOD FROM UNDER NAIL	0.83	–
11750	MATRIXECTOMY	4.16	10
11752	REMOVAL OF NAIL BED/FINGER TIP	5.84	10
11770	EXCISION CYST	11.16	90
13132	COMPLEX REPAIR	9.71	10
15574	EXCISION BIOPSY OF MANDIBLE LESION W/FLAP RECONSTRUCTION CHIN	16.39	90
15576	EXCISION BIOPSY LESION WITH FLAP RECONSTRUCTION	8.43	90
15580	CROSS FINGER FLAP	12.59	90
15952	EXCISION TROCHANTERIC PRESS ULCER	16.39	90
20205	DEEP MUSCLE BIOPSY	10.00	–
20525	REMOVAL OF FOREIGN BODY	6.09	10
20550	INJECTION TENDON SHEATH	1.66	–
20600	ARTHROCENTESIS AMALL JOINT	1.25	–
20605	ARTHROCENTESIS ELBOW	1.25	–
20615	TREATMENT OF BONE CYST	2.93	10

CPT®/HCPCS*	Description	Total RVUs	Follow-Up Days
24102	REMOVE ELBOW JOINT LINING	2.59	90
24105	EXCISION, OLECRANON BURSA	8.26	90
24110	EXCISION BONE CYST	16.86	90
24115	REMOVE/GRAFT BONE LESION	18.86	90
25620	OPEN TREATMENT INTERN FIX	17.30	90
25622	TREAT WRIST BONE FRACTURE	5.31	90
25660	TREAT WRIST DISLOCATION	6.95	90
25810	FUSION/GRAFT OF WRIST JOINT	25.83	90
27350	REMOVAL OF KNEE CAP	19.65	90
27355	REMOVE FEMUR LESION	16.72	90
27360	PARTIAL REMOVAL LEG BONE(S)	20.22	90
27365	RADICAL RESECTION FOR TUMOR	31.83	90
27370	INJECTION FOR KNEE X-RAY	1.70	90
27372	REMOVAL OF FOREIGN BODY	9.25	90
27385	REPAIR OF THIGH MUSCLE	18.38	90
27392	INCISION OF THIGH TENDONS	18.41	90
27500	TREATMENT OF THIGH FRACTIRE	12.14	90
27506	OPEN REDUC FEMORAL SHAFT	35.88	90
27520	TREAT KNEECAP FRACTURE	6.51	90
28250	REVISION OF FOOT FASCIA	11.20	90
28260	RELEASE OF MIDFOOR JOINT	13.08	90
28262	CAPSULOTOMY EXTENSIVE	26.92	90
28270	RELEASE OF FOOT CONTRACTURE	7.83	90
28280	FUSION OF TOES	7.84	90
28290	BUNIONECTOMY	11.98	90
28435	TREATMENT OF ANKLE FRACTURE	7.50	90
28445	OPEN TREATMENT OF TALLUS FX	20.02	90
28450	TREAT MIDFOOT FRACTURE, EACH	4.08	90
28456	REPAIR MIDFOOT FRACTURE	13.36	90
30120	REVISION OF NOSE	13.76	90
30125	REMOVAL OF NOSE LESION	13.77	90
30130	REMOVAL OF TURBINATE OF THE NOSE	7.01	90
30140	RESECTION, SUBMUCUOUS TURB, PART	7.01	90
30150	PARTIAL REMOVAL OF NOSE	18.40	90
30220	INSERT NASAL SEPTAL BUTTON	3.32	10
30300	REMOVAL OF F.B NOSE	1.58	10
30400	RECONSTRUCTION INTERN NOSE	14.00	90
30520	REPAIR OF NASAL SEPTUM	16.04	90
30540	REPAIR NASAL DEFECT	15.58	90
30580	REPAIR UPPER JAW FISTULA	14.02	90
30600	REPAIR MOUTH/NOSE FISTULA	10.53	90

CPT®/HCPCS*	Description	Total RVUs	Follow-Up Days
30620	RECONSTRUCTION INNER NOSE	17.17	90
30630	REPAIR NASAL SEPTUM DEFECT	13.16	90
30801	CAUTERIZATION INNER NOSE	1.62	90
31087	REMOVAL OF FRONTAL SINUS	25.15	90
31090	EXPLORATION ON SINUSES	31.70	90
31200	ETHMOIDECTOMY	13.23	90
31225	REMOVAL OF UPPER JAW	39.06	90
32800	REPAIR LUNG HERNIA THROUGH CHEST WALL	23.13	90
36262	REMOVAL INFUSTION PUMP	8.11	90
36415	VENIPUNCTURE	0.44	–
36430	BLOOD TRANSFUSION SERVICE	1.08	–
36450	EXCHANGE TRANSFUSION SERVICE	4.51	10
36471	INJECTION SOLUTION VEIN	2.03	10
36481	INSERTION OF CATHETER, VEIN	13.61	–
36821	ARTERY-VEIN FUSION	18.01	90
36822	INSERTION OF CANULA(S)	9.37	90
36832	REVISE ARTERY-VEIN FISTULA	23.97	90
36833	REVISION OF ARTERIOVENOUS FISTULA, W/THROMB. AUTO. GRAFT	23.97	90
37660	REVISION OF MAJOR VEIN	8.32	90
37700	REVISE LEG VEIN	11.26	90
37720	COMP STRIPPING VEIN	11.26	90
37760	REVISION OF LEG VEINS	6.07	90
37785	REVISE SECONDARY VARICOSITY	4.97	90
38100	REMOVAL OF SPLEEN, TOTAL	22.22	90
38101	REMOVAL OF SPLEEN, PARTIAL	22.89	90
38115	REPAIR OF RUPTURED SPLEEN	4.47	90
38200	INJECTION OF SPLEEN X-RAY	23.13	10
39501	REPAIR DIAPHRAGM LACERATION	26.18	90
39520	REPAIR HERNIA DIAPHRAGMATIC	25.54	90
39545	REVISION OF DIAPHRAGM	22.87	90
40808	BIOPSY VESTIBULE MOUTH	1.84	10
42821	TONSILLECTOMY	16.39	90
43234	ENDOSCOPY, UPPER G.I. SIMPLE	5.63	–
43453	DILATE ESOPHAGUS	3.29	–
43760	CHANGE GASTROSTOMY TUBE	1.97	–
43761	REPOSITION GASTROSTOMY TUBE	3.49	–
43800	RECONSTRUCTION OF PYLORUS	18.69	90
43825	GASTROJEJUNOSTOMY W/VAGOTOMY	26.02	90
43840	REPAIR OF SEOMACH LESION	21.03	90
43843	GASTRIC STAPLING	100.00	90

CPT®/HCPCS*	Description	Total RVUs	Follow-Up Days
43885	REVISE STOMACH PLACEMENT	20.21	90
44005	FREEING OF BOWEL ADHESION	21.24	90
45308	PROCTOSIGMOIDOSCOPY	3.42	–
45330	SIGMOIDOSCOPY	2.52	–
45333	SIGMOIDOSCOPY & POLYPECTOMY	4.91	–
45378	COLONOSCOPY	8.48	–
45380	COLONOSCOPY W/BIOPSY	9.49	–
46200	FISSUREECTOMY	7.35	90
46500	INJECTION INTO HEMMORHOIDS	2.00	10
46600	ANOSCOPY	0.85	–
46606	ANOSCOPY AND BIOPSY	1.28	–
47610	CHOLECYSTECTOMY	25.42	90
47630	REMOVE BILE DUCT STONE	12.01	90
47700	EXPLORATION OF BILE DUCTS	24.18	90
49500	REPAIR INGUINAL HERNIA	9.94	90
49540	REPAIR LUMBAR HERNIA	14.99	90
49550	REPAIR FEMORAL HERNIA	10.51	90
49560	HERNIA REPAIR ABDOMINAL	15.26	90
49565	REPAIR ABDOMINAL HERNIA	16.98	90
49570	REPAID EPIGASTRIC HERNIA	10.28	90
51800	CYSTOPLASTY	20.51	90
52204	CYSTOSCOPY	5.26	–
52240	CYSTO W/FULG OF LRG BLADDER	20.51	–
52250	CYSTOSCOPY & RADIOTRACER	8.05	–
52281	INTRA OP CYSTO W/DILATION	5.63	–
52340	CYSTOURETHROSCOPY	14.14	90
52400	CYSTOURETHROSCOPY	14.14	10
52500	REVISION OF BLADDER NECK	16.84	90
52510	DILATION PROSTATIC URETHRA	11.33	90
52601	PROSTATECTOMY (TURP)	25.86	90
52612	PROSTATECTOMY, FIRST STAGE	19.04	90
52614	PROSTATECTOMY, SECOND STAGE	14.56	90
53085	DRAINAGE OF PERINEAL URINARY EXTRA VASATION, COMPLICATED	25.86	90
53520	REPAIR OF URETHRAL DEFECT	15.46	90
53600	DILATION URETHRAL MALE	1.65	–
53620	DILATION OF URETHRAL STRICTURE BY FILIFORM AND FOLLOWER, MALE	2.26	–
53640	RELIVE BLADDER RETENTION	2.35	–
53660	DILATION OF URETHRA	1.05	–
56300	LAPAROSCOPY	15.97	–
56304	LAPAROSCOPY W/LYSIS	11.86	90

CPT®/HCPCS*	Description	Total RVUs	Follow-Up Days
57250	REPAIR RECTUM & VAGINA	15.26	90
57260	COLPORRHAPHY	19.09	90
57265	EXTENSIVE REPAIR OF VAGINA	20.21	90
57292	CONSTRUCT VAGINA WITH GRAFT	18.46	90
57330	REPAIR BLADDER-VAGINA LESION	21.88	90
57400	DILATION OF VAGINA, ANESTHESIA	1.27	–
57410	PELVIC EXAMINATION	1.05	–
57520	CONIZATION OF CERVIX	8.01	90
57530	TRACHELECTOMY	9.29	90
57540	REMOVAL OF RESIDUAL CERVIX	15.03	90
58120	DILATION AND CURETTAGE	6.03	10
58140	REMOVAL OF UTERUS LESION	18.58	90
58605	DIVISION OF FALLOPIAN TUBE	9.81	90
58611	TUBAL LIGATION IN C-SECTION	1.27	90
58615	OCCLUDE FALLOPIAN TUBE(S)	7.43	10
58660	LAPAROSCOPY WITH LYSIS OF ADHESIONS	11.86	30
58700	REMOVAL OF FALLOPIAN TUBE	14.29	90
58720	OOPHERECTOMY-SALPINGO	16.15	90
58740	REVISE FALLOPIAN TUBE(S)	16.60	90
59350	REPAIR OF UTERUS	9.81	–
59400	VAGINAL DELIVERY	26.10	90
59410	OBSTETRICAL CARE	14.13	90
59412	ANTEPARTUM MANIPULATION	3.39	90
59430	CARE AFTER DELIVERY	2.58	90
59510	C-SECTION – TOTAL OB CARE	34.41	90
59514	C-SECTION ONLY	22.30	90
59515	C-SECTION	22.30	90
59525	REMOVE UTERUS AFTER CESARIAN	11.84	90
59820	TREATMENT MISSED ABORTION	6.03	90
59821	TREATMENT, MISSED ABORTION 2ND TRIMESTER	6.03	90
61690	INTRACRANIAL VESSEL SURGERY	68.90	90
61700	INTRACRANIAL ANEURYSM	76.07	90
61703	CLAMP NECK ARTERY	32.38	90
62282	EPIDURAL INJECTION/INFUSION LUMBAR, SACRAL	0.35	–
63091	REMOVAL OF VERTEBRAL BODY	6.56	90
63170	LAMINECTOMY W/MYELOTOMY	42.50	90
63172	DRAINAGE OF SPINAL CYST	47.62	90
63180	REVISE SPINAL CORD LIGAMENTS	32.04	90
65771	RADIAL KERATOTOMY	16.59	90

CPT®/HCPCS*	Description	Total RVUs	Follow-Up Days
65772	CORRECTION OF ASTIGMATISM	10.75	90
65800	DRAINAGE OF EYE	3.93	–
66852	REMOVAL OF LENS MATERIAL	18.83	90
66920	INTRACAPSULAT EXT/LENS	21.29	90
66930	EXTRACTION OF LENS	21.93	90
67040	LASER TREATMENT OF RETINA	54.25	90
67105	REPAIR DETACHED RETINA	24.47	90
67107	PHOTOCOAGULATION	37.90	90
67112	RE-REPAIR DETACHED RETINA	35.32	90
69205	CLEAR OUTER EAR CANAL	2.44	10
69210	EAR LAVAGE	0.91	–
69220	CLEAN OUT MASTOID CAVITY	1.45	–
69400	INFLATE MIDDLE EAR CANAL	1.39	–
69620	REPAIR OF EARDRUM	18.80	90
69631	TYMPANOPLASTY	27.67	90
69632	REBUILD EARDRUM STRUCTURES	31.84	90
69641	REVISE MIDDLE EAR & MASTOID	33.50	90
70200	X-RAY EXAM OF EYE SOCKETS	0.84	–
70210	PARANASAL SINUSES	0.94	–
70220	X-RAY EXAM OF SINUSES	1.24	–
70250	X-RAY EXAM OF SKULL	0.67	–
70260	SKULL X-RAY	1.48	–
70300	X-RAY EXAM OF TEETH	0.44	–
71015	CHEST X-RAY	0.84	–
71020	CHEST X-RAY – 2 VIEWS	1.01	–
71023	CHEST X-RAY & FLUOROSCOPY	1.45	–
72050	X-RAY EXAM OF NECK & SPINE	1.30	–
72052	SPINE CERVICAL COMPLETE	1.76	–
72069	X-RAY EXAM OF TRUNK SPINE	0.53	–
73130	X-RAY EXAM OF HAND	0.85	–
73140	X-RAY FINGERS	0.65	–
73200	CAT SCAN OF ARM	7.01	–
74241	UPPER G.I. W/KUB	4.00	–
74246	CONTRAST X-RAY UPPER GI TRACT	2.87	–
74250	X-RAY EXAM OF SMALL BOWEL	2.14	–
76090	MAMMOGRAM, ONE BREAST	1.52	–
76091	MAMMOGRAPHY, BILATERAL	2.04	–
76092	MAMMOGRAM SCREENING	0.00	–
76096	X-RAY EXAM BREAST NODULE	4.36	–
76645	ECHO EXAM OF BREAST	2.00	–
76700	ABDOMEN ULTRASOUND	3.37	–

CPT®/HCPCS*	Description	Total RVUs	Follow-Up Days
76770	ULTRASOUND OF ABDOMEN BACK WALL	3.27	–
76830	ULTRASOUND, TRANSVAGINAL	2.74	–
76856	PELVIC ULTRASOUND	2.74	–
76870	ULTRASOUND OF SCROTUM	2.65	–
76872	ULTRASOUND OF PROSTATE	2.74	–
77300	BASIC RADIATION	2.74	–
77401	RADIATION TREATMENT	3.65	–
77402	RADIATION TREATMENT	6.84	–
77600	HYPERTHERMIA	9.25	10
78201	LIVER IMAGING	7.69	–
78700	KIDNEY IMAGING	7.83	–
78810	TUMOR IMAGING	6.95	–
80048	BASIC METABOLIC PANEL	2.60	–
80049	BASIC METABOLIC PANEL	0.26	–
80050	GENERAL HEALTH PANEL	3.40	–
80051	ELECTROLYTE PANEL	1.98	–
80054	COMPREHENSIVE METABOLIC PANEL	2.60	–
80055	OBSTETRIC PANEL	1.05	–
80058	HEPATIC PANEL	0.62	–
80059	HEPATITIS PANEL	0.56	–
80061	LIPID PROFILE	0.49	–
80076	HEPATIC PANEL	0.62	–
80091	THYROID PANEL	0.60	–
80418	THYROID PANEL	0.60	–
81000	URINALYSIS	1.00	–
81002	URINALYSIS WITHOUT SCOPE	0.74	–
82105	AFP TEST	BR	–
82145	ASSAY OF AMPHETAMINES	0.23	–
82150	AMYLASE	0.14	–
82310	CALCIUM	0.48	–
82465	CHOLESTEROL	0.33	–
82550	CPK	0.40	–
82800	ABG, PH ONLY	0.62	–
82805	BLOOD GASES, OXYGEN SATURATION	4.00	–
82947	BODY FLUID GLUCOSE	0.45	–
82948	BLOOD GLUCOSE	0.55	–
83540	IRON	4.75	–
83615	LDH, LACTIC ACID	0.10	–
84403	RIA ASSAY BLOOD TESTOSTERONE	1.48	–
84436	THYROXINE TOTAL	1.00	–
84437	ASSAY NEONATAL THYROXINE	1.38	–

CPT®/HCPCS*	Description	Total RVUs	Follow-Up Days
84479	THYROID TEST	0.60	–
85007	HEMATOCRIT, PLATELETS, DIFF	0.50	–
85018	HOMOGLOBIN, COLORIMETRIC	0.86	–
85022	CBC	1.00	–
85025	CBS W/DIFFERENTIAL	1.00	–
85027	CBC W/PLATELET COUNT	1.00	–
85031	MANUAL HEMOGRAM, COMPLETE CBC	1.24	–
86243	FC REPORTER ASSAY	1.00	–
86255	FLUORESCENT ANTIBODY, SCREEN	1.23	–
86287	HEPATITIS B	2.45	–
86590	STREPT-A TEST	0.18	–
86901	BLOOD TYPING & RH	0.47	–
87045	STOOL CULTURE FOR BACTERIA	0.34	–
87060	STREPT-A TEST	0.18	–
87070	CULTURE OTHER THAN URINE, BLOOD OR STOOL	2.40	–
87076	BACTERIA IDENTIFICATION	1.79	–
87184	SENSITIVITY, DISKMETH – 12 OR LESS	1.60	–
87197	BACTERICIDAL LEVEL, SERUM	0.78	–
87205	GRAM STAIN	0.60	–
87340	HEPATITIS B TEST	2.45	–
88150	PAP	1.00	–
88155	PAP W/INDEX	1.50	–
88160	CYTOPATHOLOGY	1.55	–
88300	TISSUE EXAM	1.65	–
88304	GROSS AND MICRO SPECIMEN	1.69	–
88305	PATHOLOGICAL TISSUE EXAM	1.69	–
90780	IV INFUSION, 1 HOUR	1.27	–
90782	INJECTION, THERAPEUTIC, SUBCUTANEOUS OR INTRAMUSCULAR	0.11	–
90788	INJECTION ANTIBIOTIC, INTRAMUSCULAR	0.12	–
90804	INDIVIDUAL PSYCHOTHERAPY	1.79	–
90806	INDIVIDUAL PSYCHOTHERAPY	2.58	–
90835	SPECIAL INTERVIEW	4.25	–
90845	MEDICAL PSYCHOANALYSIS	2.04	–
90853	SPECIAL GROUP THERAPY	0.72	–
90855	PSYCHOTHERAPY	2.38	–
90862	MEDICATION MANAGEMENT	2.56	–
90904	BIOFEEDBACK, BLOOD PRESSURE	1.62	–
92002	EYE EXAM, NEW PATIENT	1.60	–
92004	OPTHALMOLOGY EXAM, NEW PATIENT	2.33	–
92012	OPTHALMOLOGY EXAM	1.34	–
92014	OPTHALMOLOGY EXAM NEW REFRACT	1.71	–

CPT®/HCPCS*	Description	Total RVUs	Follow-Up Days
92015	DETERMINE REFRACTIVE STATE	1.45	–
92020	SPECIAL EYE EVALUATION	0.38	–
92070	FITTING OF CONTACT LENS	2.07	–
92083	VISUAL FIELD	1.46	–
92100	SERIAL TONOMETRY EXAM(S)	0.71	–
92960	HEART ELECTROCONVERSION	5.13	–
92990	REVISION OF PULMONARY VALVE	27.96	90
93000	EKG WITH INTERPRETATION	0.83	–
93005	EKG TRACING	0.48	–
93012	TRANSMISSION OF ECG	0.23	–
93015	TREADMILL	3.18	–
93024	CARDIAC DRUG STRESS TEST	3.98	–
93222	VECTORCARDIOGRAM REPORT	0.77	–
93224	HOLTER MONITOR – 24	5.02	–
93226	HOLTER MONITOR – 24/REPORT	2.22	–
93510	HEART CATHETERIZATION	49.46	–
93527	HEART CATH R&L	53.69	–
93545	INJECTION FOR CORONARY X-RAYS	3.89	–
93979	VISCERAL VASCULAR STUDY	4.26	–
94010	PULMONARY SPIROMETRY	0.93	–
94060	EVALUATION OF WHEEZING	1.69	–
94400	CO2 RESPONSE CURVE	1.30	–
94620	PULMONARY STRESS TESTING	3.12	–
96100	PSYCH TESTING (PER HOUR)	1.98	–
96900	ULTRAVIOLET LIGHT THERAPY	0.43	–
97018	PARAFFIN BATH THERAPY	0.53	–
97022	WHIRLPOOL THERAPY	0.40	–
97024	OV W/DIATHERMY	0.42	–
97026	INFRARED THERAPY	0.48	–
97036	HYDROTHERAPY	0.90	–
97140	MANIPULATION	0.43	–
97261	SUPPLEMENTAL MANIPULATIONS	0.24	–
97500	ORTHOTICS TRAINING	0.64	–
99000	SPECIMEN HANDLING	0.31	–
99002	DEVICE HANDLING	0.44	–
99025	OFFICE/OUTPATIENT VISIT, NEW	0.78	–
99070	MATERIAL, SUPPLIES	BR	–
99071	PATIENT EDUCATION MATERIALS	0.11	–
99199	SPECIAL SERVICE OR REPORT	BR	–
99202	OFFICE/OUTPATIENT VISIT, NEW	1.31	–
99203	OFFICE/OUTPATIENT VISIT, NEW	1.77	–

CPT®/HCPCS*	Description	Total RVUs	Follow-Up Days
99204	OFFICE/OUTPATIENT VISIT, NEW	2.59	–
99205	OFFICE/OUTPATIENT VISIT, NEW	3.22	–
99211	OFFICE/OUTPATIENT VISIT, EST	0.43	–
99212	OFFICE/OUTPATIENT VISIT, EST	0.72	–
99213	OFFICE/OUTPATIENT VISIT, EST	1.00	–
99214	OFFICE/OUTPATIENT VISIT, EST	1.52	–
99215	OFFICE/OUTPATIENT VISIT, EST	2.34	–
99221	HOSPITAL ADMISSION	1.91	–
99222	HOSPITAL INITIAL CARE	3.03	–
99223	HOSPITAL INITIAL COMP	3.83	–
99231	HOSPITAL VISIT INTERMEDIATE	1.00	–
99232	HOSPITAL VISIT EXTENDED	1.45	–
99233	DETAILED HIGH COMPLELXITY	2.17	–
99238	HOSPITAL DISCHARGE	1.74	–
99242	CONSULTATION	2.02	–
99244	CONSULTATION COMPREHENSIVE	3.66	–
99251	HOSPITAL CONSULTATION, INITIAL	1.39	–
99254	CONSULTATION	3.69	–
99255	CONSULTATION INITIAL COMPREHENSIVE	4.84	–
99261	CONSULTATION LIMITED	0.87	–
99263	CONSULTATION COMPLEX	2.17	–
99271	CONFIRMATORY CONSULTATION	2.85	–
99274	CONFIRMATORY CONSULTATION	3.13	–
99281	EMERGENCY DEPT VISIT	0.62	–
99282	EXAM EXPANDED, LOW COMPLEXITY ER	0.95	–
99283	EXAM EXPANDED, MODERATE COMPLEXITY ER	1.49	–
99284	EXAM DETAILED	2.60	–
99288	DIRECT ADVANCED LIFE SUPPORT	BR	–
99302	NURSING FACILITY CARE	1.99	–
A0300	AMBULANCE (BLS)	BR	–
A0308	AMBULANCE (ALS)	BR	–
A0427	AMBULANCE SERVICE ADVANCE LIFE SUPPORT, EMERGENCY TRANSPORT, LEVEL 1 (ALSI)	BR	–
A0428	AMBULANCE SERVICE, BASIC LIFE SUPPORT, NON-EMERGENCY TRANSPORT (BLS)	BR	–
A0429	AMBULANCE SERVICE, BASIC LIFE SUPPORT, EMERGENCY TRANSPORT (BLS)	BR	–
A4550	SURGICAL TRAYS	BR	–
H5160	READING THERAPY	1.51	–
H5220	REHABILITATIVE EVALUATION	2.65	–
H5300	OCCUPATIONAL THERAPY	0.61	–

CPT®/HCPCS*	Description	Total RVUs	Follow-Up Days
J3260	INJECTION, TOBRAMYCIN	0.12	–
J3530	NASAL VACCINE INHALATION	0.15	–
M0064	MONITORING DRUG PRESCRIPTION VISIT	0.70	–
M0075	CELLULAR THERAPY	0.62	–
M0799	PHYSICAL MEDICINE, NOC	0.84	–
P2029	CONGO RED, BLOOD	0.89	–
P9013	FIBRINOGEN UNIT	0.94	–
P9022	WASHED RED BLOOD CELLS, EACH UNIT	1.01	–
Q0040	PORTABLE OXYGEN CONTENTS, GASEOUS	2.56	–
Q0092	SET-UP PORTABLE X-RAY EQUIPMENT	0.23	–
Q9945	INJECTION OF EPO, PER 1000 UNITS	0.25	–
V2102	SPHERE, SINGLE VISION	1.76	–
V2200	SPHERE, BIFOCAL	2.00	–
V2300	SPHERE, TRIFOCAL	2.26	–
RX	PHARMACY/PRESCRIPTION DRUGS	BR	–

Durable Medical Equipment/Orthotic and Prosthetic Devices

		Rental	Purchased
A4119	SKIN BARRIER; WIPES, BOX PER K9	–	9.51
A4630	REPLACEMENT BATTERY FOR TEST UNIT	–	9.50
A5093	OSTOMY ACCESSORY; CONVEX INSERT	–	1.65
E0450	VOLUME VENTILATOR, STATIONARY	719.96	7,395.00
E0570	NEBULIZER, W/COMPRESSOR	130.00	450.00
E0607	HOME BLOOD GLUCOSE MONITOR	25.76	291.05
E0618	APNEA MONITOR	204.41	1,215.00
E1050	FULLY RECLINING WHEELCHAIR, FIXED FULL LENGTH ARMS, SWING AWAY DETACHABLE ELEVATING LEG RESTS	–	1,400.00
E1091	YOUTH WHEELCHAIR, ANY TYPE	76.16	1,761.60
L0170	CERVICAL COLLAR, MOLDED TO PATIENT MODEL	–	553.59
L0210	THORACIC RIB BELT, CUSTOM FITTED	–	32.37
L0978	AXILLARY CRUTCH EXTENSION	–	167.54
L1920	SINGLE UPRIGHT FOOT STABILIZER PHELPS OR PERLSTEIN TYPE	–	402.07

Assistant Surgeon Procedures

Following is a list of surgical procedures by CPT® code for which an assistant surgeon is considered NOT necessary. This list and is intended to be used for training and reference purposes only, as the particular company or plan guidelines may differ from those guidelines stated.

17108	19125	19126	19328	21616
23020	24101	24105	24110	24351
25295	25909	26037	26358	26516
27358	27619	27831	28290	30130
30140	30520	30620	31502	33470
36469	37700	42220	46700	52510
54110	54430	55040	55680	56304
58660	59821	61556	62142	63308
63746	64862	65155	66605	67101
67311	67875	68505	69631	69670

Network Provider List

Bart Bailey, M.D.	Luke Longwood, M.D.
Benita Bernstein, M.D.	Minnie Malorn, M.D.
B.R. Health Care	Moira Minton, D.P.M.
Broward Baxter, M.D.	Michael Mitchell, M.D.
Farmilla Fah, M.D.	Permanent Weight Loss
Foster Farminghan, M.D.	Sharla Sayers, M.D.
Fashion Medical Center	Sarah Shaw, M.D.
Folley Medical Center	Steve Sorby, M.D.
Folley General Hospital	Sharon Shaver, M.D.
Felicia Freeze, M.D.	Sharon Stack, M.D.
Harold Hamada, M.D.	Stan Still, M.D.
Herbert Harnsen, M.D.	Samuel Stone, M.D.
LA Moore Women's Clinic	Sylvia Sweet, M.D.
Lafayette General Hospital	Ted Tagliari, D.P.M.
Lafayette Surgical Center	Tessa Tamsen, D.P.M.
Lincoln Lansing, M.D.	Turnville Ambulance Service
Linda Russo, M.D.	